Free to Decide

Building a Life
in Science and Medicine

by

James A. Magner, M.D.

Lena:
I hope you enjoy some of these
anecdotes.
James Magner
April, 2016

®

2015
Russell Enterprises, Inc.
Milford, CT USA

Free to Decide
Building a Life in Science and Medicine
by
James A. Magner, M.D.

ISBN: 978-1-941270-16-5

Published by:

James A. Magner, M.D.

in cooperation with

Russell Enterprises, Inc.
PO Box 3131
Milford, CT 06460 USA

http://www.russell-enterprises.com
info@russell-enterprises.com

Cover design by Janel Lowrance

Printed in the United States of America

Table of Contents

For Glenda

My true love and partner in life

Introduction

People like to hear and tell stories. Throughout prehistory sunburned and calloused laborers, curious teenagers, and children in their young mothers' laps crowded around smoky campfires to wonder at tales of heroes and gods. Such gatherings likely occurred 50,000 years ago, and even before that. Stories help organize our thinking about the world, and their lessons shape our cultures and traditions, color our biases, and help us plan for the future. When early hunters and their families followed the migrating herd through hills, for example, they may have followed the west branch of the path instead of the more direct east branch because the ancestors had memorably warned of the ogres that might attack along the east branch. The colorful story of the ogres had a survival value based on the long and successful past hunting experience of the ancestors. The fact that there were no ogres did not lessen the survival value of taking the historically successful west branch.

Even in more modern scientific times, stories are important and extremely useful. Newton told stories of great mathematical precision describing how one massive body attracted another massive body by a mysterious invisible force. Early hearers of the theory of gravity dismissed the strange action-at-a-distance concept as preposterous, but acceptance became widespread because there was no denying the power of the story and its accompanying mathematics to correctly describe the paths of the planets, or centuries later guide the paths of spacecraft to their distant targets. Einstein revolutionized the story by telling a new tale about mass bending space-time, also with convincing mathematics and measurable evidence of validity—yet it is just another useful story that in the future may be further refined.

Author Jonathan Gottschall entitled his insightful book *The Storytelling Animal: How Stories Make Us Human*. "Stories the world over," he writes, "are almost always about people (or personified animals) with problems. The people want something badly – to survive, to win the girl or the boy, to find a lost child. But big obstacles loom…" Gottschall quotes author Christopher Morley, "Lord! When you sell a man a book you don't sell him just twelve ounces of paper and ink and glue – you sell him a whole new life. Love and friendship and humour and ships at sea by night – there's all heaven and earth in a book, in a real book I mean."

I am not certain that this autobiography can measure up as "a real book." I wrote it because I feel that I have lived an eventful life that is also an interesting story. By taking the time to write and re-write the draft chapters I mentally and emotionally processed the events of many years, and it was a good exercise for me, even if not another soul ever looks at the product. I also realized that my experiences might have useful lessons for young people who might be inclined to follow similar paths in life.

Many years ago I read the first few chapters of the irreverent and satirical book *House of God* by a Harvard physician who used the pen-name Samuel Shen. The book describes the hard work and many trials that medical interns must undergo, and shows how they can become rather callous and cynical. Notice that I say I read the first few chapters—I never finished the book. By the 1970s my personal character had been strongly shaped by my small-town Illinois background. I had been raised in a wonderful, loving family. I was religious (although not overly religious, I thought), and I was a serious but idealistic student who genuinely wanted to do good in the world. I was so shocked by *House of God* that I just could not bring myself to finish the book. I was having a stressful but invigorating training experience myself in medicine at that time, and I thought that if I ever had the chance someday, I might try to pen a more positive book about the rigors but also the wonders and satisfactions (and sometimes comedy) of training in medicine. So this motivation has partially shaped my efforts. But I wanted to do more than help trainees gain a different perspective about training in medicine. I thought that I would be able to benefit readers in other important areas of their lives as well.

I was raised in small-town America by loving parents in the 1950s and 1960s. That post-war era was a time of national confidence and prosperity in the United States, which allowed my young parents to rise economically into the middle class and thereby provide all necessities and a few luxuries for my brother and myself. Very importantly, I had access to excellent schools. I recognized by age 8 that I had a natural curiosity about the world that prompted me to work hard in school, and during elementary school I read extensively and broadly on my own time simply for the pleasure of finding things out. I was a bookworm with only a few good friends, although this was balanced to an extent by my active play in the outdoors with neighborhood children. I rode my bicycle from one end of Quincy, Illinois to the other and sometimes far out into the flat surrounding countryside that had no end of fields, woods and creeks. I went on camp-outs in the woods with the Boy Scouts and frequently got poison ivy and a little sunburn. And I watched a lot of black-and-white television (we had two channels), although this didn't seem to cause any permanent harm.

From an early age I was unusually ambitious (in the best sense of that term, I think). I wanted to be the best student in my school class, and someday a famous scientist. I wanted to make a discovery or a significant contribution that would really help humanity. Getting only 95% of the test answers correct on my elementary school quizzes was completely unsatisfactory to me. These thoughts came very naturally to me, but it was only years later that I realized that this was probably not the norm for 10 year old boys. I now see some of this early behavior as, yes, a healthy interest in the pursuit of excellence, but there were elements of introversion and compulsiveness that may have been a bit excessive.

I found that I had a very strong mind. As I came to realize this in elementary school, I told my parents that I wanted to be able to purchase books (a bit of a burden for them), and I wanted our home to have a set of encyclopedias—and they complied happily with these requests. By high school I became determined to take the most difficult subjects and I read more and more advanced books on my own. This came easily to me, and I even amazed myself at my progress.

You will see in this book how I took a zig-zag path in life, capitalizing on many opportunities and overcoming a number of crises. Like anyone I had to make many decisions, and I tried to make thoughtful and well-informed choices. That is why I entitled this book *Free to Decide*, because fortuitous circumstances started me from birth on a path that allowed me truly to be free to make positive, life-altering decisions. My many advantages included the century and nation of my birth, the support from my family, my generally good health, the culture in which I was raised that respected learning, integrity and hard work, the marvelous opportunity to obtain an excellent education, and the ability to pursue opportunities. These were considerable benefits that no one should ever take for granted or waste, yet many young people squander such advantages. Of course, at any point along the way a young person may make a bad decision that also could have life-altering consequences, but somehow my enculturation, natural aversion to unnecessary risk, and the influence of caring family members, teachers and mentors kept me from ever stumbling too badly. I also met the right girl to marry.

Since boyhood I had an interest in games that called for constant decision-making, such as chess. To prepare this book I drew freely on content that I previously published in a book entitled *Chess Juggler* (2011). That book consisted of a mix of chess along with wide-ranging personal anecdotes about family and career, and the diverse readers of that book tended to like either the chess-half of the book or the anecdote-half of the book better. So in this current effort I have largely set chess aside, and I have developed more fully the content that I think will be most instructive and helpful to a reader interested in medicine and science, but also interested in how a young man found his way forward in life.

Anecdotes have always been an important tool that I have used very effectively over the years, I think, with students and trainees. So the sort of readable style of *Chess Juggler* has been continued in this book, in part because I was very favorably influenced by the entertaining style of Richard Feynman, the Nobel Prize winner in physics, as exemplified in his book, *Surely You're Joking, Mr. Feynman*. I should add that Feynman was a man of his times, and some of his behavior is today viewed negatively because of his seeming willingness to take advantage of women in a number of ways. One really cannot forgive him for such failures. But he was truly a quirky mathematical and scientific genius. And he was a down-to-earth, slap you on the back, let's have a laugh storyteller. By the way, that book by Feynman has been included on a helpful list of excellent books in an appendix that I prepared for readers—the list has been expanded since the version that appeared in *Chess Juggler* because many readers wanted to know more of the titles that had influenced me over the years. In fact, a reader who actually reads a half-dozen of those books will have taken a major positive step.

My book has other appendices intended to be useful. There is one about general advice for life and career, and also a more focused appendix listing some of the advantages and disadvantages that a physician might find if he chooses to work for a pharmaceutical or biotech company.

Finally, there is an appendix of full-length copies of some of my publications, reproduced here with permission of the various publishers. I limited the number of the articles to be shown to provide representative examples, and a few of the papers chosen have an interesting associated personal story. I thought that having some of those articles easily available to readers was important. As one skims a book section about my experiments done with Bruce Weintraub at the National Institutes of Health, for example, a reader will be able to flip back to the publication appendix to see in more detail what we actually were thinking about and doing at that time in the laboratory or clinic. I also have prepared in that appendix a short introduction to each publication to help provide context. A current list of my publications is also provided in case a few readers want to pursue other articles that might be relevant.

One general theme of this book is that we must be rigorous, exacting, detail-oriented, logical and responsible, yes, but we also should enjoy life, love and be loved, and be fully open to chance events that might provide interesting and somewhat unexpected opportunities. We must develop intellectual and emotional strength. We must read about and reflect on life's big questions.

Another theme of this book is that difficulties are sure to arise, and we simply must recognize and understand them, and then solve or mitigate them (or just endure them) as best we can. Challenges add flavor to life, whether the difficulty involves a chess game in which one is being gradually beaten by a stronger opponent or a setback in one's career. We must be courageous, but sensible. We must always try to understand the problems we face, plan carefully using both one's head and one's heart, and then try to overcome serious challenges. We must have the maturity to recognize, however, that sometimes the problems might just be too much for us. Even if that should turn out to be the case, we should be philosophical and keep in mind Teddy Roosevelt's observation, "Far better it is to dare mighty things, to win glorious triumphs even though checkered by failure, than to rank with those poor spirits who neither enjoy nor suffer much because they live in the gray twilight that knows neither victory nor defeat."

James Magner
Woodbridge, CT
February 2015

Chapter 1

A Life of Scholarship, Adventure, Family and Broad Interests

She said nothing. I stood there as more seconds passed, and still she said nothing. That is not what I had expected. Glenda seemed about to cry. I stood there with a single red rose in my hand. She took one step forward and hugged me and put her head on my shoulder, but she remained silent. Now she was crying!

"So, is that a yes?" I asked a little bewildered since I had been sure that she would immediately say yes to my marriage proposal, but still she said nothing!

Glenda looked up at me and sighed. "Yes, yes," she exclaimed and smiled, but with tears in her eyes! We kissed.

Her delay in responding, it seems, was due to my success in executing the element of surprise as part of my marriage proposal—perhaps one should not always strive for flawless execution in such matters.

Glenda and I were both 25 year-old graduate students at the University of Chicago, and we had been dating steadily for about 3 years. It was February 14, 1977, and I had procured the red rose for the momentous special occasion. Glenda and I lived on separate floors of International House on 59th Street in Hyde Park, and we had first met in 1974 in the laundromat on the third floor. In early February I had decided that I would propose to her on Valentine's Day, and a fitting place seemed to be the laundromat where we had first met. I called Glenda that evening and asked if she could please bring her Woolite to the laundromat because I was having trouble with a stain on one of my sweaters. Perhaps slightly perturbed both by the mundane interruption and likely by what might be viewed during the late 70s as a rather sexist (and I might add, out of character) request, she apparently had grabbed the item and strode quickly down the hall to meet me. She was completely taken aback to see me standing there holding a red rose. The sudden shock was compounded by my greeting: "Happy Valentine's Day, Sweetheart! I want to know if you will marry me?!"

Glenda recovered completely within a few more seconds, and it was clear that she was very enthusiastic about our marriage. We went out for drinks with a good friend at the bar on top of the John Hancock building to celebrate. It was certainly an evening that we will never forget.

Every adult has scores of such memorable events that they can relish, if they are fortunate. We need to reflect frequently on such events and enjoy those memories. Don't let them fade!

Even very personal and idiosyncratic events can be well appreciated by others who have had similar experiences in their lives. And sometimes anecdotes we hear can do more than stimulate our own memories, or merely entertain. Anecdotes can be instructive.

In this book I am going to recount many personal anecdotes about growing up, going to school, and my experiences in science and medicine. I think the anecdotes are entertaining, but I hope that especially for persons interested in careers in science and medicine there are lessons that may be learned.

My life has not only been enriched by my family and my work, but also by my broad reading about the world, and my interest in many hobbies, including chess.

Let me share with you now a bit of an outline of how I came to chess while also doing many other things in my life. Although I could win some games, I was having trouble with stronger players. So I began to formulate my strategy of becoming a determined and tricky opponent.

I will start by showing you where I ended up, and then explain how I got there. Below is a fairly recent short game in which my role as a chess bandit is both very clear and very successful (although this opponent was rated only a bit higher than I).

Game 1
Richard Lunetta II (1565) – James Magner (1545)
Continental Open, August 12, 2007
Sturbridge, Massachusetts
Time Limit: 40/2, SD/1
Italian Game [C50]

1.e4 e5 2.Nf3 Nc6 3.Bc4 Nd4?!

Black uses an old move to set a nasty trap, but apparently it is a trap that my White opponent has not seen before!

4.Nxe5?

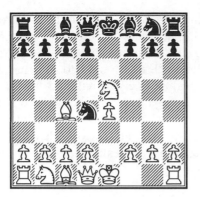

4...Qg5!

An early queen move like this is usually a big error, so even an experienced player may not be watching for it. Yet Black's queen move sets up a dangerous double attack with lots of threats.

5.Bxf7+ Kd8 6.Qh5 Qxg2 7.Rf1 Qxe4+ 8.Kd1 Qxc2+ 9.Ke1 Qxc1+ 0-1

White will have to interpose his queen, and after the queens are exchanged, White will be subject to a number of lines of attack that will cost White more material. But now let me wind back the clock and tell the tale of how I was attracted to this style of play.

Although I learned to play chess during the summer following 8th grade, in 1965, during the next four years I played only informal games with friends, and never with a clock. I bought a couple of paperback chess books, one of them by I. A. Horowitz and Fred Reinfeld entitled *Chess Traps, Pitfalls and Swindles; How To Set Them and How To Avoid Them*. This book probably left its mark deep in my psyche and may be the reason that years later I decided to emphasize trickery in my hardest games. Although the book is 243 pages long, I actually found only four or five opening tricks that could be practically applied in a pre-planned manner – the remainder of the tricks needed to appear in potential positions that might or might not happen in a given game. Yet it was good to know about those types of positions in case something similar might occur, and sometimes a trap could be constructed "on the fly."

By the way, Horowitz and Reinfeld provided useful working definitions for the terms trap, pitfall and swindle, along with many entertaining examples. I paraphrase their definitions below.

A *trap* is a situation in which a player goes wrong by his own efforts. The player is confronted by a critical choice, and for some reason (greed, fatigue, miscalculation, etc.) the player makes the wrong choice.

Technically, a *pitfall* is a trap that has been intentionally set up by a player. An imaginative player conceives a move that will create a position that allows his opponent to make an incorrect choice.

A *swindle* is a special form of pitfall. A swindle is a pitfall employed by a player who has a clearly lost game. If the opponent sees the idea and avoids it, the losing player goes on to lose. If the opponent makes a mistake and stumbles into the pitfall, the losing player is rescued from his predicament and manages to draw, or even win the game!

After high school in Quincy, Illinois, I studied biology and chemistry at the University of Illinois in Urbana, and during four years in college I played about three games on campus, and just a few informal games during the summer breaks. One of my most instructive opponents was an elderly man who lived alone in a room in a run-down hotel in Quincy, Mr. Walter Buss. He had played chess for years, and he gave me several old books, including a two volume set of *Alekhin's Greatest Games*, published (no year shown?) by Harcourt, Brace & Co. This may be a first edition, I am not sure, and it is odd today to see Alekhine's name spelled without the "e." Mr. Buss also gave me a set of weighted plastic chess pieces into which he had sealed BBs and glued felt on the bottom. Mr. Buss and I often played at the Hotel Quincy on summer afternoons, and this practice was valuable experience.

I played a practical joke related to chess on some of my Quincy boyhood friends in about 1970 when I was home from college one summer. I had played chess informally with these guys for at least five years, and now some of them were studying at University of Illinois to be electrical engineers, while I was studying biology. Their coursework included what today would be considered primitive computer science courses, and they regaled me with nightmare tales about their work with punch cards. They stood in line to have their programs run on the mainframe computer at University of Illinois, and the lines were shorter at about 2:00 am, so they often had walked to the computer center in freezing winter weather at odd hours. While waiting in line their hearts would be filled with both hope and terror—one tiny error on their punch cards would cause their program to fail. We had some discussions about whether a machine could ever be built that might be able to play chess well. We had all seen the movie "2001: A Space Odyssey" with the iconic HAL computer. (In the film HAL relates that he was built at the University of

Illinois in Urbana.) I decided that I might be able to fool my sophisticated friends with a fake chess-playing machine.

There is actually a long history of fake chess-playing machines. One famous 18th century hoax was constructed by Wolfgang von Kempelen in 1770 to impress the Empress Maria Theresa of Austria. It featured a wooden cabinet that cleverly concealed a small adult who was an expert chess player. Panels on the cabinet could be opened to reveal clockwork machinery that could be shifted to give the audience a clear view through the cabinet. But the human chess player was on a sliding seat so that as panels were opened rapidly in turn the man was quietly slipping to the left or right and was never in view. A mannequin dressed as a Turk complete with turban and robes sat behind the cabinet. The mannequin's elaborate mechanical arm, which was highly sophisticated and genuine, could move chess pieces on the board. The human inside the cabinet was able to see how the chess pieces were moved on the board atop the cabinet by a scheme involving magnets. This automaton toured Europe for decades and caused a sensation. Napoleon Bonaparte and Benjamin Franklin both played chess against it.

For my hoax in 1970 I took advantage of the fact that my father worked at Motorola, a company that built radios and televisions at that time. There were large boxes in the factory with rejected electronic parts that had been partially assembled on the work-line but then were found by ongoing inspections to be defective, so they were destined to be junked. Dad sometimes brought some of these home to show Jeff and me what different electronic parts were and how they could be wired together. After several years we had several boxes of these useless electronic scrap pieces in the basement. I also took advantage of the fact that Motorola sponsored a group of high school-aged boys as Explorer Scouts who were taught how to build their own radios. Over a couple of years I successfully built three radios, with all parts and instruction generously donated by Motorola. So I knew the basics about circuits, electronic components, and how to solder electronic parts. Two of my friends had been in this Explorer Scouts group with me, giving me some credibility in electronics.

My complicated chess machine plugged into a wall outlet to make red and green lights shine, and a clock motor turned a large dial clockwise. This large dial was the means of inputting data as well as getting desired chess moves out of the machine. Numerous toggle switches that really did nothing supposedly told the machine what bit of information was next being provided to or extracted from the machine using the dial. The key for the hoax was the single motor that made the dial turn clockwise. This dial would move but then stop and point at the name of the chess piece the machine intended to move, and then the dial would turn again and stop on the name of the square of location of that piece, and then move again and stop at the intended destination on the chess board of that piece. The only electrical wire going to my machine was the power cord, and no one was within 3 feet of the machine during operation, so there was no obvious way that a person could make the dial go and stop to indicate those perfect chess moves. All indications were that the machine was actually calculating its desired moves. My friends were flabbergasted.

The trick was that the wall outlet into which the machine was plugged could be powered or not by secret activation of a separate switch—so my machine was either entirely on or entirely off at my discretion. I could make the turning dial stop precisely over the name of any chess piece or the name of any chess board square that I desired. I had altered the wiring to the wall power outlet in our basement to have that outlet controlled by a small silent switch hidden near the floor on the edge of a free-standing book case that stood next to the chair where I was seated for the performances. My left foot could inconspicuously slide over to toggle that switch to provide power or not to the wall outlet, thereby precisely controlling the machine's dial and the content of information being communicated by the machine. My friends never figured it out, although I told them my secret a month later.

During the summer of 1972 I was awarded a scholarship to do research at the Marine Biological Laboratory at Woods Hole, Massachusetts. In addition to the wonderful intellectual climate there, and the fun of having a successful small summer project that resulted in my first published scientific abstract, I followed some of the Fischer-Spassky games in the newspaper. At Christmas, 1972, my parents gave me the paperback book *Fischer-Spassky: The New York Times Report on the Chess Match of the Century*, by Richard Roberts. I graduated from college in June, 1973.

Next came four years of medical school on Chicago's south side at the Pritzker School of Medicine. Again, there was no time for substantial amounts of chess, but I did manage to meet an intriguing girl from Houston in the laundromat in International House on 59th Street. We dated for almost three years. I later called her to meet me in that same laundromat, where I surprised her with a marriage proposal (on Valentine's Day, 1977). We were married in July of that year just as I started my internship in Internal Medicine at the University of Texas Health Science Center in San Antonio.

The three years of internship and residency left zero time for chess, however. Then followed my Endocrinology

Fellowship at the National Institutes of Health in Bethesda, Maryland from July, 1980 until June, 1983, where I may have played a dozen informal games, and I also bought a primitive chess computer on which I could practice a bit. This was before the age of the internet!

Glenda gave birth to our first child in 1981. There are many stories to tell about Erin, since she was born with severe congenital heart disease and required extensive medical interventions over several years. Thankfully, all of her medical challenges were overcome successfully, but that left little time for chess.

In June, 1983 I moved my wife and child to the Chicago area when I took a position on the faculty of Michael Reese Hospital on the south side, having done a few clinical rotations there as a medical student. As a new young doctor on the endocrinology faculty I saw patients both in the clinics and in the hospital, taught medical students and residents, ran a small research laboratory, tried to discover new things in endocrinology and publish scientific papers, and wrote long and complex proposals to obtain federal research funding. I was pretty successful at all of those activities, and in addition, our second daughter, Carly, arrived in September, 1984.

On June 1, 1985, I finally found time to play in a Saturday chess tournament in a small chess club on the north side of Chicago. My first day there I signed up for a $10 tournament as an unrated player, I joined the U.S. Chess Federation (USCF), and I played my first rated games. I had at that time a very conventional chess style, yet I won two of my four games that day. The wins were against players rated 1540 and 1429, so I felt pretty good about my showing. I next returned to that chess club on Sept. 14 and 15, 1985 for a two-day tournament. I was still unrated, of course, but in the end I won three of five games against fairly strong opponents, including the following game in the final round. My two losses during the first four games had been against players rated 1615 and 1650, so I decided that if I was going to win against this strong player, rated 1666, I was going to have to make somewhat unorthodox moves, possibly sacrifice a little material to gain development, and make threats on many moves.

Game 2
James Magner (Unrated) – J.R. Jackson (1666)
Chicago, September 15, 1985
Time Limit: G/60
Alekhine's Defense [B02]

1.e4 Nf6 2.Nc3 d5 3.e5 d4 4.exf6 dxc3 5.Bc4

White follows the strategy to seek development while sacrificing a pawn. The focus on the weak f7-square could pay dividends. Fritz says that now 5...Qd4 is the best move for Black, likely followed by 6.Bb5+ c6 7.bxc3 Qe4+ 8.Be2 Qxg2 9.Bf3 Qg6. But my opponent chose a different move.

5...cxd2+ 6.Bxd2 exf6 7.Qh5 g6

Note that White has developed three pieces, while Black has developed none.

8.Qb5+ Nc6

Fritz recommends for Black the line starting with 8...Qd7.

9.0-0-0

Always threatening.

9...a6 10.Qb3

Still another threat.

10...Ne5 11.Re1 Qd7 12.f4 h5

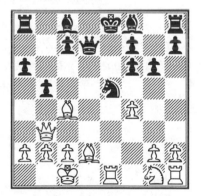

13.Bxf7+

Fritz calculates that a better choice for White here is 13.Bd5 because 13.Bxf7+ can be refuted by 13...Qxf7 14.Qxf7+ Kxf7 15.fxe5 f5 16.Nf3 Be7 17.h4 Be6 with the game then being about even.

13...Qxf7 14.Qxf7+ Kxf7 15.fxe5 Bg7 16.Nf3 fxe5 17.Nxe5+ Bxe5 18.Rxe5 Bb7

Black is trying now to get pieces developed, but the bishop on this diagonal will not provide effective defense. Instead, 18...Re8 would have been a better choice for Black.

19.Rf1+ Kg7 20.Bc3

Toying a bit. Black's position is now hopeless.

20...Kh6 21.Bd2+ Kg7 22.Re7+ Kg8

But now the king is in a trap!

23.Bc3 Bxg2

Black takes a pawn in desperation.

24.Rg7# 1-0

When I returned to that chess club for my third small tournament on October 26, 1985   I had been assigned a preliminary USCF rating of 1715. Amazing! But I was paired against players rated 2159 and 1942 and fared badly. I then won one game that day against a novice. I lost games against strong players on my next visits on April 19 and 20, 1986, and in small tournaments in June 1987 and September 1987. I just was not able to play frequently enough or to have enough time for study. I didn't play one rated game of chess in 1988, although that year I spent a week at a scientific meeting in Kyoto and then tacked on a three-week tour of mainland China. I also volunteered for a month as the lone clinic doctor in a Public Health Service Clinic in a rural area of southern

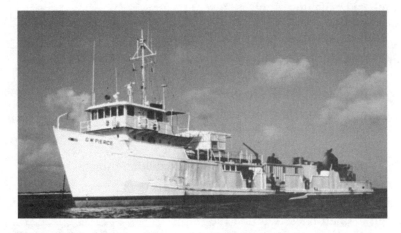

The ship G. W. Pierce used in the Marshall Islands Survey

The G. W. Pierce *was my home for a month in 1990 as a small medical team traveled in the Marshall Islands to perform health assessments on the Marshallese exposed to radioactive fallout from Bikini in a 1954 hydrogen bomb accident.*

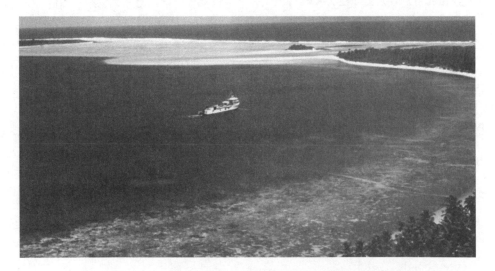

Flying over Utrik Lagoon

I took this photo of the G. W. Pierce *anchored in Utrik Lagoon in 1990 as I arrived from Majuro in a small plane. The pilot was quite a hotshot, and we landed on a very short gravel runway.*

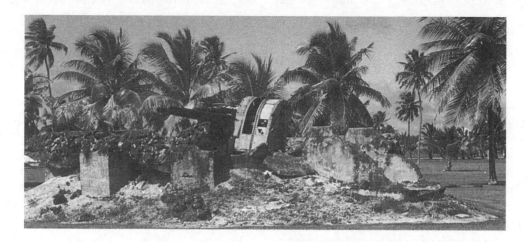

A destroyed Japanese gun from World War II

The Marshall Islands had been heavily fortified by the Japanese during World War II. Remnants of the old battles still dot the landscape. Most of the thousands of Japanese defenders were killed while they put up stiff resistance.

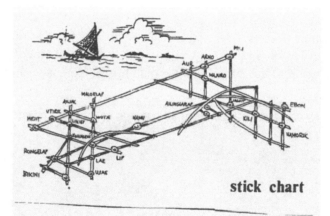

Marshallese navigational stick chart

The Marshallese have been superb navigators for centuries. The coral atolls are low-lying, so as one goes to sea in a small boat a distant island can be difficult to see. Getting lost could be fatal. Clouds can linger over an island indicating its presence, but that is hardly reliable. The relatively steady trade winds from the east create wave patterns that show subtle features to a skilled observer that reveal that an island is near but out of sight. Teenage navigators already had memorized where all the islands were and what the wave patterns looked like. Stick charts were used as teaching aids for children, and were not taken along in the boats.

Idaho. When I returned to Illinois and resumed my full-time job at Michael Reese Hospital, I also taught Sunday school for a year at my church. And my wife and young children deserved ample amounts of my time. So you see why I had no time for chess.

I played only a very few games in 1990 because I was very busy at work. I spent a month in the Marshall Islands to help the U.S. government with its study of the long-term effects of the hydrogen bomb test accident (1954 at Bikini atoll). By the way, mention of Bikini atoll in the newspaper headlines for a few days is thought to have influenced the creators of the two-piece swimsuit to adopt that name. Just as the large hydrogen bomb was detonated, the usually reliable trade winds shifted and the radioactive cloud of fallout drifted east instead of west. In addition to several isotopes of radioactive iodine, which were concentrated by the thyroid glands, the dust contained large amounts of relatively short-lived radioactive isotopes (newly created in the explosion and soon to disappear by decay) as well as strontium and cesium, so it was a rather novel mix. White dust coated people and the landscape, and caused radiation burns on the skin. The accident exposed about 245 Marshallese to radioactive fallout, which increased their risk of thyroid cancer and hypothyroidism, and possibly other cancers. The fallout also fell on some Japanese fishermen on a boat that was east of the atoll – ironically, the name of the craft was the

"Lucky Dragon." My role in 1990 was to travel by boat from atoll to atoll to examine the thyroid glands of persons who had been exposed to the fallout back in 1954 — these people had identification cards and were familiar with the periodic assessments in this long-term program, which was run by Brookhaven National Laboratory. I made sure that the individuals had a supply of thyroid hormone tablets to take, if that had been prescribed. Blood tests were checked – we had a small lab on the ship. Other physicians on the trip performed additional medical assessments on these persons, such as pelvic and breast exams. After the exposed persons all had been officially assessed, then the next days in a port could be spent providing medical care to any residents who wanted to be seen, since they rarely had an opportunity to see a physician.

In 1990 I also published a large scientific review paper in a prestigious journal, certainly the crowning event of my scientific career up to that time. In the summer I volunteered for a month at a Public Health Service Clinic in the northwest U.S.

Then in September I spent a month in Greece to give one lecture in Athens, and take some tours. Opportunities for these sorts of trips were some of the key advantages of a career in academic medicine, since a grant or the hospital paid for the expensive airfare overseas. If I wanted to tour

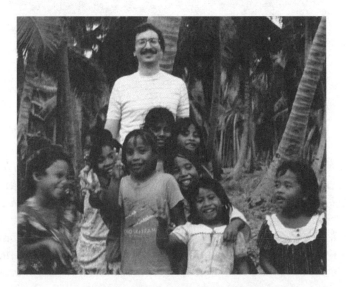

Jim with Marshallese children
The Marshall Islands is an impoverished third world country with marginal health care, simple homes and food, little electricity and very basic education. Most clothing has been donated, and it can be momentarily disorienting to see a Las Vegas t-shirt. The young children are extremely happy in their land of sun and fun, but young adults come to realize the many problems that must be faced.

for a few days of vacation, I could do so inexpensively. At least that was true in 1990.

But my chess was languishing. In June, 1991, with a rating of 1642, I decided to play in the National Open Reserve Section (entry fee $64) that was held at the Ramada Hotel near O'Hare Airport. But I was very, very rusty.

I had two wins, a loss, and two draws by the time of the final round. So I was unlikely to win any prize. In the late-morning on June 2, 1991 I went into Chicago by train to see a movie, and I thought that I would have plenty of time to get back to the Ramada Hotel before the start of Round 6, the final round. I had not counted on the possibility that on the way back out of the city my train would fill with the smell of burning rubber and come to a full stop for 45 minutes! By the time I rushed into the large tournament room, I found that I had been assigned the black pieces against a player rated 1771. He was standing near the board, and my clock was running with 15 minutes gone. I saw that he actually had not moved a white chess piece, but he said that he had moved a pawn, started my clock, and then moved the pawn back temporarily. He wanted to disguise what move he had made in case I was walking around in the tournament hall and might be spying on the board! This was probably not correct procedure on his part, but at that point, I was just happy to start playing, and I thought I would need to try some desperate measures anyway in order to have a chance of beating him. So we shook hands, I sat down behind the black pieces, and I waited a few seconds for him to reveal to me what his first pawn move had been. So here is the game.

Game 3
Stephen Wheeler (1771) – James Magner (1642)
National Open, June 2, 1991
Chicago, Illinois
Time Limit: 45/2, 25/1,15/30
Bird's Opening [A03]

1.f4 d5 2.b3

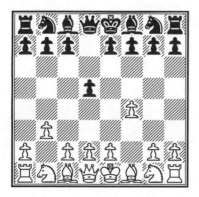

2...Bg4

Black was in an unfamiliar opening situation, and I was just trying to provoke some "out of preparation" moves.

3.Bb2 e6

Black's move was made hoping that White might err and play 4. h3? This would lead to 4...Qh4ch, and White would very soon be checkmated.

4.Nf3 c5 5.Ne5 h5?! 6.Nxg4 hxg4 7.g3 Nc6 8.e3 d4

Black's queen pawn move created a pitfall, and I had all of my fingers crossed that White would fall into the trap. The pawn on pawn action and the opposed queens possibly provide enough distraction from the real danger.

9.Na3?

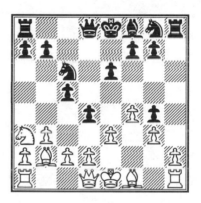

Of course, 9.Bg2 would have been much better.

9...Qd5!

Move 9 brings to mind the famous comment by Savielly Tartakower as he surveyed a chessboard with all the pieces set in their starting places, "The mistakes are all there, waiting to be made."

10.Rg1 Rxh2

Many experts recommend control of the seventh rank with a rook, but rarely does this opportunity arise on move ten!

11.Bc4

I presumed that White was not eager to play Qxg4 for fear of allowing development of my knight with a threat.

11...Qh5 12.Nb5 0-0-0

White's attempt to gain counterplay has resulted only in even more terrible pressure down the center of the board.

13.exd4 cxd4 14.Bf1 d3 15.Bg2 Bc5 16.cxd3 Rxg2

I suspect that White thought that I would take the rook, but by taking the bishop instead I have set up more immediate mating threats.

17.Rf1 Rxd3 0-1

Weary of the continuing pressure, my opponent gave up. This result gave me quite a thrill even though I won no monetary prize. I was determined that in the future I would always be highly observant in games to see what pitfalls I could create for unwary opponents.

Essentially, I had crossed an important intellectual boundary. I had resolved to become a tricky and tenacious player.

Chapter 2

Growing Up in Quincy, Illinois

I grew up in the Western Illinois community of Quincy in the 1950s and 1960s. Let me share some thoughts that will further illuminate how I started on my chess journey.

My father was a mid-level manager at the Motorola factory in Quincy, while my mother was mostly a stay-at-home Mom who worked on occasion outside the home. My Dad (Louis, born 1925) grew up in the days before TV. In the 1930s going to the movies was very sheik, and he decided as a teenager that someday he would manage a movie theater.

He graduated from high school in Jacksonville, Illinois during World War II, and a few months later had to report to the post office to register for military service. Dad reports that each boy had a very cursory physical exam, and then as they were lined up, a man counted off the boys, "One, two, three, four – you're in the Army; five, six, seven, eight – you're in the Navy!" So in one fell swoop my Dad (who couldn't swim!) found himself in the U.S. Navy. The boys later lined up on the steps of the library, and I still have the photo of the group that was published in the local newspaper. After training and a number of adventures, which will make good stories for another book, he served in Okinawa, and finally returned to the U.S. in 1946. He attended Quincy College on the GI Bill, where he met Elizabeth Metzger, a girl who lived in the college neighborhood, and they were married in 1949.

True to his teenage dreams, Dad sought employment as manager of the Belasco Theater on Hampshire Street. I'm sure it was exciting at first, but he worked long hours late into the evenings, including most holidays, Saturdays and Sundays, while other people were relaxing and enjoying the movies at his theater. One of Dad's tasks was to put the cash collected from ticket and popcorn sales into a wall safe each evening; the next morning he routinely walked the money to the nearby bank for deposit. When Mom became pregnant with me, she asked Dad to find another job so he would be home more, and with mixed feelings, he applied for a job and was hired at the new, small Motorola plant in Quincy. With a little better pay he also soon bought his first car. After a few weeks, Dad got a call at his new job with word that there was a problem with the new manager at the Belasco that day, and would he please come back to the theater during his lunch hour and open the wall safe. So at noon Dad drove to the Belasco, walked up to the safe, twirled the dial to and fro, but simply could not recall the combination. He considered that he had come to the theater by car rather than on foot, and with a different

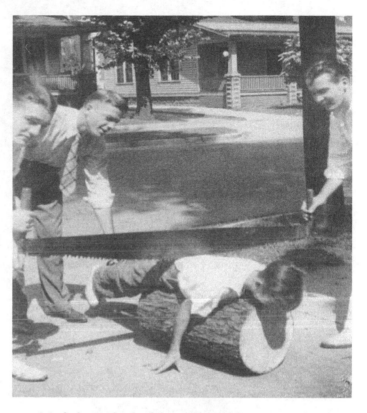

My father, who had five older siblings, was their darling. In approximately 1933 he was nearly sawed in half by his three older brothers.

mindset than a few months before. So he drove the car to where he lived and parked it, and then walked his former route from there to the Belasco, strode confidently up to the safe, twirled the dial, and without even thinking, opened the safe without any difficulty!

When I was a small child, Dad still had friends at the Belasco. He sometimes went down to visit with them, and I on occasion got to sit in the back row of the movies for free. I was a bright student in kindergarten and at St. Francis Solanus elementary school. My parents were very helpful to me with my school work, and my Mom sat with me for hours during my fourth grade year to help me learn my "times tables" and other lessons. But somehow I never learned the chess moves until a school friend taught me during the summer of 1965. During my years at Christian Brothers High School I found that I loved all subjects, and performed well scholastically. I must here insert a note of appreciation for all of the efforts of my prior teachers in elementary and high school, and elsewhere. Without

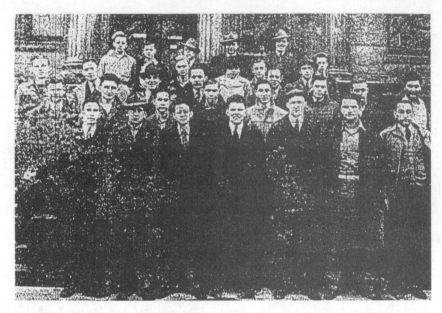

Louis Magner Goes to War
*This old photo from the local Jacksonville, Illinois newspaper,
published in November, 1943, shows my father at the left end of the
front row.*

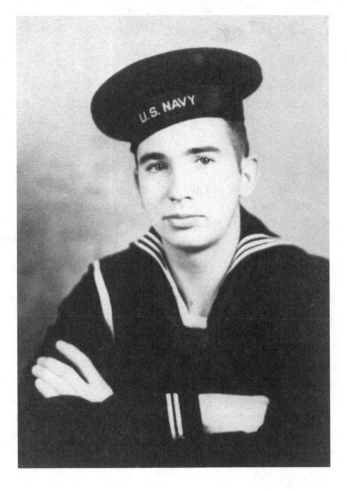

Louis Magner in the U.S. Navy

*My father served in the Navy from November 1943 until
May 1946. He slept with hundreds of men under very
basic conditions on the troop ship USS Carlson which
refueled in Hawaii and the Marshall Islands on the way
west. A weekly shower consisted of groups of naked men
on the deck being firehosed with cold seawater. They
picked dead weevils out of the biscuits. But morale was
high. He fought at Okinawa, and was awarded five
service medals, one Asia-Pacific ribbon and one battle
star. He was sleeping near the ruined city of Naha and
was being trained for the invasion of Japan when, to
everyone's great relief, the war suddenly ended in 1945.
Because of limited transportation back to the U.S., the
men had to earn points by doing various jobs to move up
the line to get a ship home. He was terminated from
service at the Great Lakes Naval Air Station and was
given a train ticket to Springfield. When he arrived at
the bus station in Jacksonville, the victory celebrations
were long over, and he had to walk home.*

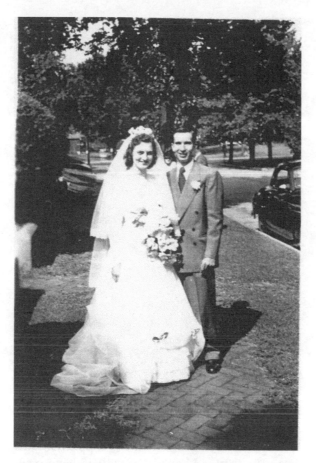

Betty and Louis Magner on their wedding day: August 27, 1949.

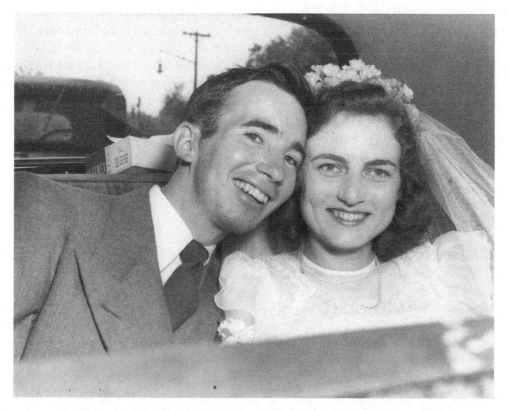

Betty and Louis Magner on their wedding day: August 27, 1949.

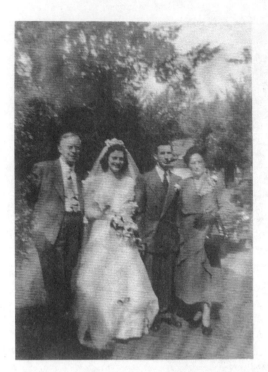

James and Rose Etta Magner, parents of the groom, stand with the happy couple, 1949.

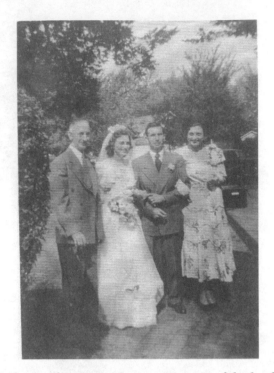

Arthur and Loretta Metzger, parents of the bride, stand with the happy couple, 1949.

excellent and dedicated teachers, the kids of my generation would have been lost. Sadly, in more recent years I have collected the obituaries of these teachers, but their contributions live on. My skilled and hard working teachers certainly made a big difference in my life! When I was in high school I was very studious and I was determined to make something of myself, most likely a research scientist in biology or chemistry. I also loved to read about astronomy. But chess was just a game to be played with a few friends for 45 minutes while waiting for the bus to take me home, or on a rainy Saturday. I went out on very few dates, and I was not very athletic. I enjoyed playing a variety of board games with my friends and my brother, Jeff, who was five years younger.

The next four photos give some flavor of happy small town life in West-Central Illinois in the mid-1960s. The first photo shows my brother and me with our prize catches from a nearby farm pond. I was 13 and Jeff was 8 in 1964. We always just dug up a few earthworms for bait. We never cleaned the fish, but instead enjoyed catching one or two fish per outing, showed them off, and then buried the fish in our small backyard garden as nitrogen fertilizer. So the fish actually gave their lives for a good purpose. Our garden had some ornamental flowers, but also a variety of ordinary vegetables, including some corn. We also had a sage bush at the side that mom used for flavoring. Jeff and I were active in cub scouts and also boy scouts, and I was pretty industrious earning merit badges in the 1963 to 1965 period, including in astronomy, geology, nuclear physics

(pretty simple non-quantitative material, of course), as well as many of the more usual boy scout topics. At about this time, I think during the summer of 1964, my parents allowed me to ride the train with the boy scout group all the way to Raton, New Mexico so that I could spend a week hiking and camping at Philmont. I had enough merit badges to make Eagle Scout in 1965, and my parents enjoyed that local awards ceremony and seeing my picture in the local newspaper. The important point is that my parents valued learning and academic accomplishment, and this message was absorbed by osmosis into the core of my personality. My parents also valued family activities and having fun, as long as the work got done, so it was a quite healthy home environment. I wish that all children might have such a wonderful experience at home, but as an adult I came to realize how many children in the world sadly are not having such a nurturing experience.

While out in the countryside I explored many creeks that often had exposed limestone with many fossils of mollusks, crinoids and corals. I took out books from the libraries and read extensively about minerals, fossils and the history of the Earth. I was astounded already by the age of 8 by the concepts of the immense age of the Earth, and that oceans had once covered our neighborhood! The thick layers of Mississippian limestone, about 300 million years old, had formed at the bottom of an ancient sea while the warm Earth had a bounty of strange plants and animals on the land. I joined the Gem City Rock Club, which had only a few children. Monthly meetings were in the basement of a nursing home. The Club had local outings to find certain minerals and fossils, and there was a three- or four-page monthly newsletter – even in the 1963 to 1965 period I volunteered to write up short articles about different fossils and geology topics for the newsletter, and I found that I really liked to see my name in print. I guess I should have realized that someday I would be a professional academic.

My grandfather Metzger died of a heart attack in March 1965, but during 1964 he had made for Jeff and me sets of stilts, and we enjoyed them.

In 1965 I got the idea to bring home some orange crates and discarded lumber to try to nail together a car. For such small projects I never asked permission of my parents, and they never were upset that I had taken apart old clocks, or had scattered junk items in the backyard. I borrowed my father's tools and scavenged the garage for junk. The wheels for the rear axle came from an ancient baby carriage and they no longer had any rubber on the rims. I took two big metal wheels off an old push lawnmower to go on the front, but it took some creativity to invent a front axle. I found a rusted three-foot iron bar that had a 90 degree bend on one end and a sharp point on the other – so the bend kept the left front wheel on the axle. But for the right front wheel I used a metal file to make a circumferential groove around the bar, which was a lot of work. Having nailed the front axle onto the bottom of the wooden cross-piece, and after slipping on the right wheel, I put several large washers on the bar and then wound tightly a copper wire within the bar's circumferential groove and then made the winding large enough so that the washers could not slip off the bar. My brother and I made many gravity runs down a nearby street with a long hill and that front wheel never fell off. The car could reach perhaps 15 miles per hour, but we then had quite a three block walk using the rope to pull the car back up the hill. One afternoon a police car stopped and the officer told us to stay out of the street. We went home immediately, but we went right back to that same hill the next day. I should mention that during all of our bicycling and other exploits we never wore helmets, which were unheard of in those days, but we survived.

The photo of our family group on our back patio was taken in June, 1965 at the time of my graduation from 8th grade.

Jeff and I also enjoyed those classic days of TV, adventures camping with the cub scouts and boy scouts, and the traditional two-week family vacation by car during

July or August every year. We saw quite a few national parks, museums and interesting places in the U.S. as we were growing up. All of those stories would make for yet another book! One of our most memorable trips was to Titusville, Florida in July, 1969, where Mom, Dad, Jeff and I slept on the beach with a million people who had come to watch the Apollo 11 moon rocket blast off in the morning. We were located just in front of the flatbed truck on which the big cameras from *Life Magazine* were positioned, so many of the views looking east that later were published in the magazine were particularly evocative for us. I will never forget the white contrail as the huge rocket rose into the brilliant blue morning sky, nor the enormous roar of that Saturn V booster as, for about three minutes, that marvelous machine exerted more horsepower (about 190 million horsepower) than all of the automobiles in some large cities!

A chance event during one of those family trips had a profound influence on my life. The family loaded up our Chevy and headed from Illinois to California. My parents always allowed me to suggest interesting sites to see during the trips, so I had plotted out the route map for Dad, who did all the driving. On the way home I had inserted a stop at Dinosaur National Monument in Utah, and we all very much enjoyed the main enclosed exhibit of numerous dinosaur skeletons that had accumulated in one location –

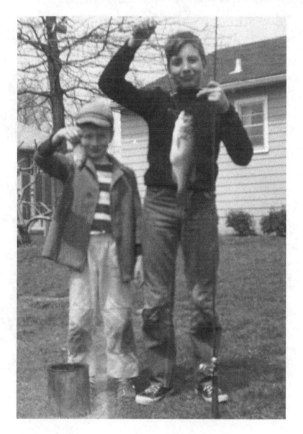

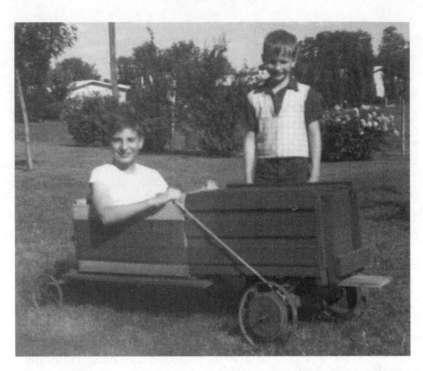

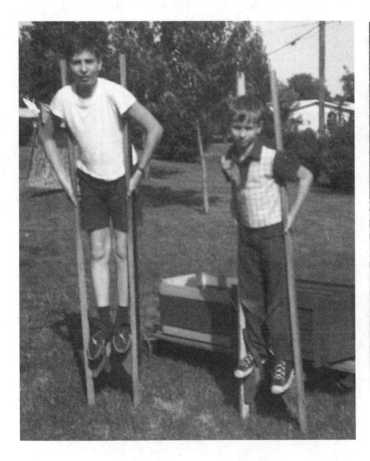

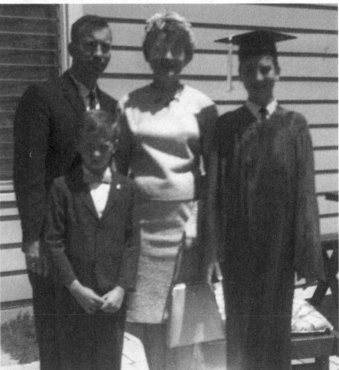

they were left for viewing still partially unexcavated. At the gift shop afterward, by chance I bought a paperback copy of Loren Eiseley's book, *The Immense Journey*, and I was enthralled. I finished it in the backseat by the time we had made a few more days progress. Over the years I purchased copies of nearly all of Eiseley's other books. An anthropologist and inspired naturalist, Eiseley has a mystic's sensitivity for the magnificence of this world, and he writes elegant prose to communicate his visions. His thinking considerably influenced my own philosophy about life. Over the years I have given his books to friends and family as holiday gifts, and *The Immense Journey* tops my list of recommended books to be read, as explained in the Appendix.

One June during those high school years I was very pleased with myself. I had planned to read several books during the summer break, and I actually had obtained them for my shelf. I was perturbed when my mother came to talk to me with the suggestion that I should get my first job during that summer so that I could "learn the value of a dollar." She was unmoved by my argument that this would disturb my reading program. So I applied for a starting job at a nearby hamburger fast-food restaurant, which was a short walk from my home, and I was hired at the astounding rate of 85 cents per hour. For several hours each day I swept floors and took out garbage, and I learned to make French fries and even milkshakes. The latter activity required subtle manipulation of the milkshake as one lowered it out of the decelerating but still spinning stirrer. The concept was that the surface of the milkshake should be broken while the stirrer was still spinning at low speed so that any bit of remaining liquid would spin off and into the paper cup. But if the milkshake was lowered while the spinner was still revolving too quickly, a brown horizontal line of chocolate milkshake decorated the front of the mandatory white shirt. During my first week on the job I returned home late each evening with a brown line on my shirt, but by the second week I had perfected the milkshake technique.

On another occasion, however, after cleaning a ceiling fixture, I stepped down the ladder and put one foot into a large bucket of spoiled tartar sauce that one of my workmates had quietly placed strategically at the bottom of the ladder. Very funny. By the third week the managers had figured out that I was pretty smart, so for most of the rest of the summer I worked the cash register. By late August I had accumulated about $250. My mother cheerfully announced "job well done" and said that I could now spend my hard-earned money on anything I wanted. So I ordered a fairly sophisticated Japanese 60mm refractor astronomical telescope, with an equatorial mount, out of the Sears catalogue. That telescope had heavy use in my backyard during the next two or three years, although I then ran out of useful objects to view with such a small instrument. I have kept it all these years, and I have used it intermittently for decades to give sky tours to family and friends. Thus, although my summer reading program had been sabotaged, I had a special benefit from my fast-food job. And in later years I did find the time to read lots of interesting books, so perhaps my brief summer job was not such an unfortunate experience after all.

Astronomical Sketches: Moon, Uranus, Comet

Like most young kids, I loved to draw. By about age 14 I found that I was a very visual thinker, and that sketching out a diagram while reading something complex quickly helped me to understand the text. I also made drawings of organisms in pond water as magnified by an inexpensive microscope my parents gave me for Christmas one year. As illustrated here, I also made a few astronomical sketches. I had a toy, poor quality 3 inch reflector telescope (also a Christmas present) during elementary school – the cheap optics and shaky mount were a nightmare, but it was fun to look at the moon. Then in 1967, at age 16, I purchased my first high-quality telescope for about $200 right out of the Sears catalogue. It was a 60 mm objective Sears Discoverer Model 4 6305-A equatorial refractor telescope that arrived packed in white Styrofoam snuggly fitted inside an impressive wooden case. I bought several useful paperback books about backyard astronomy and use of an equatorial mount, and I was in love! The telescope came with three eyepieces, some filters, barlow lens, diagonal prism, and a sun projection screen. Compared with my toy 3 inch reflector, this was a real Cadillac, and the optics produced very sharp images that were best with the low-power Kellner eyepiece, which also was very comfortable to use (your head might drift side to side a bit but you could still see the object easily).

I made this sketch of the moon on the evening of August 24, 1967, probably after having the telescope for only a week. During that month I systematically made numerous sketches of sunspot patterns. (Note: the sun's image was projected – one never looks through a telescope toward the sun! Galileo did the same sorts of observations.) During the next several months I sketched M42 and M43 in Orion, a number of bright star fields, M31 in Andromeda, Saturn, and Jupiter with its shifting pattern of moons. Note that Christian Huygens at his home near The Hague in The Netherlands had made many observations of Saturn, and had discovered its largest moon, Titan – years later I toured his house. Galileo had first discovered the four main moons of Jupiter, and years later I visited Florence to see many sights that included some of his instruments, and reputedly a bone from a finger of Galileo retrieved when they had to repair his grave.

By 1969 Sky and Telescope magazine provided the information that I needed to find and sketch Uranus – the planet was clearly a small disc rather than a point like surrounding background stars. This was the same type of observation that had allowed William Herschel to discover Uranus while standing in his backyard in Bath, England in March, 1781. Then he noted movement of the planet over subsequent weeks. More than 40 years later I had the privilege of standing at that exact spot in Herschel's yard, and I also toured the small basement workshop in which he had constructed his telescope.

My telescope had less use when I was away at the University of Illinois in Urbana, although I made sketches in January, 1970 of Comet Tago-Sato-Kosaka (1969g) as it passed through Aries.

Sketches also helped me in high school in biology and physics classes. During college I frequently used many sketches to make the methods and results sections of my laboratory reports more clear. So it was natural for me when doing my first real science at Woods Hole, and later at the National Institutes of Health, to have many sketches in my laboratory notebooks, as these made complex, multi-step directions very clear in my mind. So I suppose I would recommend students to take up the practice early on of making drawings – these not only are fun, but they actually can help you to think better.

<u>Moon</u>: Area between 10°-20° S. Lat. and 20°-30° E. Long.
     August 24, about 11:00 p.m., various powers, type C, cond: very good
     note: moon filter not used

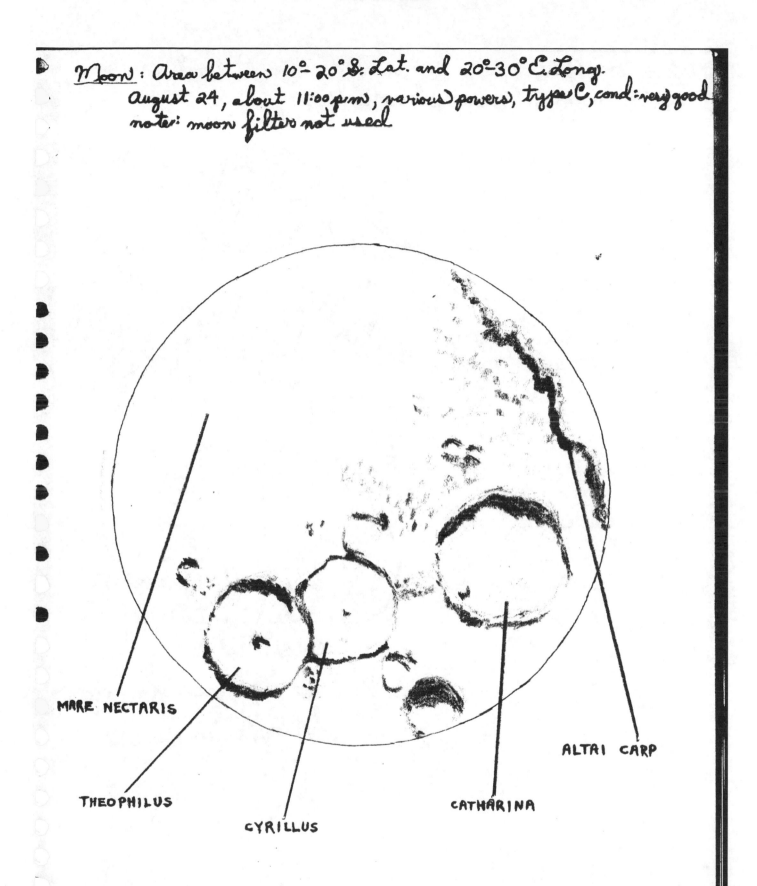

MARE NECTARIS

ALTAI CARP

THEOPHILUS

CATHARINA

CYRILLUS

<u>Uranus</u> : June 7, '69; 10:12, 41X, type A, cond: very good
note: no moon, very clear skies

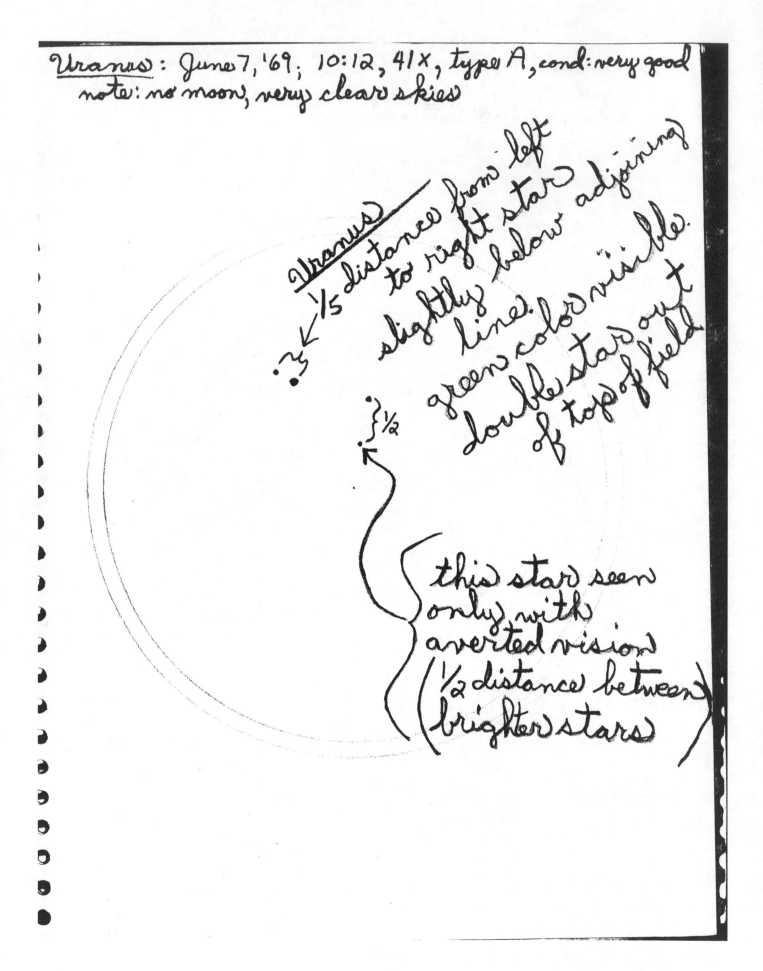

<u>Uranus</u>

.3 ←¹/5 distance from left
to right stars adjoining
slightly below adjoining
line. green color visible.
double stars out
of top of field

}½

{ this star seen
only with
averted vision
(½ distance between)
(brighter stars)

COMET TAGO-SATO-KOSAKA
(aries)
(1969g)

Sky + Telescope, 1/70, p. 64
predicted 1^h 29^m, +9°.2 for 1/28/70

at 6×30 and 41×60 no tail
was visible, and 1969g
looked somewhat like a
bright yet unresolved
globular cluster.

1/29/70
7:25 pm

comet

3
3
2
2
1

6×30
View finder

a few misty patches
hung in the south but
for the most part the
sky was very clear,
and there was no moon.
the trapezium was easily visible.
The comet was high in the sky during
the observation, and there was only
a slight breeze.

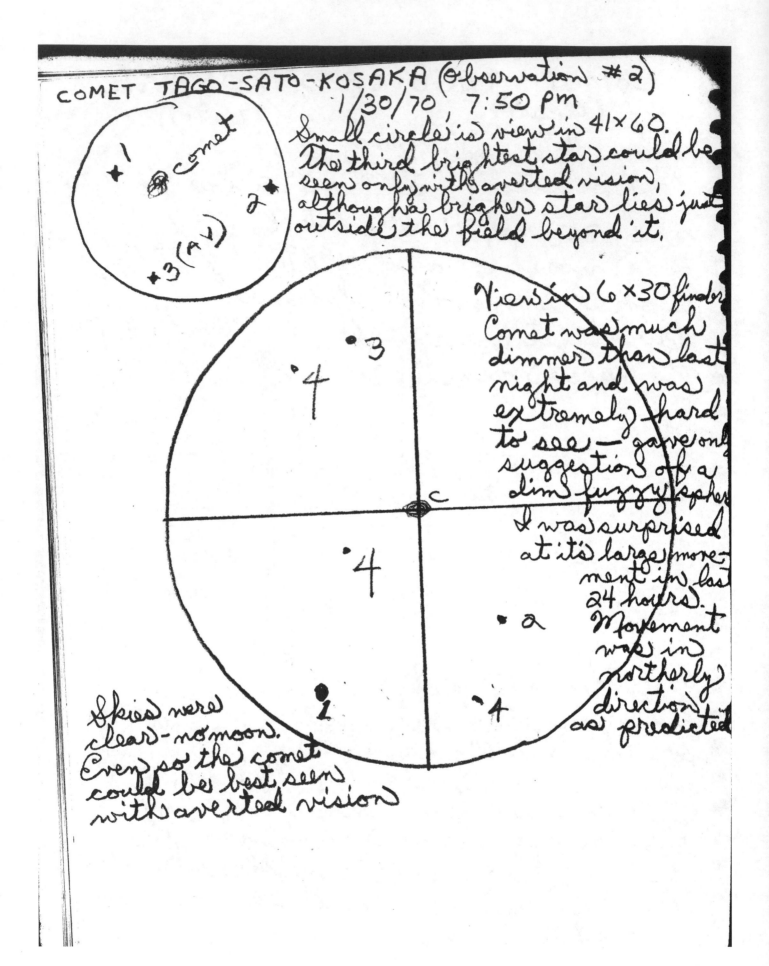

COMET TAGO-SATO-KOSAKA (Observation #2)
1/30/70, 7:50 PM

Small circle is view in 41×60.
The third brightest star could be seen only with averted vision, although a brighter star lies just outside the field beyond it.

View in 6×30 finder. Comet was much dimmer than last night and was extremely hard to see — gave only suggestion of a dim fuzzy sphere. I was surprised at it's large movement in last 24 hours. Movement was in northerly direction as predicted.

Skies were clear — no moon. Even so the comet could be best seen with averted vision

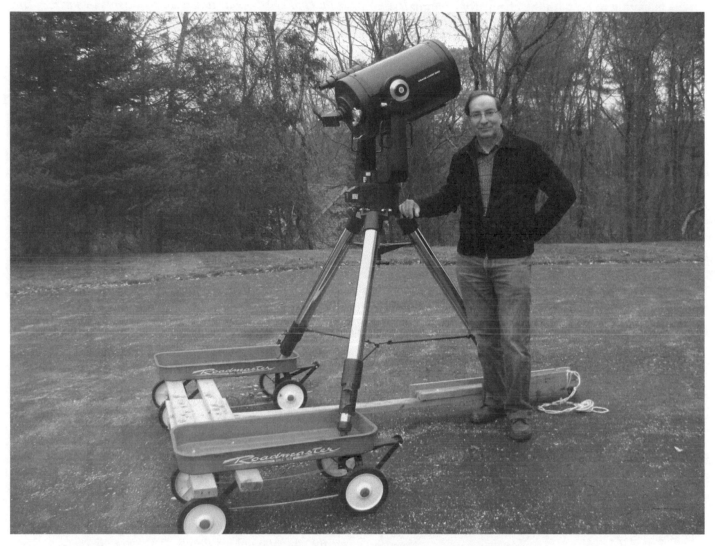

Jim and Amateur Astronomy: Fast Forward 47 Years!

One may fast forward 47 years to consider how my current interest in amateur astronomy compares with my fledgling efforts in 1967 when I made the first sketches shown in this book. I have graduated from a 2.4-inch objective to a 12-inch objective telescope! My Meade LX 200 EMC Schmidt-Cassegrain telescope has a small viewfinder (seen in this photo just at the top) that has an objective lens only a little smaller than the main objective lens in my first refractor. Note that the Meade scope is heavy, so I constructed a home-made contraption from two toy wagons and spare lumber so that I can easily transport the telescope out of my garage. I guess I did pick up a few tricks when I made that orange crate car back in 1965!

During the summer after my junior year of high school I attended the University of Illinois in Urbana for a few weeks on a special scholarship. I lived in Barton Hall and worked at Burnsides Research Laboratory on some simple projects having to do with the chemistry of human serum lipids. I was favorably impressed by the University of Illinois, which also would be a relatively inexpensive choice for me since I was a state resident, so during my senior year of high school I applied to attend college there and was accepted. I had already taken calculus in high school (at the public high school across town), and I had lots of "advanced placement credits" acquired by reading books in my spare time and then sitting for the formal tests to get the college credits. I had decided that I would become a scientist of some type, and more importantly, I had decided that I would become very good at whatever I chose to do – actually, my goal was to become the best in the world in my narrow field, if possible.

So as I started my freshman year in Champaign-Urbana, I took a heavy load of classes and spent nearly every hour studying. I did the same during the next three years. Like Eisenhower preparing for D-Day, at the start of each semester I mapped out on a large sheet of paper and on calendars when the term papers or projects were due, when the quizzes and exams would occur, and when the final exams would be given. Then I prepared a battle plan to not only learn all the material but also perform optimally on all tests, projects, papers and final exams. My system worked beautifully. But there was a price. I went to only one sporting event in four years, I watched no TV for months at a time, I rarely went out with friends, and I had only about three dates in four years. Needless to say, I played only a few games of chess during the summer vacation periods.

I made use of opportunities to add extra classes in areas of particular interest, such as higher mathematics (differential equations), physical chemistry, astronomy, anthropology, the history of science, and courses related to biblical redaction criticism. I earned more credits doing a research project in a biology lab on campus with Dr. Phil Carl. We tried to detect and study bacterial DNA-RNA hybrid molecules that seemed to be present very transiently during the early steps of DNA replication. By senior year my academic advisor, Dr. Judy Willis, was astonished to see that I had acquired so many credits that I qualified to graduate with two B.S. degrees, one in biology and the other in chemistry. My Dad was pleased, however, and at my graduation ceremony he quipped to the family, "Jim has two college degrees, but I only paid for one!"

Doing Well in College – a Case Study

I offer here my own college transcript from University of Illinois at Urbana as a helpful case study. My sincere wish is that college-bound students, or students in earlier years at college, can learn some key lessons from my good experience so that they can make the most of their college years. (This transcript was slightly altered to obliterate my social security number.) So here are the general lessons I want to emphasize, along with a bit of detail explaining how I applied these principles.

Get a running start in high school:

I was a serious student in high school. More than that, I used my free time to read many books, and it was fun. I also did targeted reading – I found out what College Board Advanced Placement Program tests could be taken in my town to get college credits, then I read textbooks on those topics and took the tests so that I could start college with a lot of college credits already earned. I also decided to take calculus at a nearby school during my last year in high school to give me a head start in advanced math. On my first day at University of Illinois I already had 25 credits on my transcript by passing the following tests back in Quincy: Analytic Geometry, Calculus, Principles of Biology I, Principles of Biology II, Freshman Rhetoric and Composition, and Descriptive Astronomy.

As a senior in high school, identify your weak areas and plan to mitigate them:

I did great in high school Spanish, but I could tell that it took tremendous effort to get the A grades. I just was not good at foreign languages, whereas math and science came easily. In college I would need to take four semesters of a foreign language, and I estimated that if I took Spanish I might make Bs or Cs; if instead I took German or French I likely would get C grades. I was not happy about those prospects – I wanted to get a good graduate position in biology or chemistry someday, and I did not want even one C on my college transcript. Fortuitously, after I had been accepted to attend the University of Illinois I received a letter from Arts and Sciences there saying that in the fall they were going to have a new program in Scandinavian languages – the classes would be small and supportive as the program was just beginning, and there would be one semester each of Norwegian, Swedish, Danish, and finally readings in all three languages. I reasoned that I might be able to do well in a small group with lots of attention, because I certainly was weak in languages. I signed up for the program with the hope of, yes, learning something, but mostly I just wanted to get through the four required semesters of foreign language with a real chance of getting a B each semester. In fact, there were the same 20 or so students in class with me during the two years, there was lots of personalized instruction, and I actually made grades in those four semesters of A, A, B and "Pass." I could never have done that in Spanish or German. Sadly, within a few years I retained only a little proficiency from those classes – hardly unexpected for a young American living in Illinois. But I had identified an academic weakness that I feared might affect my overall life goals in science, and I found a way to mitigate it.

Take many courses in the key areas you want to learn, and work very hard:

Because I believed I was inclined to biology or chemistry, I decided at the start to take during my four years many, many courses in biology and chemistry. I had no idea what my major should be, but I knew what subjects I wanted to emphasize over four years. So I agreed to be in the Honors Biology Program, a special program for about 30 highly skilled students interested in biology. And I started with the usual Freshman semesters of elementary chemistry, followed by lots more biology and chemistry in my third and fourth years. During my Senior year I took two advanced courses in physical chemistry, which was particularly challenging since a lot of mathematics is involved. But I was great at algebra and calculus – I started Freshman year taking Calculus II, and then that spring as a Freshman I had taken an advanced course in mathematics in Differential Equations and Orthogonal Functions, so I was not afraid of math. Note, however, that for that Differential Equations course while a puny Freshman, I did mitigate the risk by taking that course pass-fail. It was interesting to be mixed with the high-powered upper level students, and I passed. The lesson here is to push yourself and learn, learn, learn – but also get good grades.

Enjoy and learn in your other required courses, and find a way to make the As or Bs:

Rhetoric as a Freshman, and later two semesters of Physics were some of the other required courses for me, and I managed to do well. Note that for all my courses like Physics in which today a hand calculator would be used, I actually used a slide rule. Hand calculators were primitive and hugely expensive in the early 1970s. I still can close my eyes and recall the scent of bamboo that filled the air as I worked my slide rule, which I still have as a souvenir of a vanished era. For a social science I took a

semester of Anthropology as a Sophomore, and then to meet the requirement for a second semester I passed the Advanced Placement Test in Cultural Anthropology by reading the textbook on my own time. Four semesters of Physical Education were required, and I was not athletic. I also was afraid of injury. But I did well in my four required semesters by careful selection of the Physical Education courses: Swimming, Bowling, Tennis and Figure Skating – I suffered no broken bones or concussions.

Take advantage of electives to expand your mind and deepen your core skills:

I loved exploring courses of interest to me at a major university. I took two biblical redaction courses, Old Testament and New Testament, during my Junior year. I had passed Descriptive Astronomy by testing when I had first entered the university, but while in college I read an astronomy textbook and took the Advanced Placement Test to get credit for another semester of more advanced aspects of astronomy, which had a little more math involved. I then took a graduate seminar with readings: Astronomical Topics. I took Honors Seminars in Biology with wide-ranging readings and discussions in that field, and I also took an excellent course in immunology. I enjoyed a high level course in the History of Science that focused on the years 1543-1727. During the spring of my senior year I took special research courses and worked in the biochemistry laboratory of Dr. Philip Carl. I continued that laboratory work for two additional months even after I graduated in June, 1973. During that summer session in 1973 I also read a textbook of genetics that would be required for my upcoming matriculation at University of Chicago, and then I took the Advanced Placement Tests required by the University of Chicago in Genetics, and also in Biochemistry, so that I would start in the autumn of 1973 at University of Chicago already with credits on my transcript – I was following the same "running start" plan as I had done four years before.

Evolving a major:

Regarding a formal major designation at the University of Illinois, this did not really worry me too much since I knew that I was hitting all the right categories anyway to be certain that I would get a degree. So my official major drifted during my college career. I started as General, within six months changed to Teaching of Biology, and then in six more months I was formally something called Arts and Sciences. I ended up with two majors: Chemistry, and also Honors Biology.

September 1969

UNIVERSITY OF ILLINOIS
OFFICE OF ADMISSIONS & RECORDS

NAME		DEGREE AND DATE

ADDRESS AT TIME OF ADMISSION	Magner, James Arthur
	
	3008 College Avenue
	
	Quincy, Illinois 62301
		B.S.(L.A.S.)Major-Honors Biology
		  see other side June 9, 1973
		B.S.(L.A.S.)Major-Chemistry, see other side
		        June 9, 1973

PLACE AND DATE OF BIRTH	RESIDENCE CLASS.
Quincy, Illinois, May 30, 1951	Resident

EDMUND J. JAMES SCHOLAR
1969-70 , 1970-71 , 1971-72 ,1972-73

PARENT, GUARDIAN, OR SPOUSE
Louis R. Magner

HONORS DAY RECOGNITION
1970 , 1971 , 1972, 1973

ADDRESS AT TIME OF STUDENT'S ADMISSION
3008 College Avenue, Quincy, Illinois 62301

ACCEPTED FROM:
Christian Brothers High School
Quincy, Illinois 5/69

HIGH SCHOOL UNITS

ENGLISH	4	LATIN		U.S. HISTORY	1	PHYSICS	1	AGRICULTURE	
ALGEBRA	2	GERMAN		OTHER HISTORY		CHEMISTRY	1	HOME ECONOMICS	
GEOMETRY	1	FRENCH		OTHER SOCIAL STUDIES	2	ZOOLOGY			
TRIGONOMETRY		SPANISH	2			BOTANY			
CP Math	2					BIOLOGY	1	MUSIC EXAM.	
						OTHER SCIENCES		MISC. SUBJECTS	3½

RANK: 2-111   99 %ILE

Descriptive Title of Course	Course Number		Credit	Grade
L.A.S. - SCIENCES & LETTERS				
TO GENERAL				
College Board Adv. Placement Prog.:				
Analytic Geomtry	Math.	123	5	-
Calculus	Math.	132	5	-
Prin. of Biology I	Biol.	110	4	-
Prin. of Biology II	Biol.	111	4	-
FRESH RHET & COMP	RHET	101	3.0*Pass	
DESCRIPTIVE ATRONOMY	ASTR	101	4.0*Pass	
1ST SEM 1969-70				
GENERAL CHEMISTRY	CHEM	107	5.0	A
ELEM SCANDINAVIAN I	SCAN	101	4.0	A
FRESHMAN SEMINAR	BIOL &198		3.0	A
CALCULUS II	MATH	143	5.0	A
INTERMED SWIMMING	P E M	108	1.0	A
Ave: 17-85-5.000				
TO TCHG. OF BIOLOGY				
2ND SEM 1969-70				
GEN CHEM EQUAL ANAL	CHEM	108	5.0	A
RHET-SUPERIOR STUD	RHET &108		4.0	A
ELEM SCANDINAVIAN II	SCAN	102	4.0	A
BOWLING	P E M	137	1.0	A
Ave: 13-65-5.000				
DIFF EQUAT & ORTH FUNC	MATH	345	3.0*Pass	
TO SCIENCES & LETTERS				
DESCRIPTIVE ASTRONOMY	ASTR	102	4.0*Pass	
1ST SEM 1970-71				
ORIGIN MAN-CULTURE	ANTH &102		4.0	A
INTERM SCANDINAV I	SCAN	103	4.0	B
THE CELL	BIOL &151		5.0	A
BASIC ORGANIC CHEM	CHEM	136	3.0	B

Descriptive Title of Course	Course Number		Credit	Grade
STRUCTURE -SYNTHESIS	CHEM	181	2.0	A
TENNIS	P E M	135	1.0	B
Ave: 18-83-4.611				
2ND SEM 1970-71				
INTERM SCAND II	SCAN	104	4.0	P
THE ORGANISM	BIOL &251		5.0	A
ORGANIC CHEMISTRY	CHEM	336	3.0	B
ORGANIC CHEMISTRY	CHEM	337	2.0	A
FIGURE SKATING	P E M	145	1.0	A
Ave: 10-47-4.700				
INTROD TO CULT ANTHRO	ANTH	103	4.0*Pass	
1ST SEM 1971-72				
GEN PHYS-MECHANICS	PHYCS	106	4.0	A
INTRO OLD TESTAMENT	HUMAN	201	3.0	A
HONORS SEMINAR	BIOL &203		1.0	A
POPULATION BIOLOGY	BIOL &351		4.0	A
ANAL OF DEVELOPMENT	ZOOL	367	3.0	A
Ave: 15-75-5.000				
2ND SEM 1971-72				
GEN PHYS-HT-ELEC-MAG	PHYCS	107	4.0	B
SCI REVOL 1543-1727	HIST	349	3.0	A
INTRO NEW TESTAMENT	HUMAN	202	3.0	A
HONORS SEMINAR	BIOL &203		1.0	A
GENERAL BIOCHEMISTRY	BIOCH	350	3.0	A
Ave: 11-51-4.636				
(SEE OTHER SIDE)				

IN GOOD STANDING

KEY TO TRANSCRIPT ON BACK

Magner, James Arthur

Descriptive Title of Course	Course Number	Credit	Grade		Descriptive Title of Course	Course Number	Credit	Grade
1ST SEM 1972-73								
ASTRONOMICAL TOPICS	ASTR 8110	2.0	A					
IMMUNOLOGY	BIOL 307	4.0	A					
BIOCHEMISTRY LAB	BIOCH 355	4.0	A					
PRIN-PHYSICAL CHEM	CHEM 340	4.0	P					
Ave: 10-50-5.000								
2ND SEM 1972-73								
SPECIAL PROBLEMS	ENTOM 306	4.0	A					
RES AND SPEC PROB	MCBIO 207	5.0	A					
PHYS CHEM OF MACROM	CHEM 346	3.0	A					
Ave: 12-60-5.000								

B.S.(L.A.S.)MAJOR-CHEMISTRY, HIGH HONORS
IN LIBERAL ARTS AND SCIENCES   JUNE 9, 1973

B.S.(L.A.S.)MAJOR-HONORS BIOLOGY, HIGH
HONORS IN LIBERAL ARTS AND SCIENCES
WITH HIGH DISTINCTION IN HONORS BIOLOGY
JUNE 9, 1973

TO IRREGULAR

SUMMER SESS 1973								
INDIVIDUAL PROBLEMS	MCBIC 490	2.000	A					
Ave: 8-40-5.000								

IN GOOD STANDING

Getting the degree:

A student needs to pay attention and stay in touch with a good academic advisor during the college years. I was blessed to have Dr. Judy Willis as my formal advisor, a caring, energetic and brilliant biologist. The advisor can help a student make sure that he is meeting degree requirements, and will finish the requirements on time. And the advisor can also make the student aware of interesting opportunities inside or outside of the university. That's how I applied for a summer biology course and research experience at Woods Hole, Massachusetts after my Junior year. Judy Willis met with me at intervals during the college years, and in my Senior year as we were meeting to check that I had met degree requirements, she looked up at me from her paperwork with a startled expression and informed me that I had so many academic credits and so many courses in biology and also chemistry that I was eligible to be awarded two B.S. degrees! That was fine with me, although I only needed one degree to move on in my career. I also received a number of academic honors during my college years, including admission to Phi Beta Kappa. But the real treasure I gained at the University of Illinois was a huge fund of knowledge and experience that would serve me well and be a strong foundation for additional learning for the rest of my life.

During the summer of 1972, after my junior year of college, I was awarded a small scholarship to live and study in Woods Hole, Massachusetts. I was to take the summer biology course and complete a well-defined research project in a few weeks, if possible. I joined a group of a dozen bright students from around the U.S., and we had a great time both at work and play. During the first week, Dr. Holger Jannasch invited the students to spend an informal evening at his home. We had some lively discussions about biology, science and Woods Hole when, at about 10:30 pm, one of the young ladies from California stood up and shouted, "Let's go skinny dipping!" Everyone immediately agreed and we raced out the front door to the nearby beach – although I'll admit that this shy and studious boy from Illinois, land of endless cornfields, was trailing in the rear and was quite bemused by this sudden turn of events! On other evenings we had outings in small boats to nearby islands for clam bakes, or spent time sitting around a campfire while Ken Nealson strummed on his guitar. Years later Dr. Jannasch would become world famous after his participation in the explorations that discovered the unusual life forms near deep-sea hot water vents. His expertise in the complex microbiology of the oceans became widely recognized.

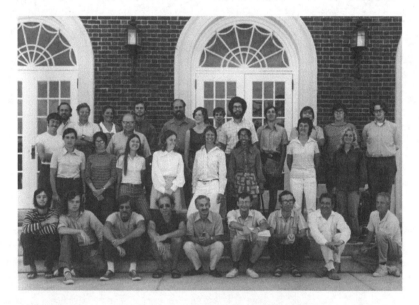

A Bright Group at Woods Hole Marine Biological Laboratory

This 1972 photo taken in front of the library shows the group of students who had won scholarships to study for the summer at Woods Hole, as well as several of our teachers. I am the enthusiastic-looking student with the notebook in the back row, fourth from the right, and Ken Nealson is next to me in that row, third from the right. Dr. Holger Jannasch is in the back row, second from the left, with his wristwatch showing prominently. Notable in the front row, starting from the right side, are instructors Ralph Wolfe, Bruno Battaglia, Anatol Eberhard, Edward Wilson and Ralph Mitchell.

On a couple of weekends I took the big ferries out to Nantucket and to Martha's Vineyard. On Nantucket I was fascinated by the round cobblestones in some of the streets. As the 18th and early 19th century whaling ships left port they were loaded down with supplies, and as they journeyed for months the supplies were consumed. Although the sailors did collect some whale oil and other products, they often had to add ballast to keep the sailing ships stable. The spaces in the lowest parts of the ships where supplies had been removed were filled with local smooth round rocks, and when the ships returned to Nantucket (or to nearby Gloucester, Massachusetts), the rocks became paving stones. While visiting Nantucket I toured the home of one of the earliest female astronomy buffs, Maria Mitchell, who discovered a comet in 1847, and who later became the first female professor at Vassar College. I do recall that during the ferry ride back I read an article in the newspaper about the ongoing Fischer-Spassky championship match.

On one day while on Martha's Vineyard, a couple of my fellow students and I rented one-speed bicycles and rode the complete circuit of the island. Older adults often overestimate what they still can do physically, and this bicycle episode was the first instance in my young life when I had fallen into that misconception. I was never very athletic, but I had been riding bicycles for years, I was 21-years old and reasonably fit, so what could be the difficulty with riding a bicycle for a day? In fact, I made the circuit of the island with my friends, but I was barely able to walk onto the ferry that evening for the trip back to the mainland, and the next day I could hardly move!

My research project at Woods Hole was about bioluminescent bacteria found living freely in seawater. I characterized them based on their inducers of luciferase synthesis. With the help of my mentors, Anatol Eberhard and Ken Nealson, the project was a success, and resulted in my first published scientific abstract. Also while at Woods Hole I was able to interact with Wolf Vishniac, who was designing his "Wolf Trap," a device he hoped would be flown to Mars and that might succeed in finding bacteria or other tiny life forms in the frozen Martian environment. Tragically, after the summer program ended, Dr. Vishniac was killed in Antarctica when he fell into a crevice while trying to do an experiment.

I also met the great naturalist E.O. Wilson, who loved to come to Woods Hole for the summer and was well known for his expertise on ants. Over many years he spent countless hours on his hands and knees watching and learning from his beloved ants. It is said that after one public lecture about ants, a woman asked rather practically, "Well, Dr. Wilson, if I have ants in my kitchen, what should I do?" His answer: "Get a good magnifying glass so that you may watch them more easily." Other scientists, some from the University of Illinois, also were at Woods Hole during the summer of 1972, and I learned a lot about science and life from this wonderful experience.

Critical Experiment!

9/8/15 MAV

41

MAV

	1	2	3	4	5	6	7	8
4ml SWC								
MAV PREP'D	4ml	3ml	3ml	3ml	4ml	3ml	3ml	3ml
41 USED	0ml	1ml	0ml	0ml	0ml	1ml	1ml	0ml
MAV USED	0ml	0ml	1ml	1ml	0ml	0ml	0ml	1ml

MAV PREP'D } MAV grown in SWC to oD .23, centrifuged, and millipored (.45μ), autoclaved 15 min. 8/15

41 USED } 41 grown in SWC to oD .32 etc., (NOT AUTOCLAVED!) harvested 8/15, pH = 6.8

MAV USED } MUST BE USED IMMEDIATELY!

MAV

SWC 4ml 4ml → put on shaker at 250 RPM room temp at 5:00 AM, grow till oD .5 (approx 7:00 AM) then centrifuge at 4°C (10,000 xg 10 min.) and millipore filter (.45μ)

cells will be approx. oD 0.6 by time to make inoculation

start 41 preinoculum at 12:10 AM to be ready by 7:30 AM should be 0.1oD by 5:00 AM

8/16 41 growing faster than estimated oD .6 BY 8:45
MAV " slower " oD .19 BY 9:40

Woods Hole Laboratory Notes, 1972

Here are a few pages from my laboratory notebook at Woods Hole that show how I often used sketches to avoid confusion when performing multi-step laboratory procedures

8/16

3	4	5	6	7	8	9	10
(.57) .855	(.59) .75	(.29) .435	(.23) .345	(.29) .435	(.24) .36	(.65) .975	(.31) .465
(.50) .75	(.47) .705	(.28) .42	(.23) .345	(.30) .45	(.24) .36	(.55) .81	(.33) .495
(.48) .72	(.43) .645	(.25) .375	(.20) .30	(.27) .405	(.21) .315	(.50) .75	(.30) .450
(.48) .72	(.43) .645	(.24) .36	(.20) .30	(.25) .375	(.20) .30	(.44) .66	(.25) .375
(.48) .035	(.44) .025	(.21) .315 .025	(.17) .255 .02	(.23) .345 .02	(.19) .285 .395	(.50) .75 .032	(.06) .39 .022
(.44) .045	(.39) .585 .035	(.19) .285 .39 .035	(.17) .255 .305 .025	(.22) .33 .40 .022	(.19) .285 .285 .02	(.40) .60 .036	(.22) .33 .45 .031
(.34) .51 .052	(.33) .495 .045	(.59) .295 .046 .22	(.51) .255 .03 .19	(.68) .34 .032 .25	(.53) .265 .025 .20	(.38) .57 .055	(.76) .38 .035 .28
(.24) .36 .41 .07	(.22) .33 .41 .06	(.12) .18 .48 .24 .042	(.29) .195 .035 .145	(.52) .26 .04 .195	(.46) .23 .032 .175	(.27) .405 .073	(.60) .30 .45 .225
(.78) .147 .086	(.61) .915 .083	.15 .06	(.26) .13 .10 .052	(.45) .225 .17 .072	(.34) .17 .13 .052	(.42) .21 .12 .16	(.40) .20 .075 .15

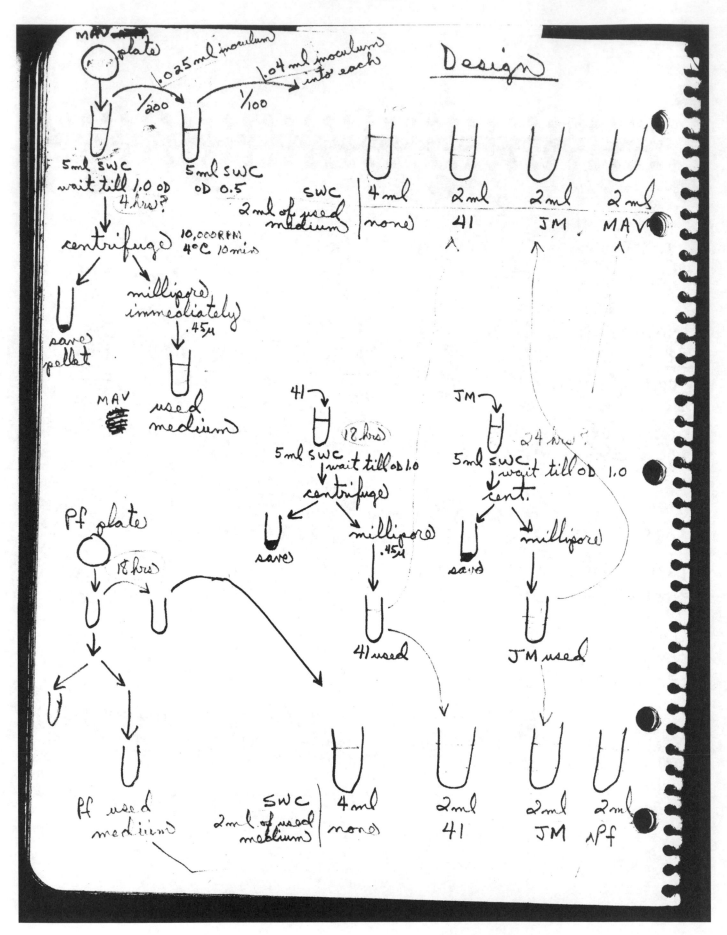

Pf. MAV Conditioned Media Experiment

7/28

Pf plate

.02ml → 4ml SWC media → centrifuge 10,000 × g 10 min 4°C filter

25ml SWC media
WAIT TILL OD 1.0 (7 hrs)

4ml SWC media
WAIT TILL OD 0.5 (5 hrs)

Pf Pf 41 JM MAV

supernatant	0	3ml	0	3	0	3	0	3
SWC	4ml	1ml	4	1	4	1	4	1

MAV plate

.02ml → 4ml SWC → centrifuge 10,000 × g 10 min 4°C filter

25ml SWC
WAIT TILL OD 1.0 (5½ hrs)

0.4 ml

4ml SWC
WAIT TILL OD 0.5 (4 hrs)

MAV MAV 41 JM Pf

supernatant	0	3ml	3ml	3ml	3ml
SWC	4	1	1	1	1

Pf
4ml SWC (2½ hrs) WAIT TILL OD 0.1 → inoculate experimental tubes 0.20ml

.04 ml

MAV
4ml SWC (2½ hrs) WAIT TILL OD 0.1 → inoculate experimental tubes 0.20ml

41 plate
17 hrs → 4ml SWC WAIT TILL OD 1.0 → .02ml (10 hrs) → 4ml SWC WAIT TILL OD 0.5 → .04ml (2½ hrs) → 4ml SWC WAIT TILL OD 0.1 → inoculate experimental tubes 0.20ml

JM plate
4¾ hrs → .02ml → as above (3hrs) → .04ml → (1¾ hrs) → 0.20ml

Ship Sketch, Woods Hole, 1972

I had seen few sailboats while growing up in Illinois, so during my 1972 summer experience at Woods Hole, Massachusetts I often spent time near the sea. Our group of students was invited to go sailing one afternoon, and I sketched the ship. We also had many outings in smaller boats to make specific ecology measurements, or just for fun.

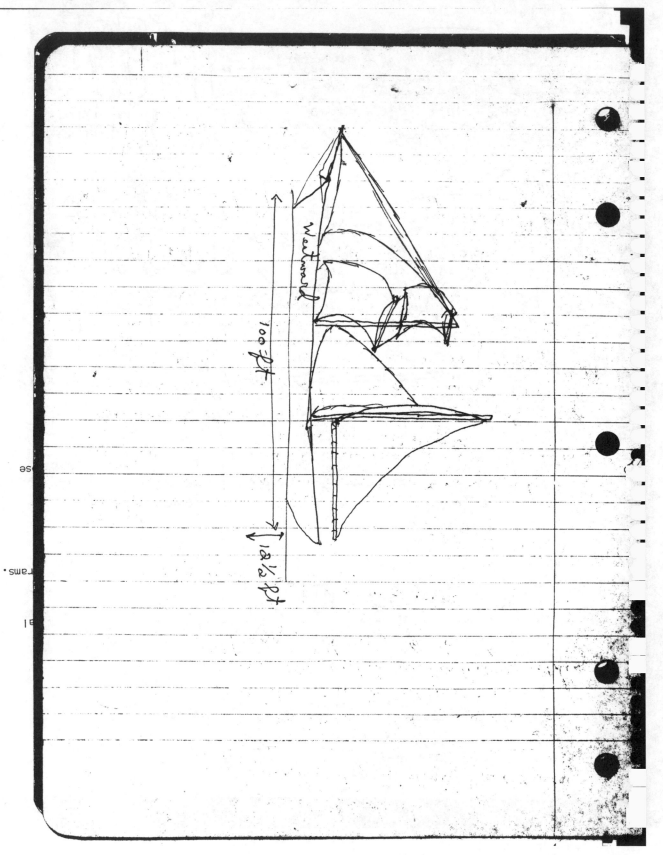

UNIVERSITY OF ILLINOIS AT URBANA-CHAMPAIGN
DEPARTMENT OF ENTOMOLOGY
320 MORRILL HALL
URBANA, ILLINOIS 61801
U. S. A.

July 5, 1972

Dear Jim:

I'm delighted you're enjoying the course and Woods Hole. Does the course ever get up to a eukaryotic ecology?

I sent your recommendation in to the Health Professions Information Office several weeks ago, and called this morning to make sure it was there - it is. If you are interested in an MD-PHD program you should look into some others too. Illinois produces very few of such but Chicago produces a lot and so do some of the Eastern Schools. You should be able to find people at Woods Hole who know about other programs. Many other places have stronger research faculty than the U of I medical school. Don't hesitate to apply to some of the other places, there may even be fellowship money in abuddance for some of the joint programs.

The easiest and most direct way to find out who would know best, is to check where different people now at Woods Hole come from - all of the instructors will be in American Men of Science. People love to give advice so you should have no toouble getting information. If you insist about going on to med school, at least choose one with a challenging faculy, if you want the research.

Best regards,

Judy Willis

A Valuable Note from a Caring Mentor

While I was at the University of Illinois as an undergraduate, Dr. Judy Willis helped me in many ways. She had suggested that I apply for the course at Woods Hole in 1972, for example. While at Woods Hole I wrote to her to ask her advice about medical schools, and she promptly replied with an informal and extremely helpful note. This was a life-changing letter for me, because I quickly decided to apply to the Pritzker School of Medicine at the University of Chicago. Not only did I get superb training at the University of Chicago, but I met the girl there who later would become my wife. Little things in life can sometimes make a huge difference. During my careers in academic medicine and in industry, I always made an effort to be a good mentor to others, thereby following the excellent examples of the mentors who helped me.

A few months before attending the Woods Hole program, I had decided that rather than becoming a PhD in Biology, I probably should become an MD/PhD, or at least an MD who could do both medical practice and basic scientific research. I was cautious about the need to win grants year after year, and the MD would be insurance that I could still make a living if the research projects failed. I was uncertain about this MD idea, however, so I decided that I would apply only to one medical school and see if I was accepted – if I were rejected, I would just go with the PhD-in-biology plan. Since most of my undergraduate experience was with the University of Illinois, I considered applying to that medical school, which is located in Chicago. While at Woods Hole I corresponded with my academic advisor back in Urbana, Dr. Willis. She wrote that the University of Illinois is a fine medical school, but mainly turns out skilled practicing clinicians. If I was actually inclined to research and a career in academic medicine, she advised, I should instead apply to the University of Chicago, which had much stronger basic science credentials. This seemed quite sensible. So I shortly obtained the paperwork, and one day I sat in the Woods Hole Marine Biological Laboratory library and filled out that medical school application. To make this paperwork task (and potentially life-changing activity) particularly memorable, I filled out my application using a black pen while sitting in the old wooden desk that had belonged to the famous Swiss-American paleontologist and geologist, Louis Agassiz (1807-1873), the discoverer of the Ice Ages, who had spent time years before at Woods Hole. I know that in the twenty-first century his old desk is still at Woods Hole, but it has been moved and is now part of a special exhibit, so no one can actually do paperwork while sitting there anymore. But for me, this has been a special memory. I made a photocopy of my application, applied the stamps and mailed it off to Chicago. A few months later I was called to interview at the University of Chicago, and a few weeks after that I was accepted to start in medical school there in the autumn of 1973.

Chapter 3

Medical School: Stimulating and Exhausting

In early September, 1973 I loaded up the family car with some clothes and a few boxes of items and books. I was going to have a small radio for my room, but certainly no TV, stereo, refrigerator, and – unimaginable to the modern reader – no computer. My father drove me north from Quincy to Chicago on a sunny morning, and we found International House on 59th Street, a substantial building from the 1930s with a comfortable lobby area for socializing, a cafeteria, and two major wings of dormitory-like rooms for residents, all graduate students. Residents shared large bathrooms on each floor, both all-male and all-female floors.

I had applied to have a shared room. My new roommate, Jeff Glick, who was from California and was studying for a masters degree in Social Services Administration, happened to be in the room when we went upstairs to the fourth floor. He was a very friendly and outgoing person, and he immediately offered to walk us around the campus to orient us to the main sites. The university buildings set among the grassy quadrangles were gorgeous, and we also stopped by the monument commemorating the site of the first "atomic pile," built by Enrico Fermi and his team on the squash court under the university sports stadium bleachers. This was where the first controlled nuclear reactions were studied. A few hours later my father headed back to Quincy, and my adventures in medical school had begun.

During the prior summer I had taken the formal advanced placement tests in both biochemistry and genetics, and easily passed both, so I was able to construct for myself a somewhat unique starting class schedule. I loved biochemistry, but it was important to me to avoid the usual starting biochemistry courses for the first year medical students because some instructors really push for a lot of memorization of formulas, structures and other details. I had never been a fan of rote memorization. The real value of education is not memorization of details, but instead it is gaining true understanding of the material, and developing the ability to think critically and creatively. One is then able to properly judge new and controversial ideas, and contribute novel concepts in an area of learning. For the most part, this is the standard University of Chicago philosophy. This approach is important in science, and particularly in medicine, since the fields are constantly changing and advancing. With my freed-up class time I took a special reading course about evolutionary biology and a class about New Testament redaction criticism in the Divinity School. Of course, I also took some required classes, including the quite challenging and memory-straining course in human anatomy.

Transcript in Medical School

It was my privilege to attend the Pritzker School of Medicine of the University of Chicago (1973-1977). College students today, especially pre-med students, could probably learn several valuable lessons by reflecting for a few minutes on my four years of medical school experience.

My class had very bright young men and women who were verbal, enthusiastic and friendly. We also had great teachers. All of the 100 students were quite scholarly, so it was great that the key medical classes and rotations were "Pass-Fail" since some other sort of grading system using a "curve" for this highly skilled group made no sense.

To get a running start, I took advanced placement exams in Genetics and also in Biochemistry and passed those a few weeks before I matriculated, so I did not have to sit for those courses. I replaced them with electives: Readings in Evolution in 1973, and Christology and the New Testament (in the Divinity School) in 1974. My goal has always been to try to take full advantage of learning opportunities in topics I have interest in, so being at a major university was fun as well as very beneficial.

The first two years of medical school were classroom lectures and some laboratories for hands-on experience. My academic advisor who helped me stay on track was Dr. Steven Lerner, an infectious disease specialist. He later also informally performed a routine tuberculosis skin test on his several advisees, and he found that mine had become positive; he advised me to have a chest x-ray at the Health Center and then take a year of oral daily ionized treatment, which I tolerated well.

In the autumn of 1975, when it was time to start clinical rotations, I was thinking that I was inclined eventually to go into internal medicine as a career. So the smart strategy would have been to take first other clinical rotations of lesser importance to me, perhaps obstetrics, to gain clinical experience. I should have taken the internal medicine rotation later. This strategy to delay the most important rotation had to do with learning clinical basics in settings where if one fumbled around a bit drawing blood or reading an EKG, the spotty performance wouldn't matter as much as the necessary high-level performance in one's chosen area. This demonstration of high competence had to do with getting very high quality letters of recommendation from attending physicians who would see me perform in internal medicine. I would need those letters when I applied for internships in internal medicine.

Well, many of my classmates also were inclined to internal medicine, so the required 25% of my class who must agree to take internal medicine first as greenhorns so as to distribute the class logistically into four equal parts was not forthcoming. After a couple more class meetings with teachers pleading for a few more students to volunteer to be the guinea pigs and take internal medicine first, I raised my hand and agreed. That spirit of volunteerism was certainly a reflection of my small-town helpful nature, but it was a mistake, although the term mistake might be a bit too harsh a word. I had so many very elementary things to learn in my first three months of clinical rotations that I naturally appeared to my superiors to be a true greenhorn, as I actually was. I was on a steep learning curve for various procedures and even basic routines of how a busy hospital ward functioned. One young attending physician who saw my performance was known to be a genuinely good man and very frank in all things. He had a routine private meeting with me at the end of a medicine rotation and told me that I presented orally in a timid fashion and had many practical skills to perfect. Clearly he was genuinely worried about my self-effacing and mild-mannered personality. He asked me if I really thought I was cut out for medicine. "Do you really think that you can make it?" he asked in a brusque manner, certain in his own mind that I was not tough enough or competent enough to succeed. But I replied, "Yes." I knew in my heart that I was fully capable, just inexperienced and honestly unassuming.

As I performed along with the bright, friendly and highly competitive fellow students, I noted that many of the young men adopted an alpha-male confidence in their manner of speaking and interacting. I began to perceive that my small-town behaviors and cautious approaches were making me appear to be less competent. An alpha-male student would crisply present the facts of a case verbally to the group, make definitive conclusions and a plan of action, and always seemed certain of everything he said. My mind did not work that way – I saw uncertainty and risk in all things, and when I presented a case to others I sounded that way. I often presented clinical findings not as facts, but as observations that might be incorrect or

incomplete in important ways. My weighing of details in that way made me seem overcautious and tentative. What I only realized some years later was that my insights and concerns about the many uncertainties and risks actually were a reflection of my seeing much more deeply into many issues than most of my classmates, but my sort of intellect did not serve me well as a third-year medical student. In a bit I will return to the story about the attending physician who thought that I would never make it in medicine.

I survived that first rotation in medicine with a lackluster performance, and gradually gained more competence as I rotated through obstetrics and gynecology, ophthalmology, ear-nose & throat, surgery, pediatrics and psychiatry. In fact, I had progressed so much by the time I did surgery that the top university surgeons viewed me as a promising young star and thought I certainly should become a surgeon because I scored nearly perfectly on all written examinations and by then had excellent clinical and procedural skills – I smiled and kept quiet because I knew that I had no long-term interest in becoming a surgeon. I liked the puzzle-solving aspects of internal medicine too much. Ironically, the surgical attending physicians were so impressed with me that it was the Chief of Surgery who proposed that I receive at graduation in 1977 a coveted place in the exclusive Alpha Omega Alpha organization awarded to only a few top students in the entire class each year. At the awards banquet with various faculty and those few top students, I could tell as I shook hands that several of the internal medicine attending physicians whom I had known in the earlier days were flabbergasted to see me get that award! They made no such comment, of course, but it was actually pretty funny to me at the time, and this was a demonstration as to how one must be careful about superficial first impressions of people, especially of bright and determined students who are learning rapidly.

Coming back to my final year (1976-1977), however, I decided that since I did want to target internal medicine as an internship, I took some of the most difficult and rigorous medical rotations as elective choices during the last year of medical school – whereas other students that year signed up for less stressful choices. I elected to take very taxing rotations in cardiology and hematology, for example, during which I would encounter desperately ill patients with many problems and high mortality rates – and I would be able to demonstrate my high competence in those difficult situations. This strategy accounts for how I eventually got those vital excellent letters of recommendation – as well as one glowing letter from the Chief of Surgery.

By 1976 I was planning after graduation to marry my girlfriend, a Texan, so in the autumn of 1976 I took two rotations away from University of Chicago (at San Antonio and at Dallas) so that I could better evaluate those Texas programs as potential internship choices, and also develop a track record at those institutions that might aid a potential application for internship. I eventually favored San Antonio and made that my first choice during the application process, and I was accepted to begin the internal medicine internship there in the summer of 1977.

Turning back now to the young attending physician who asked me when I was a bumbling student novice if I was really cut out for medicine, there is a follow-up story. In 1983 I applied for a faculty position at the University of Chicago, certainly one of the best medical schools in the world, and I got that job with stationing at Michael Reese Hospital, a prestigious private institution in its day. A faculty reception in honor of the several newly appointed young faculty members was held at the University of Chicago Hospital so that the full medical faculty could welcome the new members. It was a great honor for me to be so introduced. As I mingled, off to the side I saw that attending physician, now a professor, who had asked me rather pointedly years before, "Do you really think that you can make it?" Casually, I walked up to him at the reception and shook his hand, and the light of recognition instantly flashed in his eyes, followed by a look of astonishment. I simply smiled and said, "Well, I made it."

HE UNIVERSITY OF CHICAGO
OFFICE OF THE REGISTRAR
CHICAGO, ILLINOIS 60637

OFFICIAL ACADEMIC RECORD

A transcript is official when it bears the Registrar's seal and signature. Unless otherwise indicated, Honorable Dismissal is granted. Consult the accompanying notes for an explanation of this record.

Institution last attended B.S. (Biol.) Univ. of Illinois 1973 Urbana, Illinois
B.S. (Chem.) ibid. 1973
Entered: 10-1-73 DIV. OF BIOLOGICAL SCIENCES AND THE PRITZKER SCHOOL OF MEDICINE

Transferred To:

NAME JAMES ARTHUR MAGNER
HOME ADDRESS 3008 College Avenue, Quincy, Illinois
BIRTH PLACE Quincy, Illinois
Birth Date 5-30-51
Student Number 705374

SUBJECT		COURSE TITLE	UNITS	GRADE
AUT 73 FILE # 705374 ACAD.STAT. 2 DEPT. 710				
ANAT	301	GROSS ANATOMY	150	P
BIOCH	300	INTRO TO RSCH-BIOCHEM	100	P
CLINIC	300	CLIN ORIENTATION PROG	000	P
EVBIOL	333	READINGS IN EVOLUTION	100	A
WIN 74 FILE # 705374 ACAD.STAT. 2 DEPT. 710				
CLINIC	300	CLIN ORIENTATION PROG	050	P
MEDBIO	301	HISTOLOGY	100	P
MEDBIO	302	INFECTION & IMMUNITY	100	P
MEDBIO	303	CELLULAR/ORGAN PHYSIOL	100	P
SPR 74 FILE # 705374 ACAD.STAT. 2 DEPT. 710				
SOCMED	309	SOCIAL MEDICINE	050	P
MEDBIO	304	ORGAN PHYSIOL/ENDOCRIN	100	P
MEDBIO	305	NEUROBIOLOGY	100	P
DIV NT	479	CHRISTOLOGY NEW TESTMNT	100	P
AUT 74 FILE # 705374 ACAD.STAT. 2 DEPT. 710				
MED	466	INTRO TO HISTORY OF MED	100	P
MEDBIO	306	CELL/GENERAL PATHOLOGY	100	P
PATHOL	327	NEOPL DIS-CLIN PATH DGN	050	P
PHAPHY	306	PHARMACOLOGY	050	P
WIN 75 FILE # 705374 ACAD.STAT. 2 DEPT. 710				
CLINIC	301	HIST TAKING/PHYS DIAG	050	P
MEDBIO	307	PRINCIPLES OF PATHOPHYS	250	P

SUBJECT		COURSE TITLE	UNITS	GRADE
SPR 75 FILE # 705374 ACAD.STAT. 2 DEPT. 710				
CLINIC	301	HIST TAKING/PHYS DIAG	050	P
MED	343	FNDMNTLS OF ELECTROCARD	050	P
MICROB	331	MICROORG IN INFECT DIS	100	P
PATHOL	327	NEOPL DIS-CLIN PATH DGN	050	A
PHAPHY	307	CLINICAL PHARMACOLOGY	050	P
SUM 75 FILE # 705374 ACAD.STAT. 2 DEPT. 710				
MED	303	JR EXT INPAT MED SERV	300	P
AUT 75 FILE # 705374 ACAD.STAT. 2 DEPT. 710				
MED	304	EXTERNSHIP IN MEDICINE	050	P
OB&GYN	303	EXTERNSHIP IN HOSPITAL	150	P
OPHTH	316	OCULAR EXAM & DIAGNOSIS	050	P
SURG	330	BASIC ENT	050	P
WIN 76 FILE # 705374 ACAD.STAT. 2 DEPT. 710				
SURG	303	EXTERNSHIP IN HOSPITAL	300	P
SPR 76 FILE # 705374 ACAD.STAT. 2 DEPT. 710				
PEDS	303	JUNIOR EXTERNSHIP	200	P
PSYCHI	303	CLERKSHIP IN PSYCHIATRY	100	P
SUM 76 FILE # 705374 ACAD.STAT. 3 DEPT. 710				
MED	340	CARDIOLOGY-CLINICAL	125	P
MED	356	INFECT DIS SR CLRK-MRH	125	P
MICROB	471	NON-THESIS RSCH MICROB	050	P

OVER

THE UNIVERSITY OF CHICAGO – OFFICIAL ACADEMIC RECORD

			UNITS	GRADE
AUT 76 FILE # 705374 ACAD.STAT. 3 DEPT. 710				
MED	321	STUDY AWAY FROM U OF C	175	P
MED	390	INPAT HEMATOLOGY CLRKSP	125	P
WIN 77 FILE # 705374 ACAD.STAT. 3 DEPT. 710				
MED	345	CARDIOL-HEART STATION	100	P
MED	421	NEPHROLOGY SERVICE-CLIN	100	P
NEUROL	459	NEUROL CONSULT SERV-MRH	100	P
SPR 77 FILE # 705374 ACAD.STAT. 3 DEPT. 710				
MED	375	LIVER & GI DISEASES	125	P
MED	416	RDNGS GEN INTERNAL MED	050	P
MED	422	RENAL/ELECTROL PATHOPHY	050	P
MED	465	MED ETHICS PRACT PHYSCN	100	P
DEGREE MD		DOCTOR OF MEDICINE		
		AWARDED JUNE 1977		
ELECTED TO		BETA OF ILLINOIS		
		ALPHA OMEGA ALPHA		

Anatomy instruction was given in lectures, and also by practical dissection of a human cadaver. I had heard that one reason that there were so many medical schools established in Chicago in the 19th century was because of the more ready availability of cadavers, but I am not really certain that is true. Our cadavers were preserved in formaldehyde, and were laid out individually on metal tables. Each cadaver was covered by white plastic sheeting to retain formaldehyde vapor to prevent the tissue from drying out.

My starting medical school class had exactly 100 beginning students. In alphabetical order, four students were assigned to each cadaver, and we were to work as partners during the course. A manual set out what dissection procedures were to be done, and what structures were to be identified, at each dissection session. What I found particularly interesting was the cadaver to cadaver variation in structures, including significant variations in very important blood vessels, nerves and organs. Humans are not products of an assembly line process with strict quality control measures in place. Instead, there is a general plan, but also a fantastic amount of variation of details among individuals. This also is true on the biochemical level, and, as we all would learn decades later as molecular biology techniques advanced, it is also true on the genetic level.

Permit me to digress momentarily to comment on this individual variation in our genetic information. As discovered in the 1990s, the basic DNA sequences of all human individuals are very nearly the same. The DNA sequence can be viewed as an extremely long string of letters, but the alphabet of these letters is very restricted, since the sequence makes use of only the four letters: ATGC. These are one-letter abbreviations for adenine, thymine, guanine and cytosine, so-called DNA bases, which are molecules that are linked in a linear sequence in a strand of DNA. These four molecules can be arranged in any order, so the letters may be written in any order, including repeating the same letter once or more than once. The four DNA bases are like specially shaped links in a long chain. The complete DNA molecule actually has two chains wound around each other in a spiral known as a double helix, with the specific individual links of one chain actually fitting precisely into the specific individual links on the other chain to make a ladder-like structure. An A on one chain must be paired with a T on the other chain, while a G on one chain must be paired with a C on the other chain. So if one knew the letter sequence of one chain, one could construct the letter sequence of the other chain — this actually is the basis of the ability of a DNA molecule

to reproduce itself by unzipping the two chains, followed by each chain serving as a template to construct a new chain partner.

If the long strings of the DNA letter sequences from any two persons were set side by side and compared, about 999 out of every 1,000 letters would be exactly the same in the two sequences. Of the approximately 3 billion letters in each long string, the inheritable differences in each person thus would consist of just 0.1 percent of the sequence. In contrast, chimpanzees are approximately 7 to 10 times more genetically diverse. Moreover, the genetic differences between a chimpanzee and a human are 20 times greater than the differences between two average humans, even though the overall DNA sequence of an average chimpanzee is about 98.5% identical to that of an average human.

The high similarity of the DNA sequences among individual people is evidence that all humans descended from a relatively small group of ancestors, perhaps because many thousands of years ago the human population went through a so- called "bottleneck" because of famine or disease or lack of resources. The "bottleneck" concept would be more believable if our ancestors were living in a relatively small region, so that a famine, for example, could affect the entire location where the ancestors lived. Intriguingly, our direct ancestors possibly moved out of Africa about 50,000 to 100,000 years ago and, after stopping for awhile in the Middle East, they spread over a wide area. They followed in the footsteps of other hominids who had exited Africa in prior waves of migrations, and these human-like creatures who had migrated earlier shared a common ancestor with us, but the ones who had emigrated earlier from Africa were not (for the most part) our direct ancestors. In fact, there may have been a little breeding between these separate groups under special circumstances.

Recent studies of complete modern human and Neanderthal genomic sequences suggest that these groups did interbreed outside Africa. The genomes of modern humans outside Africa consist of about 2% Neanderthal sequences, and there is a slightly higher percentage in some modern populations. But native Africans have no Neanderthal sequences. After this interbreeding the Neanderthals became extinct, but this raised the questions as to where the interbreeding had occurred and how long the overlap of Neanderthal and modern human populations persisted. The timing question is very difficult to answer because radiocarbon dating techniques to study human bones or sea shells are operating near the edge of their reliable range when examining specimens that are about 40,000 years old, which is the period of interest. Specimens no longer contain the necessary radiocarbon after 50,000 years, whereas a 40,000-year-old specimen that contains 1% contamination with recent biological material will provide an erroneous date about 7,000 years younger than the real age. In August, 2014 an interesting paper by Higham et al. appeared in *Nature* entitled, "The timing and spaciotemporal patterning of Neanderthal disappearance." The authors dated specimens from 40 sites across Europe and a few sites along the east coast of the Mediterranean and the Black Sea. An important detail is that for bone specimens they purified collagen for the analysis of a specific amino acid to help exclude contamination. Accelerator mass spectrometry dating was conducted at the University of Oxford. It was found that some Iberian sites that had been believed to be evidence of fairly late survival of some groups of Neanderthals actually were older than had been previously thought. The main conclusions were that modern humans and Neanderthals overlapped in Europe for a period of about 2,000 to 5,000 years, and likely no Neanderthals survived in Europe later than 39,000 years ago. Of note, additional dating studies are now planned for specimens from Eastern Europe and Asia.

In February, 2010, a paper appeared in *Proc Natl Acad Sci USA* by Huff et al. from the University of Utah in which the study of "mobile elements" in human DNA sequences confirmed mathematically that there was at times a very small population size of our human ancestors. Even though these researchers compared in detail the slightly different sequences of only two persons, they were able to calculate that the effective population size of human ancestors living at about 1.2 million years ago was only 18,500 animals. Other workers have found that *Homo* after that time may have had some good years, and had a more expanded population by 200,000 years ago. But then there was another drastic reduction in human population at about 70,000 years ago, possibly due to very unfavorable climatic conditions or volcanism. The timing is slightly different according to Curtis Marean of Arizona State University, who writes in *Scientific American* in August, 2010 that in his view the bottleneck occurred earlier. He has focused on a very cold and dry ice age called the Marine Isotope Stage 6 period, which lasted from 193,000 to 123,000 years ago. Sea levels were lower during that period, and many areas of Africa could not continue to support the early human population which lived there. But an area along the coast of South Africa had abundant shellfish and numerous plants that stored carbohydrates in their roots that provided a reliable food source. Caves there have yielded evidence that humans survived that unfavorable era there, perhaps with a total living population of only a few hundred individuals, and these later gave rise to all of us. But whatever the precise timing of the ancient crash in human population numbers, it seems that our species barely made it into the present.

In spite of the fact that all humans share nearly the identical DNA sequence, there are genetic differences between people, of course. A change of a single base of DNA, more technically called a single nucleotide polymorphism (SNP), is commonly possible in many genes. Such a small change of a single letter, if it occurs in just the right place, can make a normal cell become a cancer cell, for example, a discovery that truly was a jaw-dropping surprise to biologists a few decades ago. Some larger scale structures of the genome, such as haplotype maps, gene copy numbers, numbers of repeats in repetitive sequences, etc., also vary among people. These variations allow DNA testing to be used to identify criminals based on crime scene samples, for example. The near genetic identity of human individuals, yet with the types of variability just mentioned, may seem like contradictory concepts, but the interested reader should pursue this further for a more in-depth explanation.

Returning now to my experience with Anatomy class, my three classmates and I named our cadaver "Fred." This was not at all intended as some sort of joke or disrespectful gesture. We decided that we wanted a nickname for our corpse to personify him a bit, rather than just having to conceptualize him as a slab of meat. We were very grateful that generous people had signed the necessary paperwork before their deaths to allow their bodies to be used for this purpose. Fred had been a well-muscled man in late middle age. The causes of death were not revealed to the students, and it was not our job to discover those causes – it was our task to systematically learn human anatomy.

Week by week we did learn. Exams to test our knowledge were given both on paper in a standard classroom, and also by "walk-throughs" of the anatomy lab during which we had to walk from cadaver to cadaver and write on our exam sheet the name of the structure highlighted by a carefully placed small paper arrow. This was not a trivial undertaking, but was manageable with proper study and a little experience. Still, this was particularly stressful for me since I am not good at memorizing large quantities of information.

All my classes at University of Chicago were "pass-fail," which relieved some of the pressure about grades. I always easily passed all my classes. At the university, specific letter grades were viewed as unnecessary because the students selected for entry were already the very top students from their colleges, so they were well-proven scholars. (I later learned that for every seat filled in my entering medical school class in 1973 there had been 39 applicants.) We were there to learn the material and how to think, rather than compete against classmates for a few top letter grades.

During the first two years of medical school, most of the instruction was in the lecture classroom setting, or in a group laboratory setting, such as when we viewed tissue preparations by microscope to learn histology. But during years three and four we actually put on white coats and worked alongside interns and residents in the hospitals and clinics to learn the practical day to day skills of being a doctor. We learned how to perform a rigorous medical history and physical examination, and how to look into the eyes with an ophthalmoscope. Drawing venous blood, starting intravenous lines, drawing a sample of blood from an artery to measure blood gases, and performing spinal taps were all skills we learned by the tried and true code: "See one, do one, teach one." Of course, one needed practice to get good at these procedures.

We also learned how to diagnose and take care of various medical, surgical, gynecological and pediatric conditions. And we learned logistical and other skills, such as how to write hospital orders in a chart, how to write progress notes, how to make rounds, how to perform consultations, how the paging systems work, how to run an ECG machine, how to read basic x-rays, how to look at urine under a microscope, and literally hundreds of other things.

Working with people during their times of pain and crisis was a special privilege, and I was very fulfilled and moved by it. As a medical student I would not be doing the big colonic surgery, for example, that the patient needed the next day, but I had more time than did the attending physician. So for many patients I was able to sit down for a few moments to explain things as best I could, and answer questions. I found that I actually enjoyed these aspects of medical practice more than doing the procedures or assisting with surgery.

I preferred analyzing laboratory results, solving medical diagnostic mysteries, or explaining things to patients more than actually doing the technical things, such as assisting with a cardiac surgery or doing invasive procedures. My key interests remained biochemistry and physiology in medical school. Since my personality also was that of an introvert and bookworm, it quickly became clear to me that I would be more inclined in the future to the practice of internal medicine, rather than neurosurgery, for example. A key task for any medical student during school is to learn one's interests and become comfortable with one's future career options.

During the third and fourth years of medical school I generally changed rotations each month. What that means is that I might have been assigned to a three month block of internal medicine rotations, and for one month I would do general internal medicine, the next month I would follow around the cardiologists, and the next month I would follow around the gastroenterologists, for example. During the two years of clinical training I also did rotations in gynecology, obstetrics, psychiatry, pediatrics, ophthalmology and surgery, including various subspecialties. This pattern of changing jobs each month was generally also true for the young doctors in training, the interns and residents. So it was very true then, and still is true today, that, due to the learning curve, a patient admitted to a medical service on the 25th of the month generally had a slightly more skilled and better organized team than did a patient admitted to a medical service on the first of the month. At least on the general medicine inpatient services, the intern was the doctor who wrote the orders and was responsible for integrating all important information about a patient, and she also dictated the discharge summary.

The intern was supervised in a very hands-on way by a doctor only slightly older, a resident. The medical students basically assisted the intern. The attending physician met with the intern, resident and medical students daily, usually at 10 am, for about two hours, to hear verbal presentations about newly admitted patients, and to learn follow-up information about other patients. The attending would then briefly speak with and examine each patient, usually make some didactic comments to impart some wisdom, and then sign all the charts. The attending would certainly weigh in on any big decisions being made, and was legally responsible, but the intern had the authority to proceed with most day-to-day routine activities, with help from the rest of the team.

I had been an Eagle Scout in my hometown of Quincy, so as part of my scouting experience I had learned to shoot a small caliber rifle. But I had never seen a gunshot wound. Many patients with knife and gunshot wounds were brought to the emergency room of the University of Chicago Hospital, and one evening, as I was following a surgical resident around on call, his beeper went off and he was asked to come to the E.R. right away to see a young man who had been shot. I rode down on the elevator with the resident and I was rather uncomfortable since I had no idea what this was going to be like.

The two of us were directed to an examination room, and I held my breath as we stepped through the door. There on the exam table sat a 25-year-old man looking more annoyed than traumatically injured. He wore a bright purple vest over a lime green shirt, and sported a large grey felt hat with a small orange feather on one side. He looked up at us and pointed to his left thigh. The nurses had removed his pants and had applied pressure bandages where a small caliber bullet had entered and also exited his thigh. We unwrapped the bandages to examine the small tears in the skin where the bullet had passed clean through. After a brief medical history, the resident showed me how he could tell that the path of the bullet had not hit the bone, the pulses in the leg were normal, and the neurologic examination of the leg also was completely normal. As I watched with a suppressed smile, the resident expertly applied a Band-Aid to both the entrance and exit wounds, shook the man's hand, and pointed him to the check-out desk. Sadly, not all of my experiences with gunshot wound patients were as lighthearted.

By the time of my fourth year surgical rotation I had established myself as a smart student who was very precise, well organized and highly competent, but, unfortunately (in the eyes of my surgeon supervisors), clearly inclined to internal medicine instead of surgery. They brought me one evening to the surgical intensive care unit where a middle-aged woman lay intubated on a respirator with multiple IV lines, a foley catheter, a chest tube, etc. She had been shot in the chest and abdomen four times by her husband, and had been stabilized in surgery that day.

The surgeons told me to watch her all night, keep track of all the central lines, IVs, medications, blood transfusions, urine flow, chest tube output, vital signs, respirator settings, blood gases, etc. and give them a call if I had any serious problems. I was thrilled by this opportunity to manage a complicated and very ill patient along with a skilled nursing staff, and, characteristically and quite understandably, the surgeons were thrilled to leave these medical tasks to a bright student so that they could get back to the operating room. Different people are just naturally inclined to different sorts of challenges. All went well until midnight, when a hospital security officer peeked into the intensive care unit to see me.

"Hey, doc, got to talk to you," he whispered, and, although I was wearing a white coat, I was not a doctor, just a fourth year student. "We just got a call that this lady's husband found out she is still alive, so he has grabbed his gun and is on his way to the hospital to finish her off."

"Oh," I replied numbly while holding two clipboards and three flowcharts.

"Just wanted to let you know, doc, so that you can be ready if a man comes in here." He shrugged and then added, "The chief asked me to sit down the hall for a couple hours, so I'll be there."

Not feeling much better about the security situation, I kept the IVs running, the blood transfusing, the chest tube draining, the respirator pumping, the urine flowing and the blood pressure stable all night until I was relieved in the morning. The angry husband never showed up.

While studying pediatrics, I cared for a thin white teenager who was being treated for pneumonia, and he had had many prior admissions for respiratory infections and other problems. He had been born with cystic fibrosis, a genetic disease caused by an abnormal "pump molecule" located in several types of membranes. Because the abnormality causes less chloride, sodium and water to appear on the outside of certain membranes, some passageways in the body easily get clogged with the thicker than normal secretions. These clogged areas can become sites of chronic infection in the lungs, for example, and the recurrent infections also cause local tissue damage. The ducts from the pancreas also can become clogged, resulting in painful inflammation of the pancreas. This can result in so much damage locally that the insulin-producing cells within the pancreas become depleted, and the patient can then develop diabetes.

My poor young patient struggled for a couple of weeks to improve, and at first seemed to get a bit better. He was on powerful antibiotics given directly into the veins, and several times daily he would hang over the edge of the bed with his head nearly touching the floor as the nurse clapped on his back to try to help him bring up the sticky pulmonary secretions. But he gradually grew worse and died one afternoon, probably from an overwhelming bacterial infection that was spreading from his lungs into his blood. That evening I walked slowly from the hospital along 59th Street back to International House pondering the mystery of human suffering.

During a general medicine rotation I cared for a number of young black adults with sickle cell anemia. These patients had a different genetic disease, in which the amino acid sequence of the hemoglobin molecule had been altered by a natural mutation. Hemoglobin is highly concentrated in red blood cells, which circulate between regions in the body rich in oxygen (the lungs) and regions in the body with lower oxygen levels (most other tissues, such as liver, heart, brain, muscle, etc.). The normal hemoglobin molecule changes its shape slightly, almost as if it is breathing, so that it can pick up oxygen molecules if many are present in the environment, and then later release those oxygen molecules in regions of the body where oxygen is deficient. This wonderful trick of nature was one of several that allowed larger organisms to evolve, since there had to be a mechanism (circulation of red blood cells) to allow oxygen to penetrate tissues that were far from where oxygen could be obtained by simple direct diffusion. The mutated hemoglobin molecule in sickle cell anemia changes shape even more extremely than does the normal hemoglobin molecule, however, such that in areas low in oxygen the molecule becomes more elongated, causing red cells to become sickle- shaped, sometimes with sharp points that cause the cells to clog small vessels in oxygen-poor areas. Of course, the clogging causes these oxygen poor areas to become even more depleted in oxygen, resulting in an unfortunate feedback cycle making the clogging even worse.

Clinically, this manifests as a "sickle cell crisis" with pain and abnormal function of many organs. The crisis can be treated with intravenous fluids, oxygen, pain medications, and blood transfusions, but susceptible patients may have many hospitalizations per year for such crises. Because of prolonged anemia, and the subsequent chronically active hormonal signaling to the marrow to grow and work harder, some of the patients develop characteristically tall thin heads, termed "tower skulls," reflecting an expansion of the marrow areas in the skull where a few more red blood cells could be manufactured. Experts have found that the sickle trait, essentially mildly affected persons who carry a single mutated gene, have a partial protection against malaria in their home regions. But if by bad luck an infant gets a full complement of two mutated genes, the child will develop full-blown sickle cell anemia. This disease thus reflects an evolutionary balance in which a single mutated gene gives a survival advantage, but with the price that the occasional unfortunate child with two mutated genes might not survive to adulthood.

I was also struck by patients who were suffering from subacute bacterial endocarditis, nicknamed SBE. Many of these patients were addicts who prepared illegal drugs in non-sterile containers, and then injected the mixture intravenously. Bacteria could travel in the veins to the right side of the heart, and probably most of the time caused no serious problem, but after an injection the bacteria might adhere to a frayed edge of a heart valve, most often the tricuspid valve. There the bacterial colonies would slowly grow, and then release from time to time small particles of the bacterial colony into the rapidly flowing blood. The repeated showers of bacteria in the blood cause episodes of fever and chills, and sometimes lung problems. The bacteria might also pass all the way into the arterial circulation and then lodge in capillaries in many tissues, such as the retinas, brain, etc. Such arterial distribution can result in visible changes in the back of the eye (small marks in the retina showing where debris traveling in the bloodstream has been deposited), neurologic signs, trace amounts of blood in the urine due to kidney damage, etc. SBE in prior decades was almost uniformly fatal, although by the 1970s powerful antibiotics could sometimes cure a patient if given intravenously for weeks. Cardiac valve surgery is sometimes required to replace a valve damaged by the local bacterial growth. Unfortunate persons who are not drug addicts can acquire SBE after a dental procedure, for example, which can spill bacteria into the bloodstream.

I decided to write up a short paper about SBE just for my own education, and I showed it to one of my medical advisors, "Dr. L." He thought my summary was quite good, and I was very taken aback when he asked if I thought I could publish it. That had never occurred to me, and I immediately declined to even consider publication – I thought that there were many textbooks and other sources already available that would be much more definitive. It was only a year or so later that I realized why he had asked this question. Dr. L., who was a superb clinician, a gifted teacher and a very smart man, was running into trouble in the University of Chicago system because he was told that he was not publishing enough. This was my first real-world exposure to the phenomenon of "publish or perish" in academia.

With the passing months, I was gaining a broader view of the world. I came to realize what a sheltered existence I had led in the small town of Quincy, Illinois and during my studious days at the University of Illinois. I previously had never seen drug addicts, prostitutes, tattooed gang members, alcoholics, criminals in handcuffs, and stabbing and gunshot victims. And I also previously had never seen a person with tuberculosis. This disease, known as the great imitator since it can cause so many types of clinical problems, has been a scourge of mankind since antiquity, although great progress had been made at reducing the numbers of patients in the USA and some other countries by the 1970s. But as a student, I diagnosed and took care of several indigent patients with the disease.

Months later I had my annual skin test, and this time my reaction was positive. This showed that, unfortunately, I had been exposed to some TB germs (likely by inhalation), although my chest x-ray was normal. My doctor advised a course of daily isoniazid, an oral tablet, for about one year to eliminate the few TB bacteria that likely were sleeping quietly in my lungs, waiting for my body to weaken as a result of another illness, malnutrition or age before launching their attack. I complied with this regimen and had no difficulties. Some patients develop abnormal liver tests while on the drug, but my doctor wisely chose not even to test for liver problems (unless I actually had become ill), since he wanted me to take the full course of medication and not stop it just because of some asymptomatic mildly abnormal liver tests. This reinforced in me the clinical dictum that by then I had already learned – don't measure a test in the clinic if it is not going to change what you are going to do.

On one occasion a young physician was visiting from England, and we walked him around the ward. While standing at the bedside I presented to him a case of a man who was improving on anti-TB medications. The young doctor was incredulous that we still were seeing cases of TB commonly in the United States, since during his training he had not seen one case in England. I explained that our impoverished urban areas still had malnourished or alcoholic or other down-and- out persons with TB. With typical British humor, he responded adamantly, "Not in our slums!"

During the summer of my third year of medical school I developed high fever, a very sore throat, swollen lymph nodes in my neck, and a very enlarged spleen. This constellation of symptoms was not very mysterious to the Student Health Center physician, and a blood test confirmed the diagnosis of mononucleosis. In fact, he told me that my heterophile test result was the highest titer ever seen as of that date at the University of Chicago. As you may imagine, I was not very pleased by that distinction.

I wondered if I somehow could have picked up this disease from a patient, but usually salivary contact, such as by kissing, was the common mode of transmission. I did have a girlfriend, Glenda, who was not ill, and then it quickly dawned on me where I likely had picked up mono. A few weeks previously a girl whom I sometimes saw around International House asked me if she could look something up in one of my medical books. I had eaten dinner with her in the cafeteria on several evenings, along with other students at the table, so we knew each other superficially. I invited her up to my room that Saturday afternoon to look at my bookshelf.

She looked at a few books, then we sat down to talk a bit. After a minute or two she suddenly leaned forward from her chair and planted her lips firmly on mine! I was so surprised that I was momentarily speechless, although I also was quite flattered. Nothing like that had ever happened to me before. We laughed, and then I escorted her back to the lobby. In my own mind I knew that I was quite happy with Glenda, who was home in Texas for the summer. I actually had not thought about that surprise kiss again until I was told that I had mono! In fact, I was pretty weak and ill for about a month, and I missed about three weeks of clinical rotations during my third year of medical school. Even when I returned to school, I felt that I had no stamina. I had always needed a lot of sleep, and now I needed even more – a high price to pay for an unexpected kiss.

Some of my student rotations were at Michael Reese Hospital located north of the main campus of the university. I took an infectious disease elective there, and daily kept fever and white blood cell charts on quite a few patients being seen by the consultation service. Many patients were on lifesaving but potentially toxic antibiotics, and had to have blood samples drawn at certain times just before and after a dose of antibiotic was administered to capture the trough and peak levels. Bacteria isolated from individual patients were cultured in the laboratory, and were tested on agar plates onto which had been placed small paper discs containing differing amounts of the antibiotic being given to the patient.

Many of the bacteria were resistant to an antibiotic below a certain level, so this information was a good clinical guide as to what the trough blood level needed to be in the patient in order likely to cure the infection. This intellectually satisfying service, using lab results to directly guide patient care, was attractive, and I thought that I might someday specialize in infectious disease. My attending physician, "Dr. J. G.," remembered me eight years later and put in a good word for me when I applied for a faculty position at Michael Reese Hospital as an endocrinologist in 1983.

One patient being followed on high levels of powerful antibiotics was an unfortunate young man, about 20 years old, who had been riding a motorcycle at high speed and who sustained open injuries to his cervical spine. He survived neck surgery, but developed meningitis, and remained unconscious. He was a powerfully built young man with a beautifully muscled body, and he must have been about 6 feet 4 inches tall since he barely fit in his bed. His dominating physical appearance was even more striking as he lay in his helpless unconscious state. We added antibiotics and raised the amounts to the maximum, but within a week he was dead from his meningitis. I guess he had believed himself indestructible, but this is never the case.

One wonderful aspect of training at the University of Chicago was that many of the attending doctors were experts in their areas, were doing basic science research or clinical research, and were publishing important medical articles in journals. We heard about very new information, the latest discoveries, and we tried to apply these when appropriate to the patients we were seeing practically in real time. I had always been interested in research, and I began to understand what it would be like to have a career in academic medicine.

One disconcerting aspect of medical school was the very long work hours. Our introduction to this fact was a comment made to our class on my very first class day at the school in September, 1973 – "I hope that you all have enjoyed your very last summer vacation!" And it was true, of course. Starting in September, 1973, we worked 12 months a year, with just a week off here and there, through all the rest of medical school, and through internship and residency training, and anticipated this through all the rest of our working careers, for life! Moreover, we often slept in the hospital while on-call, frequently awakened for this or that problem, so it was difficult ever to feel properly rested. For the first time in my life I began routinely drinking coffee, and I soon became dependent on it daily to keep going.

This was a bigger problem when I was an intern and resident, because I was then making key decisions, or performing minor but invasive procedures, while I was literally exhausted. But even in medical school I was chronically tired, and I feared that I was not properly thinking through some of my patient's cases. Was it really necessary to work such long hours, and try to evaluate and treat patients when so fatigued? Various arguments supporting and condemning this method of training were heard now and again, and years later there were formally agreed limits for work hours placed on students, interns and residents. But during my training there were no formal limits. We did have various call schedule schemes, but the hours were still long, and could be even longer in a rather unpredictable way if some problem came up.

In 2010, a large prospective study of 1271 young doctors in training was published in *Archives of General Psychiatry* by Srijan Sen of the University of Michigan, and colleagues. They found a marked increase in depressive symptoms among new clinicians, from 3.9% at baseline to 25.7% during internship. Many were having trouble sleeping, or were having difficulties in their close personal relationships. More than 40% of the trainees met criteria for major depression at one or more quarterly assessments. Medical specialty and age were not parameters that were associated with the development of depression. The three key variables that were associated were work hours, reported medical errors, and noninternship stressful life events.

The investigators also used the stress of internship as a model to assess the relationship between a genetic marker and the development of depression during the experience. In other words, did a medical trainee who genetically had a slightly different nerve cell molecule in his brain show a greater risk for depression? A caveat is that some of these analyses by the authors were post-hoc explorations of the data, which somewhat weakens the ability to draw firm conclusions. It was known that a relevant critical molecule in brain cells actually differed slightly among people on a genetic basis. The slightly different structures of this molecule caused it to be able to do its usual job in a nerve cell either with low-function or high-function. Each person has two gene copies or alleles, so for this gene, a person could have two low-function copies, a low and a high, or two high-function copies. One could imagine nearly identical cars lined up side by side for a race, but their engines contain slightly different types of carburetors that are a bit better or worse than a normal carburetor for passing fuel into the engines. In this case, the slightly different carburetors are altered molecules resulting from different DNA sequences in a particular gene, a serotonin transporter promoter. In fact, in the study of the medical trainees, a variant of this gene was found to be related to the response to stress among European-American subjects. Subjects carrying at least one low-functioning gene reported a 43% greater increase in depressive symptoms than did subjects with two high-functioning alleles. Thus, a person's underlying genetic makeup can be a factor that accounts in part for how they adjust to a stressful experience.

Back in the 1970s, near the end of my fourth year of medical school, our class began rehearsals for the traditional senior skit, during which it was permissible to poke fun at some of our teachers and at the university. Each year the production drew a large crowd, and we intended to do our part to put on a quality skit. I played a number of roles, including Abraham Lincoln, with beard and stove-pipe hat, as famous characters in history roasted an ambitious gentleman who during our senior year had accepted a position as a dean, but within a few weeks he resigned that position to take what he regarded as a better position elsewhere. Naturally, in everyone's opinion at the university, this person was quite safe to roast! The dangers of this type of ambition also were portrayed in a rendition of *Macbeth* that proved to be highly popular in our skit. One of my fellow witches in one scene was Steven Lukes, one of the brightest and nicest students in our class, and we did a bang-up job on the heath. Regrettably, within six years Steven died when an unsuspected brain aneurysm ruptured during his sleep in March, 1983. It was a tragic loss for his family, and for the thousands of patients he would have served.

I made it through the four years of medical school, performed well, and was well trained. I had good letters of recommendation, so I was able to secure an internship slot at my first choice institution, which for various reasons which will be explained was in San Antonio. Space does not permit me to share here very many of the fascinating and entertaining stories that I could tell about my medical school experience. Overall, my experience was much more positive than negative. I am proud to be a 1977 graduate of the Prtizker School of Medicine.

Chapter 4

A Surprise Girlfriend and a Miracle Wife

I don't think that there was anything wrong with me biologically, but I always had higher priorities than meeting girls. During the high school years I attended an all-male school, and I made few efforts to meet many girls. I loved school, reading, watching TV, family activities and a number of hobbies (somewhere far down the list was chess). In college I was fanatical about doing well in all my classes, and learning as much as I could. During a four-year period I took three or four girls out for an evening in Urbana, but there was no special chemistry. Many years later I received a letter from the alumni association at the University of Illinois requesting me to update my profile, and they asked me to complete a sentence starting, "If I could do things differently during my college years, I probably would…" I thought seriously about completing the sentence with the phrase, "…go to more parties and school events, and meet more girls!"

In May, 1974, I was finishing up my first year of medical school at the University of Chicago, and final exam week was approaching. I ran into a girl at the laundromat on the third floor of International House. I lived on the fourth floor and she lived on the third. She was from Houston and was on a track that, if she chose, could lead to a Ph.D. in English. We went out for a beer later that evening at a dance being held on the first floor of International House, and we had a great time. Predictably, however, for the next week or ten days I was all business as I prepared for and took several final exams. Later, with nearly all of that out of the way, I phoned her, and she was a little surprised (in view of the delay) and very happy to hear from me again. Clearly, we had hit it off. Glenda became my surprise girlfriend, and truly the only serious girlfriend I ever had.

I have already recounted how I proposed to her in 1977 in that same laundromat, after which we went out for a drink at the top of the John Hancock Building. I started my internship in Internal Medicine at the University of Texas Health Science Center in San Antonio in late June, and I took a light rotation my first month so that we could have a few days off in July, 1977 to get married in Houston. We rented a small apartment in San Antonio near the medical center, and things on the home front were great. The heavy work load of the internship, followed by a two-year residency program in Internal Medicine, was stressful, but we managed. Glenda continued writing her dissertation

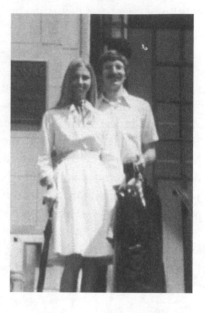

**A Couple In Love and
Departing International House**

In 1977, Glenda and I were moving a few more things out to the car before meeting friends. Within hours we would complete our move out of International House in Chicago, where we had met in the laundromat, and we would begin our long drive to Texas. Little did we know when this photo was snapped that shortly we would be running into Merle.

for her PhD. She used the University of Texas library in Austin, and there were sometimes piles of papers and notecards lying about in our apartment, which I just stepped over when I came home and collapsed into bed. In this computer age, it may be hard for readers to imagine how scholarly work once was done using paper and notecards, while typing on an electric typewriter.

We sometimes visited on a Sunday with her mother in San Antonio, her grandfather in Houston, or my parents in Seguin, TX. One Sunday evening we returned to our apartment to find the front door ajar and a note taped there saying, "Please see the Manager." It turned out that during the day when we were away someone backed a truck up to our ground-floor sliding glass door, pried the door open, and starting loading any items that looked valuable into the truck. When we first found the door ajar, I stood there speechless for a few seconds, but Glenda's reaction was immediate and quite different. She

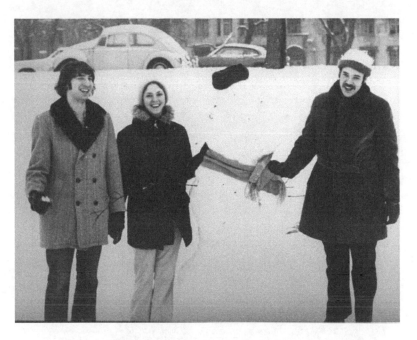

Building a Snowman in Chicago

Glenda was from Houston and had never built a snowman. We met in the spring of 1974,
and by the winter of 1975 I was teaching her my snow sculpting techniques on the Midway
along 59th Street in front of International House. I am at the left holding Glenda's hand;
another student, Steve Coombs, joined our fun. A passing student unexpectedly wanted to
take our photo with his fancy camera, and he kindly gave us a print the next week.

frantically ran around the ransacked rooms shouting, "Where's my briefcase?!" She had her key notes and notecards in manila file folders in a particular briefcase. It turns out that the crooks had dumped the contents of the briefcase, found only English literature notes inside, and quickly threw it back in the corner as obviously being of no value! Luckily for Glenda, the burglars had not been well-educated! She eventually finished her thesis and was awarded her Ph.D. from the University of Chicago in June 1979.

In early 1980, I was accepted into an Endocrine Fellowship at the National Instititutes of Health (NIH) in Bethesda, Maryland, and we moved to a two bedroom apartment there in late June, 1980. And as we moved, Glenda was pregnant with our first child!

At about 6:00 am in the morning of Jan. 23, 1981, Glenda went into labor. We were both so excited and happy! I actually jumped up and down with glee. After the momentary peak thrill had passed, I explained to Glenda that we would go to the hospital soon, but her labor probably would take several hours. With some trepidation,

I asked if she would permit me 45 minutes to run back to my laboratory at NIH to turn off an electrophoresis machine and retrieve my valuable experimental samples, which otherwise would be ruined. It is a reflection of how well she knew me, and how much she loved me, that she replied, "Of course, but come back quickly!" As a footnote, let me add that in actual fact those experimental results turned out to be vitally important, and provided the basis for my first major scientific publication.

Our little girl, Erin, was born that afternoon, and all seemed well. In the section of this book about Erin, I will detail some of the tragic and miraculous events that subsequently transpired.

Our second child, Carly, was born in Illinois in September 1984. Carly presented breech and it was hoped that the baby would turn, but she did not. The obstetrician explained that a C-section was almost always done in this situation for fear that something could go wrong during the delivery, but that with just the right conditions, a breech delivery might be in order. He suggested checking

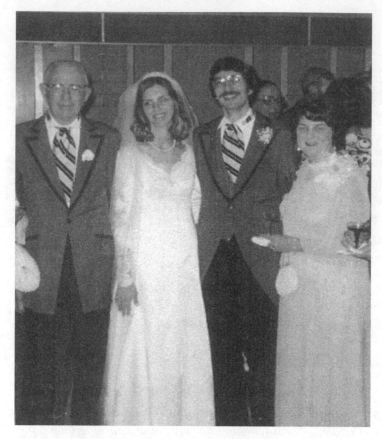

Glenda and Jim at their wedding reception, 1977
Glenda is standing beside her maternal grandfather,
Milby Iiams, while I am with my mother.

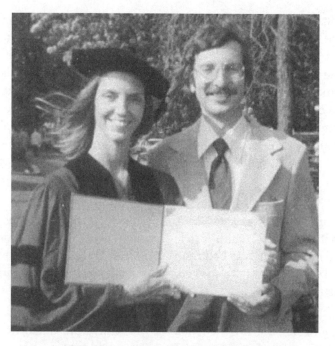

Glenda gets her Ph.D. in 1979
After years of effort, and a brilliant defense, Glenda was awarded her
Ph.D. in English at the University of Chicago.

Glenda's pelvic dimensions, and the baby's cranial dimensions, using a single x-ray, and we agreed. He found that Glenda's pelvis would easily allow the delivery – in fact, he said, "Your wife has a great pelvis!" I of course thanked him for that compliment. Being aware that we were in a teaching hospital and with Glenda in labor, I suggested that any medical trainees who were available might benefit from observing this unique delivery. With a glance that was a mixture of disbelief and – frankly – dismissal, as if she had far more important things on her mind, Glenda bravely delivered Carly at about 3 pm that afternoon, and I'm sure that a half-dozen trainees will remember that event to this day.

There is so much more that I could say about Glenda, especially about her Herculean efforts, day and night, during the years of our first daughter's critical medical illnesses. I could praise her for her remarkable teaching career at several different colleges and universities as she followed me from city to city. And there is so much more, including how she allowed me often to steal back to my laboratory to work on an experiment, or even to have an afternoon to myself to play chess, of all things! But Glenda is a very private person, so perhaps I will leave all of that for another book. I have no doubt that my life would have been greatly diminished had we not met by chance and hit it off so well in that laundromat in Chicago.

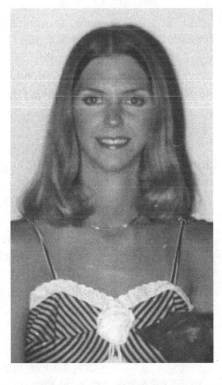

Glenda Dressed for Dinner

In July, 1978, Glenda and I were about to go out to dinner in San Antonio to celebrate our one year wedding anniversary, and I thought that she was so stunning that I insisted on taking a photo.

Tell me I'm wrong!

Chapter 5

Internship and Residency: More Stimulating and More Exhausting

Things were looking up. I was finishing medical school in 1977, and I was engaged to be married that summer. I had also been accepted at my first choice hospital for my internship in Internal Medicine. This had been accomplished in the prior months by interviewing at several institutions, then participating in the somewhat famous "internship match." Glenda and I packed up boxes of books, which made up about half of our possessions, and mailed them to Texas. We had found a small apartment on Fredericksburg Road east of the medical center. Then we loaded the rest of our items into Glenda's blue Dodge Charger. The car was a little banged up and well worn after four years and multiple trips between Houston and Chicago, but it was usually reliable. So we headed south out of Chicago.

The drive went well until we were about 30 miles outside of Little Rock, Arkansas. We were on the four-lane highway, and the Charger started coughing and losing power, so Glenda pulled it over to the side of the highway. We sat stunned for a moment as cars and trucks whizzed by, each one slightly rocking our stalled car. It was still light, although dusk was coming, and there were pine trees as far as we could see. We stood outside the car and I raised the hood. Of course, this was before cell phones. For several minutes the cars sped by, but after a quarter hour one old small station wagon passed us but slowed, pulled to our side of the highway, then backed up 50 yards to reach where we were parked. A clean-cut man in his 30s walked back toward us. "Out of gas?' he asked.

"No, the car just lost power," I replied, "so I guess we will need a tow truck."

We shook hands and I was certainly glad he had stopped. He said to grab anything valuable out of the car and then he would give us a ride to the next exit where he thought there was a filling station, and someone could probably arrange for a tow from there. He smiled and then handed me a newspaper he had carried with him: a pro-Communist newspaper with large red letters in the headlines, and a big red hammer and sickle in the top corner. "I also want to give you this," he said earnestly, "and I really want you to read it and think about it."

I was now more stunned than when the car had died. I realized that I was in the woods in Arkansas talking to someone who should be feeling a little out of place in this county. But I took the newspaper, thanked him, and when I reached into the Charger to collect a small travel bag, I tossed the newspaper into the back seat.

The ride to the exit took less than three minutes, and we hopped out at the filling station and waved goodbye. I really did appreciate his help. The station owner said that we were in luck, since Merle was just bringing the tow truck back to the shop right now, and he would be happy to tow us into a place he knew in Little Rock that could fix our Dodge. In a half hour a very large tow truck pulled in driven by a very muscular young man. I helped Glenda up the high step into the front seat next to the driver, then I stepped up, slid onto the seat, and shut the door. Off we went to retrieve our sick car.

Merle told us to take any other valuables out of the car, since he would drop the car at the dealership, and then drop us at a nearby motel. This time as I reached into the Charger, I had a couple of minutes to stuff the Communist newspaper into one of my small bags out of sight. I didn't want that in the car where the workmen would see it. Merle raised the front wheels of the Charger and hooked it up, we climbed back into the front seat, and off we went to Little Rock.

It was now dark, and within a couple minutes I realized that we were going about 85 mph. I looked back and, yes, our car was still dragging along behind. Next I realized that on the dashboard in front of our driver was a large black pistol without a holster, and next to that there was a three-inch thick stack of bills secured with a couple of rubber bands. "I guess you are ready for any trouble," I said in a loud voice to be heard above the roar of the truck as I pointed at the gun.

"Yep," said Merle. "OK if I put on the radio? My favorite show is on now," he added.

Not being in an argumentative mood, I agreed, and he clicked the button. The church choir was just starting "Holy, Holy, Holy," and Merle turned the volume up higher as the engine roared. I think he also picked up the pace to 90 mph. Our car, remarkably, was still attached. The next few minutes were quite memorable as we raced along the highway in the dark, swerving around slower traffic, with the gospel choir on the radio at full blast. Soon we were at the dealership where we dropped the car by the front door. A few blocks away at the motel we bid farewell to Merle with our sincere thanks and a small tip, since at that point we barely had any money in our checking accounts. Merle did his job well, and he did it in style – Arkansas style! The next afternoon we had a repaired car and an interesting story to tell.

I was very excited and slightly wary as I started my medical internship. I knew that the work hours would be terrible, but I was pretty sure that I could manage it.

Bexar (pronounced "bear") County Hospital was a big, busy place on the northwest side of the city. The hospital had many sick, indigent patients, many of whom spoke only Spanish. Nearly all of our nurses and many other workers at the hospital also spoke Spanish, and they were always willing to help me understand a frightened, ill patient who was trying to tell me what was wrong. I had taken Spanish in high school, so I knew a little conversational Spanish, but for all important medical work I always grabbed an employee nearby to help me understand properly. The V.A. Hospital across the street was relatively new and well-equipped, and also had lots of ill clients, most of whom spoke English. In July, the first month, I had arranged for a light elective and one week of vacation, since Glenda and I were to be married in Houston on July 23. But that meant that the remaining eleven months of my internship would be very hard work without a significant break.

The wedding and honeymoon were great, and I could write another book about all that. Glenda, a Protestant, agreed to be married in a Catholic church but with the proviso that it not be old-fashioned and dark with lots of statues! Speaking with some of her friends in Houston, she learned that there was a modern Catholic church, St. Michael's, on the west side of the city. In early 1977 I had phoned the pastor and explained that although I was not from Houston, Glenda and I would like to be married at St. Michael's in July, if possible. He replied that it was a bit of a problem since I was not a member of that parish, but that he would "pencil in a date" in July, although he might later have to take that date away if someone else needed the church. Of course, we could not plan a wedding under those circumstances, so I phoned the Bishop's office in Galveston – I did not want to seem to be pushy, but I hoped to see if perhaps a more stable and predictable arrangement could be made with the pastor at St. Michael's, or perhaps at a similar Catholic church in the Houston area.

The next day the Bishop's office called me back and said that all was worked out about the July date I had requested, and I should phone the pastor at St. Michael's once again. I phoned him, feeling a little uncomfortable because it had not been my intention to seem to apply pressure; I just needed to figure out how and where to get married. The pastor was pleasant, reported that July 23 would be fine, and that he wanted to meet with Glenda and me soon after we arrived in Texas. That meeting subsequently went well, Glenda liked the architecture of the church, and we arranged for use of the reception hall next door for a small fee. During that brief meeting we worked out many important things about our marriage, but one small detail that eluded me was that I did not specifically request that there should be chairs placed in the reception hall. We were not having dinner or music at the reception, just snacks, drinks, a champagne fountain, and of course the wedding cake. It turned out that on July 23 the wedding ceremony was perfect, and the reception was pleasant, but there were no chairs for the guests! So a piano bench had to be located so that a couple of the older ladies could rest their legs. It all went by as a blur to the groom, of course, and after a few hours at the reception Glenda and I were off to a Houston hotel where we would spend our wedding night.

Since we had no money, we drove to New Orleans for a four-day honeymoon at a modest hotel, and on the way back, stopped in a small town where one of our big expenses was to rent a rowboat for an afternoon. True love is a beautiful thing.

In August I was back to work, this time serving in the rather run-down and exceedingly busy outpatient emergency area that then operated in the old Robert B. Green Hospital in downtown San Antonio. Some patients stumbled in very, very sick, while others were there with a minor complaint, and they were all jumbled together. Although I had gained some insight during medical school, one of the key skills that I developed in a hurry during August was to learn, after only a very minimal history and exam, which patients were very sick and which were not. If a patient had to be admitted to an intensive care unit, then I would ride in the ambulance with him up to Bexar County Hospital to keep an eye on the cardiac monitor, the vital signs, and the IV, and to give medical treatments during the trip as needed. As an intern in my second month I had very limited experience, but I was learning very fast on the job, which has been the traditional approach in medicine for centuries.

Some patients who had had chest pain for a few hours revealed when they took off their shirts in the emergency room that they had several clippings of herbs Scotch-taped to their chest. These patients had presented first to the neighborhood healer, the *curandero*. The healer had a waiting area in her front room, often decorated with lots of religious pictures and statues. She then saw patients individually briefly and gave out advice, herbs or other items to help. The *curandero* actually served a useful role for us since the anxious person who had had a fight with his spouse often responded well to the herbs, whereas the true heart attack victim failed to improve much, so the healer would wisely refer that patient to the emergency room.

Mildly or moderately ill patients presented to the emergency room with a wide variety of complaints, and would have simple testing done, a diagnosis made, and treatment begun by starting a medication or issuing a prescription. Patients were given an outpatient appointment in our weekly internal medicine clinic to be followed up personally in most cases, and sometimes other outpatient testing was scheduled, such as a barium enema. My personal clinic was soon full to overflowing after my first weeks on the job, but the patients generally were wonderfully tolerant of any inconvenience. They patiently waited for their turn to see me, and at Christmastime the older ladies often brought me tamales or other treats. We tried to prescribe very inexpensive generic drugs, which may sound like a bad thing, but actually for the most common illnesses the tried and true older drugs seemed to work pretty well. In 1977 the care of the Type 2 diabetes patients, for example, was quite primitive by modern standards. It is a bit shocking, now that I am in my late 50s, to take note of how much has changed in medicine between 1977 and 2010.

Some moderately or severely ill patients had to be admitted to the inpatient service each day, and that required that I discuss the case with my supervising resident, and then phone the medical resident on call up at the big hospital and explain why we wanted to admit this patient. The harried and sometimes exhausted resident, no matter how much of a humanitarian he was, often would not be very happy to hear about another proposed admission that he and his intern would have to carefully examine and get settled on the ward with proper treatment. But we always took care of the patient, even if the resource-stretched county system did not make it very easy.

In September, the shoe was on the other foot. Another intern and I staffed a part of the inpatient medicine ward supervised by a medical resident one year our senior. Each intern had 10 to 15 inpatients at a time, and on our "long-call" admitting night we each could admit 0 to 10 new patients, with an average of about 5. So you can see that we were always trying to get patients stabilized within a couple days if possible so that they could be discharged and continue treatment and any needed further testing as outpatients. We had to discharge patients in a reasonable time because we were always getting more admissions. We worked on a four-day cycle: "long-call" (example: Monday 7 am until Tuesday 7 am, and then continued to work Tuesday until about 6 pm, but with no further new admissions after 7 am on Tuesday); "post-long-call" (Tuesday, as described); "short-call" (Wednesday, accepted hospital admissions between 7 am and noon); "non-call day" (Thursday, do routine work on ward and/or clinic). The weekly outpatient clinic was pre-set on a certain weekday, so while serving on the in- patient ward the clinic duty was sometimes occurring on each of the four types of call days, the worst situation being when it occurred on a "long-call day." Interns presented new admissions, and follow-up information, to a senior physician, the attending physician, each morning, seven days per week, including Christmas. The attending physician offered useful insights and advice, visited each patient briefly, and signed the charts.

One night a 24-year-old Hispanic woman was admitted with sudden onset a few hours before of sharp terribly cramping pain in the right flank and blood in the urine. She had been healthy and had never had such an episode before. It sounded like a kidney stone. She admitted to working in a hot environment and not drinking much water routinely, so that her urine often was darkly concentrated. I ordered routine blood and urine tests, including a pregnancy test, and I administered IV fluids and pain medication. The medication took the edge off the pain, and in the morning the urologist agreed that it was probably a kidney stone, and ordered an intravenous pyelogram, an IVP, a test in which some x-ray dye is given in the vein to be cleared into the urine. A series of abdominal x-ray pictures is taken to try to visualize a dilated ureter, or a stone. In fact, she had a small kidney stone that had lodged in one ureter, and the dye was building up behind it. We gave more IV fluids, and periodically took another abdominal film, and we could see that the stone was moving down the ureter. Finally the pain lost its sharp edge and became dull and steady, and the next film showed that the stone had passed out of the ureter. The patient collected her urine to try to capture the stone for chemical analysis, but we never found it.

Within another 24 hours the young woman felt much improved, and she was discharged with strong advice to drink more water, and keep her appointment in the urology clinic. I thought that was the end of her internal medicine story, but a few weeks later she unexpectedly phoned me. She had just learned that she was pregnant, and she calculated by the intercourse history that she might have been 2 or 3 weeks pregnant when she had all of the IVP x-ray films performed! The urine test done at that time possibly was not sensitive enough to detect her early pregnancy. She was very worried about the radiation to her fetus. Her question – should I have an abortion? She was married and desperately wanted to keep the baby if I thought it was safe. I told her I would call her back in a day.

I spoke to several colleagues, but no one could offer any relevant information. Textbooks and articles seemed not to be definitive. Clearly, she had had about 6 abdominal x-rays, but the dose of radiation and its implications for a 2 or 3 week- old embryo really were not clear. I called her back the next day and explained that there certainly was some risk of a congenital defect from the radiation, and that there is always some risk of a congenital defect in any case, even without any known extraneous radiation exposure. I told her that the risks were real but also probably small, although not minuscule. I couldn't put a precise number on it. I added that if it were my wife's baby, that I would recognize that there would be a small additional risk of a problem, but that I would advise my wife to keep the baby. It was a very open and thoughtful conversation, and in the end she thanked me and said that she would think about it. She didn't call me back that week, so I had no idea what she had decided. Pressed by many patients and responsibilities, I returned to my hectic duties as a medical intern.

A year later I was running between patients in my weekly medicine outpatient clinic, and the name of the next scheduled patient seemed vaguely familiar, but I couldn't place it. I walked into the room and found my young kidney stone patient sitting there smiling holding her three-month-old son!

"I'm well and the baby is well," she beamed, "and I just wanted to stop by for a minute to thank you and to allow you to meet my handsome son!"

I was momentarily stunned, but then overjoyed and, I must admit, very relieved. It was a strange series of emotions that swept over me wave after wave for about 30 seconds. This was certainly a unique experience in my life.

Interns and residents also worked for a month at a time on various consultative services, such as cardiology or pulmonary. They also spent a month at a time in the intensive care unit setting, which was mentally, physically and emotionally challenging, but certainly provided a wealth of experience.

During internship I had three experiences related to medication errors in hospitalized patients. These were frustrating, sad and very memorable experiences for me, and were reminders of how many things can go wrong in spite of the best of intentions. A few errors of various kinds, at low rates, are unavoidable in any complex system, so people should remember that hospitals can be very dangerous places. The first case involved a 60-year-old man who had angina and who had been placed in the intensive care unit for testing and medication adjustments. He was having a variety of extra heartbeats, so an anti-arrhythmic medication was started by the cardiologists. Tests ruled out a myocardial infarction, he was transferred out of the unit to me, and he was placed in a bed that had a cardiac monitor to keep an eye on his extra heartbeats.

The pulse remained irregular, so the cardiology consultant suggested switching the anti-arrhythmic drug to a different medication. Using pen and paper (this was 1977) I wrote on one line of the order sheet to stop medication A, then on the next line I wrote to start at "x hour" the new medication, medication B. The next day his irregular heartbeat seemed improved, but he had mild nausea, which was not particularly noteworthy. When I came in the next morning I was told that during the night he started vomiting and then suddenly suffered a cardiac arrest and died.

After rounds that morning, my attending physician asked me to sit down with him to do a thorough review of the case, and found that the pharmacy had continued to send to the hospital floor the medication A, which the nurses dutifully gave to the patient several times daily, in addition to medication B, as noted on the nurses' dispensing record.

My supervisor and I sat stunned for a moment – clearly the patient had received two anti-arrhythmic drugs instead of one, and likely had a fatal intoxication. As I sat silently, my attending physician sorted through the stacks of chart papers and found the physician's order sheet for the date that the change in medication had been ordered – he was going to see if my order had been in error or was written in a confusing manner. Finally finding the right page, he paused and pointed at the suspect written lines: "Stop medication A" followed immediately on the next line by "Start medication B at x hour." My orders were perfect and quite readable, somewhat to his surprise, I think. He just looked up at me and sighed – the error clearly had been in the hospital pharmacy.

Several months later a usually healthy 20-year old woman was admitted to the medicine ward with a devastating new illness consisting of fever, disorientation and seizures. Examination of the spinal fluid and other tests suggested that she probably had viral encephalitis, most likely in this case due to herpes virus. Only 1 in 500,000 Americans develop this serious central nervous system infection each year. This can be a fatal problem in some cases, and a neurosurgical procedure soon was done to obtain a small piece of brain tissue that, in fact, confirmed the diagnosis of herpes encephalitis. It was at that point that I became involved with this patient's care, and I worked quickly with consultants to decide what therapy to give, as anti-viral therapies were a relatively new concept in 1977.

A patient in her current state was thought to have a 70% fatality rate if no treatment were offered. Even if a patient recovered, persistent significant brain damage was possible. The herpes virus often entered the brain along the nerves of smell, and the virus thereby was steered to the temporal lobes of the brain, where damage often caused very unfortunate behavioral changes – the Kluver-Busey Syndrome. Patients who survived but who had sustained such focused temporal lobe damage often needed to be institutionalized and exhibited lack of emotion, hypersexuality, fearlessness and a desire to put things in their mouths. I stood by the bedside of this innocent young woman and was filled with great sadness as she faced death, or a fate arguably worse than death, with only a slim chance of coming through this serious illness reasonably intact.

An article by Whitely *et al.* had just appeared in the *New England Journal of Medicine* in 1977 in which intravenous infusion of arabinoside-A showed some benefit for patients with herpes encephalitis. Accordingly, the infusions were begun, although the patient seemed little changed during the first few days. Her white blood cell count had been elevated because of her infection, and that returned to the normal range, a possibly encouraging sign, but to everyone's shock and surprise, the white blood cell count then continued to decline. Was she having a toxic reaction to one of her drugs, such as the relatively new anti-viral drug? The small plastic bags containing the arabinoside-A for intravenous infusion were prepared downstairs in the hospital pharmacy, and a quick check of the bags in use showed that each label had the correct patient's name, the correct drug name and the correct dose.

A careful investigation in the pharmacy then turned up a horrifying error. The pharmacist had been putting arabinoside-C into each bag instead of arabinoside- A, although he thought that he had been placing arabinoside-A into the bags, so he had labeled each bag with the correct dose of arabinoside-A! Even the most thorough nurse could not have discovered this error up in the patient's room as she was giving the medication intravenously. Arabinoside-C is a powerful chemotherapy drug sometimes used for hematological malignancies, and it certainly will lower the number of white blood cells. The patient was immediately switched to the correct medicine, and seemed to improve a bit thereafter, but she continued to have severe drowsiness and abnormal mental function at the time I rotated off of the team taking care of her.

A third example of significant drug error occurred when an elderly woman was admitted for my care – she was having a brainstem stroke with weakness on one side of her body and characteristic neurological signs. After appropriate testing was done during the first hour in the hospital, it was decided to thin her blood by giving her intravenous heparin. This is done by giving a somewhat large bolus of heparin intravenously over a minute or two, and then running an IV solution containing a continuous low amount of heparin over several days. I wrote the order for the bolus dose of heparin, and the pharmacy sent it up in a syringe about 15 minutes later.

I walked over to the patient's room and stood by the bedside slowly pushing the contents of the syringe into the patient's IV line over about two minutes time. As I withdrew the now empty syringe, my beeper went off and I walked back to the nurses' station, called the pharmacy, and was stunned to receive the injunction, "Don't give that bolus, it might be ten-times too much!" I quickly determined that the patient seemed unchanged, but I did not hang the slow infusion of heparin, and instead just checked some blood tests during the next 24 hours. The patient's anticoagulation tests were sky high – the syringe probably had contained far too much heparin. This case has a happy ending, since although the patient remained anticoagulated for several days without further heparin, her stroke signs gradually resolved. After a few days she was entirely normal neurologically, and her anticoagulation status again was completely normal. She went home in fine shape with appointments for further neurovascular and cardiac assessments.

Several years later my own four-year-old daughter, Erin Magner, would be seriously ill while sharing a hospital room with another four-year-old with a similar cardiac diagnosis, and with a similar name, Erin Mandley. I knew from experience that this was a prescription for trouble. So although I had to go back to my job each day, my wife, who camped in the hospital room day and night, and who was on very friendly terms with the nursing staff, was under strict orders from me to recheck the label on every drug that was about to be given to our daughter. Over several days each administered drug was targeted perfectly with the exception of a single intravenous dose of digoxin that had been intended for Erin Mandley but which almost found its way into Erin Magner.

An aspect of internship that was routine in 1977, but seems very peculiar now, relates to simple laboratory assessments that were commonly done by the intern personally. As I saw patients in the emergency room or up on the hospital ward, I often took blood, urine, vaginal or sputum specimens to a small room with a microscope, centrifuge and a few test reagents to do my own personal testing. I could easily and quickly see what the hematocrit was, or if there were cells in the urine specimen, or if the mucus coughed up from the lungs had pneumococci, staphylococcus or tubercle bacilli. A skilled intern could get a quick diagnosis within a few minutes, and this laboratory assessment essentially cost the patient nothing, since no specimen might have been sent in parallel to the main hospital laboratory.

The modern reader will immediately recognize the pitfalls here. What about quality control for the reagents – were they out of date? What really is the competency of the intern to make these observations and diagnoses? Has training on all of this been documented? In 1977, the simplistic view was that if a sub-par intern could not see the pneumococci on the gram stain of the sputum, resulting in a missed diagnosis of pneumonia, for example,

this fell into the same category of error as a sub-par intern who during his physical exam failed to notice a heart murmur, or failed to notice slight weakness on the left side of the body. By the 1990's, however, the interns were forbidden from doing their own laboratory assessments both for practical quality control reasons, as well as because of litigation risk. This change also enhanced capture of revenue by the centralized hospital laboratories. I was always comfortable in the lab, however, and made many quick and useful diagnoses with my own hands. When I later volunteered to work in some rural Public Health Clinics in the US, and when I worked in the Marshall Islands, this spirit of independent laboratory work was actually quite helpful and was practically very useful.

After the internship year in San Antonio, I worked two additional years as a resident physician, during which I served in a supervisory capacity to interns while I rotated to a new duty each month and saw patients in my weekly outpatient clinic. During these residency years I honed my medical knowledge and skills to get ready to take the big exam, the Board Examination in Internal Medicine.

As a resident I also had more supervisory responsibilities in the emergency room during some months. At 6 am one Christmas morning I took over an understandably very quiet medical E.R., and I was pleased to have time to sit down and have a cup of coffee. But at 6:15 am the "squawk box" that relayed the radio traffic from the in-coming ambulances announced a warning. They were in-bound with a 35- year-old woman who had just been stabbed in the chest that Christmas morning in her living room by her husband. The patient would not see me, but would be shuttled to the trauma side of the emergency room. Nothing shocked me anymore, but I still was greatly saddened by such a report.

Not all was terribly sad in the emergency room, however. One afternoon a 70- year-old Hispanic man was brought in who had collapsed at home and injured his knee when he hit the floor. He was alert and had no chest pain or neurologic signs, and complained only of slight dizziness and his bruised knee. The fall was sudden and unexpected, and his blood pressure of 120/80 seemed a little too good to be true, so I was suspicious of a silent heart attack or some other underlying problem. Within a minute the EKG was done, and was completely normal, and his spun hematocrit was normal. He was a smoker and had once been told that he had high blood pressure.

On a hunch, within five minutes of his arrival, I ordered

a cross-table lateral abdominal x-ray to see if he had a calcified aortic aneurysm, although I was not certain of that finding on his physical exam. Basically, to obtain this x-ray picture, the patient lies quietly on his back on the stretcher while the x-ray equipment is positioned to pass the x-rays through the abdomen from the side, so the developed film would have the spine at the bottom and the front of the abdomen at the top – the aorta would be imaged above the spine. Within another five minutes I had the film in my hand, and the arc of calcium of an apparent abdominal aneurysm was clear even to me. I postulated that it had begun to leak, had dropped his blood pressure, and thereby caused his slight dizziness and fall.

I walked the x-ray next door to the trauma side of the emergency room and showed the young surgeon. I suggested that he call upstairs and send this patient directly to the operating room for emergent vascular surgery. The surgeon seemed incredulous, but heard the urgency in my voice and made the call. The patient was whisked right to exploratory abdominal surgery. Two weeks later the head vascular surgeon phoned me to thank me for sending him a great case. Once a large aneurysm starts to leak, he said, few patients survive, but this man had just walked out of the hospital with his family!

One winter night I was the only resident on the medical side of the emergency room when the "squawk box" carried word from an ambulance that multiple patients of various ages had been overcome by fumes when they tried to heat their small house by lighting barbeque briquettes in the living room without proper ventilation. Two young children and eight adults had headache and nausea, and some were vomiting. A series of ambulances would be delivering them to the emergency room within 20 minutes. I phoned the pediatrician on call to come down from the ward to meet the children in the emergency room, and I phoned the Respiratory Therapy Department to supervise installation of ten hydrated 28% oxygen lines with masks along the hallways of the emergency room. I also alerted them to my need soon for ten measurements of carbon monoxide levels because I suspected based on the history that the people were experiencing carbon monoxide poisoning.

Carbon monoxide binds more tightly to hemoglobin than oxygen, so once a carbon monoxide molecule sticks onto a hemoglobin molecule, it takes some time for it to come off. While carbon monoxide is attached to hemoglobin, that molecule of hemoglobin cannot carry oxygen, so it is essentially the same as if the hemoglobin molecule is not even there at all to help carry oxygen! If most of the hemoglobin molecules had bound up carbon monoxide, a patient would quickly die from lack of oxygen even if he were breathing 100% oxygen, since none of the oxygen could bind to the hemoglobin. Luckily, most alert patients with headache and nausea will do well if the carbon monoxide exposure is ended and an excess of oxygen is provided because over time the oxygen will slowly displace the carbon monoxide. I started getting ten stretchers lined up in position by each oxygen line. All was ready within 20 minutes, and the several ambulances arrived within a 10-minute span. Each patient got an oxygen mask while I performed a brief history and physical exam, and each had an arterial blood gas sample sent for carbon monoxide measurement – luckily the pediatrician took care of the kids. No one seemed severely ill, and the carbon monoxide values came back easily detectable but not worrisomely high. The pediatrician admitted the youngest child to the hospital for observation, but after about eight hours of rest and breathing oxygen, we sent the nine other patients home, and all were feeling much improved by that time.

I prided myself on handling multiple cases simultaneously and successfully, while at the same time taking care of many other "customers," and by the end of my shift I thought that was the end of my story. A week later I received a call from a neurologist who wanted me to attend a case presentation he was going to give the next day. The patient to be discussed was one of the adults I had discharged! It turns out that the middle-aged man had been fine immediately after discharge, but within a day he began to have neurologic signs and symptoms. The anoxia he had sustained during the carbon monoxide exposure had caused a delayed demyelination syndrome in his central nervous system. This syndrome apparently was commonly seen in the late-nineteenth century when gas was used for home lighting. A gas leak would produce anoxia that caused some of the myelin- producing cells in the brain to die, although if the damage was not too severe the patients could recover. Of course, once the anoxia had occurred, there was no real treatment for this syndrome, just supportive care. Still, I felt badly that one of the patients had suffered problems after discharge, although I remained certain that I should not have just admitted every patient to the hospital.

I had other great cases while serving on the inpatient services. One 75-year-old fair-skinned man with white hair and blue eyes had had worsening memory and mild confusion for a year, and now had anemia and other problems. He had large red blood cells as a component of his anemia, rather than the small red blood cells seen in iron deficiency. Those larger than normal red blood cells were a hint that he was missing a critical vitamin that was needed to make red blood cells properly, and was also needed for optimal brain function. I sent off the blood test, and two days later his vitamin B12 measurement returned very low. He had a disease called pernicious anemia, a very treatable condition. This auto-immune disease comes about when the body produces immune system molecules (antibodies) that interrupt the mechanisms that allow B12 to be absorbed from food. This auto-immune phenomenon is more common in fair-skinned people with blue eyes for genetic reasons. Proper treatment, the injection into a muscle every few weeks of vitamin B12 (since the patient can't absorb oral vitamin B12) likely would not only cure his anemia, but would restore his mental function to normal. One lesson for me from this case was that oral potassium replacement has to be done early and often as the intramuscular B12 injections are begun because potassium is a vital component of new red blood cells. Rapid synthesis of red blood cells can be so vigorous that the serum potassium level can fall to a dangerously low level. I avoided this potential problem only because another resident warned me about this when he heard about my patient, and the gentleman did very well. Pernicious anemia should be sought and ruled out in any older patient with significant mental changes because it is so easy to cure.

As you can tell, during my internship and residency training there was a huge amount to learn and experience, and my brain literally was running at 100 miles per hour most of the time. You can understand that there was no time to think about chess, and barely time to think about my wife. It was very gratifying to be directly responsible for figuring out what was wrong with someone, and actually being part of the immediate team that cured the patient. Even if a patient could not be cured, there were many ways to help make things a little better, including careful attention to pain relief.

During my years as a resident, my reading and thinking tended to gravitate more and more toward hormones and glandular diseases. The physiology was fascinating, and there was a substantial amount of biochemical work being done in the field. I had been enthralled by biochemistry since college. So I decided that when I finished my internal medicine training, I would take up specialty and research training in endocrinology.

One of the best places in the country for that training was at the National Institutes of Health in Bethesda, Maryland, so I completed an application. In March, 1979, I was invited to interview at Building 10 at the NIH. This was the month that applicants visited staff who were looking to take on a new clinical associate (also known as a fellow). I was given a schedule to meet one-on-one for about 45 minutes with each of a half-dozen top endocrine clinician-scientists at NIH, during which time they assessed me and I assessed them as a potential mentor. At the end of the day I ranked my interviewers 1 to 6 while each of the interviewers ranked the applicants they had seen that day. Other cohorts of applicants visited the doctors on other days. A few weeks later there was a big match process, and I happened to match with a highly verbal and rising young star investigator named Bruce Weintraub, whose specialty was thyroid diseases. I was thrilled to be accepted into the program. Since at that point I liked all of the different hormone areas about equally, I was happy to study thyroid diseases with Dr. Weintraub.

Weintraub Letter: NIH Acceptance

We all have gotten life-changing news at infrequent intervals. After interviewing with about six doctors at the National Institutes of Health in Bethesda in 1979 to seek a fellowship training position, there was a matching process. I ranked the six doctors and each of those doctors ranked the scores of applicants they had met. Dr. Weintraub and I selected each other, and were destined to work together from 1980 – 1983. I was quite excited to receive his phone call of acceptance, and then this letter a few days later.

DEPARTMENT OF HEALTH, EDUCATION, AND WELFARE
PUBLIC HEALTH SERVICE
NATIONAL INSTITUTES OF HEALTH
BETHESDA, MARYLAND ~~2001~~ 20205

April 16, 1979

Bldg. 10, Rm. 8N315

Dr. James Magner
5534 Fredericksburg Road, Apt. 67
San Antonio, Texas   78229

Dear Jim:

It is a pleasure to offer you the position as Clinical Associate in my laboratory beginning July 1, 1980. As we discussed by phone, my commitment to you is firm and I expect that your acceptance of this position is also a firm commitment. All paperwork regarding your appointment will be forthcoming from Ms. Rachael Peabody (Bldg. 31, Rm. 4B04, phone 301 - 496-2427).

I am sending along some recent reprints that you requested. However, I don't believe we need to make a final decision on your research project until you arrive.

I look forward to having you in the laboratory and am sure it will be a mutually profitable experience.

Sincerely,

Bruce D. Weintraub, M.D.
Clinical Endocrinology Branch
National Institute of Arthritis,
    Metabolism and Digestive Diseases

BDW/jt

At an evening dinner ceremony in San Antonio in late-June, 1980, each of the internal medicine residents received his/her completion certificate. Glenda and I packed up our new Chevy and started the drive across the country to Bethesda, Maryland. Glenda's sister, who lived in Maryland, had located a two-bedroom apartment for us on Battery Lane just south of the NIH campus so that I would be close enough to walk to work each day.

In the 21st century, such cutting through the fence line to enter campus would be impossible because of tightened security, but in 1980, as we placed our belongings in our new apartment, that type of short-cut was still possible. All seemed right with the world. Glenda was pregnant with our first child, and I was about to embark on an exciting new voyage of discovery.

Chapter 6

Fellowship at NIH: A Dream Experience

I was inclined toward science since earliest childhood. And now, after seven years of medical training, I was a clinician. So it was quite natural for me to take well to the environment at the National Institutes of Health, which was a particularly stimulating place for clinician-scientists. The main clinical building, Building 10, had upper floors designed such that the north half of each floor was a suite of research laboratories while the south half of each floor was an inpatient ward in which patients with various diseases could be admitted for research investigation. One could literally walk back and forth between the scientific world and the clinical world. The clinical building did not have a full emergency room, since it was not really a true hospital. All the patients who were admitted were following a pre-specified experimental protocol to test out some new type of medicine or procedure, or have samples obtained to try to learn more about their diseases. Some patients developed unexpected problems from the experimental drugs, or problems from their underlying cancer or other illness, so there certainly were some very ill patients in Building 10, and we did have intensive care units.

Bruce Weintraub, aged 40, was just starting to gray a little. He loved to speak quickly while waving his hands, and always had a sparkle of enthusiasm in his eye. He also loved to play tennis and golf, and was viewed as a rising star among experts interested in the thyroid gland. I had ranked him as my first choice as mentor because he seemed smart and personable, and was doing interesting biochemistry. But I also knew that Bruce was young enough so that he would be critically interested in whether my experiments worked or not. He would be willing to spend time and effort to help me if I ran into difficulties in the lab. If I did well, then he would do well. He was primarily studying a hormone made in the pituitary called thyroid-stimulating hormone, or TSH. This hormone traveled in the bloodstream and was the most important "go signal" for the thyroid gland to work harder to make its hormones.

I was assigned a small desk and was given some bench space. I was going to do my experiments in the same room (and on the same laboratory bench tops) in which Marshall Nirenberg had done his important experiments in 1961 to elucidate the "language of DNA." He clarified how three

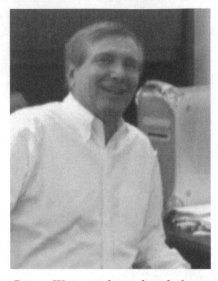

Bruce Weintraub, undated photo.

DNA letters at a time were properly translated into certain amino acids so that specific proteins (which are long chains of amino acids in a carefully specified order) could be synthesized. In other words, the long DNA sequence made up of four different letters (ATGC) was known somehow to provide a code to allow the 21 different types of amino acids to fall into line to make specific proteins, but no one understood how that worked. The situation was somewhat comparable to a man who had been handed a coded instruction sheet and told to place five different automobile 'makes' in line in a parade in a certain order. The man was to learn later that the answer to his puzzle was Chevy, Dodge, Ford, Honda and Toyota, but he did not know that answer yet, and he had a parking lot with hundreds of cars (with 21 different 'makes' of cars) waiting to be chosen to go into the parade. The Master Organizer of the parade had quickly handed him the instruction sheet with a string of letters written in a single line with no spaces or punctuation, and told him to just follow the instructions and place the specified cars in the parade in the correct order. The letters on the paper were TGACCCAATGGGACG. He puzzled over this, and then realized that the first three symbols of each car's license plate were letters. TGA was on the license plate of every Chevy in the parking lot, CCC was on the plate of each Dodge, etc., such that three sequential letters in the instructions identified a unique "make" of car. The linear reading of the string of letters, three letters at a time, allowed the types of cars to be properly placed in line in the parade as desired by the Master Organizer. In this crude example, the string of letters on the paper represents the DNA code, the metal license plate represents a special type of "conceptual linker," analogous to transfer RNA, that allows the DNA code to be associated with a specific type of amino acid, while each automobile represents an amino acid. The reader who is knowledgeable about biology will recognize that my oversimplified analogy does not really mirror exactly how this works, or how the experiments actually were done to break the code, but he will understand that I want to communicate to a general reader the key concept of a three-letter code. A phrase often used in science about models applies also to analogies: All models are wrong, but some models are useful. In 1968 Nirenberg was awarded the Nobel Prize in Physiology or Medicine for establishing that DNA used three letters at a time, in sequence, to code for specific amino acids.

During July, I shadowed Bethel Stannard, Bruce's main lab assistant, to learn some of the new techniques in the lab, how equipment worked and where things were located. I had set up "play labs" in my basement as a teenager, and I had a little more experience at the University of Illinois and at Woods Hole. But now I had been assigned space and resources in a real biochemistry laboratory! With proper supervision and lots of advice, I was going to do my own experiments and make new discoveries. I easily and quickly picked up what I needed to know, and by August I had started my first experiment using pulse-chase radioactive labeling, subcellular fractionation, immunoprecipitation, and SDS gel electrophoresis. I was having a ball. I also saw endocrinology outpatients on Tuesday afternoons, but the clinical load was light. Most of the other trainees (who worked for other mentors) and I were there to focus on science rather than clinical medicine – we hoped to wed the two, but we were going to approach the wedding predominantly from the scientific side.

In September I sat for an all-day very thorough written examination, and passed, so I was then board certified in internal medicine. This step put the finishing touch on all the internal medicine training I had had in San Antonio. A few years later I passed another big test to become board certified in endocrinology.

The weeks passed in 1980, but the lab work was not going smoothly. I was using special techniques to label with radioactivity the parts of the TSH molecules that were being made by mouse pituitary tumor cells. I wanted to learn how the TSH molecule was being built up over time,

like watching automobiles being assembled in a factory. Let me explain in an analogy how pulse-chase labeling works. Imagine that an automobile assembly line is run automatically by robots in a totally dark factory. Parts are added gradually to autos as they flow along the assembly line for 10 hours, and a complete auto comes out at the end. I want to understand the step by step assembly process during those 10 hours, because just looking at the completed car does not tell much about the steps by which it was put together. But my allowed access to the factory to make my observations is very, very limited, reflecting the great technical limitations of working with complex biological systems. A crude, somewhat silly, but permitted technique in this factory is to install a hose dangling above the first 10% of the assembly line (and the hose technically must stay there over the start of the assembly line, and cannot move elsewhere because of natural restrictions). One could use the hose to "bomb" the very first 5 to 10% of the assembly line (which is in total darkness) with fluorescent paint for a few minutes, then shine a searchlight containing an ultraviolet bulb over the entire assembly line (it is not technically possible to use the light to illuminate just one portion of the assembly line the light covers all or nothing). In this "early pulse experiment," only the auto parts being assembled in the first 10% of the assembly line become visible, and all of the cars further down the assembly line remain invisible. Photographing the glowing partially assembled "first precursor cars" will allow the first steps of the process to be understood. In a different experiment, if instead the first 5 to 10% of the assembly line were "bombed" with fluorescent paint, and then the flow of paint ceased and the assembly line was allowed to continue running in the dark for 5 hours (a "pulse- chase"), then when the fluorescent light was suddenly turned on, the only cars that could be discerned would be the ones about half-way down the 10 hour assembly line. Photographing those half-assembled cars, with some glowing parts in spots here and there in each car, would provide information about how an auto looked when it was about half assembled. Using a very short pulse of fluorescent paint, perhaps covering only the first 1% of the assembly line, would provide more precision for understanding the early steps of the assembly process, but that very short burst of paint would provide a weaker and more difficult signal to detect.

In addition to labeling molecules being assembled using radioactivity (employing pulses and chases), I was trying to further improve the experiment by breaking cells and carefully separating them into parts for analysis, as though I had wisely chosen to observe the long auto assembly line portion by portion to make the overall auto assembly process even more easily understandable. By October I had done three experiments during which I had incubated mouse tissue for short periods with a radioactive amino acid, 35-S methionine. To use more technical terms briefly, I then had performed subcellular fractionation to isolate ribosomes that might have carried very early radioactively-labeled precursor forms of the hormone TSH. I tried to isolate these early precursors using specific antibodies, and then ran SDS gel electrophoresis to identify their molecular weights. I wanted to understand the first steps of the biosynthesis of TSH, just as the RNA was being translated into the two peptide chains of the hormone on the ribosomes. It was novel research, and the method should have worked, but three times I had ended up with blank gels. I saw nothing. This was a worrisome turn of events for an enthusiastic young scientist who might have only a year or so to prove his abilities. My lab resources could be given to a more promising trainee.

During Columbus Day weekend, Glenda and I stayed in a quaint bed and breakfast in the beautiful Virginia countryside, but in the back of my mind I was calmly and carefully rethinking my research project. When I returned to the lab, I refined my methods and adjusted the project. Instead of trying to find very low-prevalence precursors still attached to ribosomes, I decided to look for slightly later biosynthetic precursors that would be in various subcellular compartments, such as the endoplasmic reticulum and the Golgi apparatus. I was going to examine a bigger segment of the automobile assembly line at a later stage of assembly. There should be a higher quantity of labeled molecules in those cell compartments. I tried various radioactive pulse-chase experiments, but still could not detect labeled TSH molecules. Over Christmas and New Year's I looked over the experimental designs again, and set up a very important experiment in January 1981. I desperately needed a success, and I could not understand why my experiments were not working.

As noted previously, it was during the SDS gel electrophoresis analyses of this January experiment that Glenda went into labor with our first child. Well aware that first labors usually proceed slowly, my wife gave permission for me to return *briefly* to the lab to rescue my precious specimens. Very fortunately, those samples showed beautiful results, and formed the basis of my first important scientific publication. The interested reader could seek out the publication to see the graphs of data that almost were lost to history: Magner and Weintraub, *J Biol Chem 257*: 6709, 1982. Later data suggested that my prior experiments had not worked simply because the tissue used as source material had not been synthesizing enough TSH, whereas for the January experiment, I had used by chance starting tissue that was a particularly rich source of TSH. With this successful experiment in hand, my work in the laboratory during the next years was quite productive. I thereby had established myself as a promising young investigator worthy of government funding, which I received through the 1980s.

While at NIH I also worked with Bruce on clinical investigations of rare patients with the syndrome of thyroid hormone resistance. This syndrome had first been described by Dr. Sam Refetoff at the University of Chicago, whom I had met during medical school. Bruce and I brought patients into the NIH for several days at a time to perform metabolic testing. We published descriptions of the clinical features of patients found in one particularly large kindred. Later it was found that this syndrome was due to mutations in the genes for the nuclear thyroid hormone receptors.

NIH also was special because there were so many bright and interesting people around, and scientific visitors from everywhere were frequently giving lectures and presenting novel research. As you will hear in the next chapter, there were challenging issues in my home life. But as a young scientist, my productive and stimulating time at NIH was truly a dream experience.

NIH Laboratory Notes

Here are a few pages of my NIH laboratory notes that illustrate how I struggled with my project in 1980. I chose to show pages that had sketches that allowed me more easily to follow the various steps in my experiments. My notes were always full of helpful sketches.

— 5 —   MOST WIDELY USED

B.) <u>Dallner method</u> (Methods in Enzymology 52: 71, 1978
   1.) Homogenization buffer should be 0.44M
      sucrose (higher sucrose minimizes
      aggregation). (Unclear what other ions present,
   2.) Layer post mitochondrial supernatant
      (which contains <u>no</u> CsCl) on top of
      two layers of sucrose - CsCl, as shown:

4ml PMS in .44M sucrose

0.5ml of 0.6 M sucrose -15mM CsCl

2.0 ml of 1.3M sucrose -15mM CsCl

Beckman 40.2 rotor
102,000 g
90 min

← SER
← pellet RER

The SER collects at 0.6M/1.3M interface.
The Cs+ specifically aggregates RER.

C.) <u>Melchers method</u> (Biochem 10, 653, 1971).
   1.) Homogenization is carried out such that
      post mitochondrial supernatant is 0.25M sucrose
      0.05M Tris-HCl, .025M KCL, .005M MgCl₂, pH 7.5
   2.) PMS is layered as shown:

sample — 2ml

0.4 M — 3ml

1.4 M — 3ml

2.0 M — 2ml

2.3 M — 2ml

Beckman L2-50B
SW 41 rotor
14 hr 40,000 RPM
OR
SW 27 rotor
24 hr 25,000 RPM

} SER

} RER

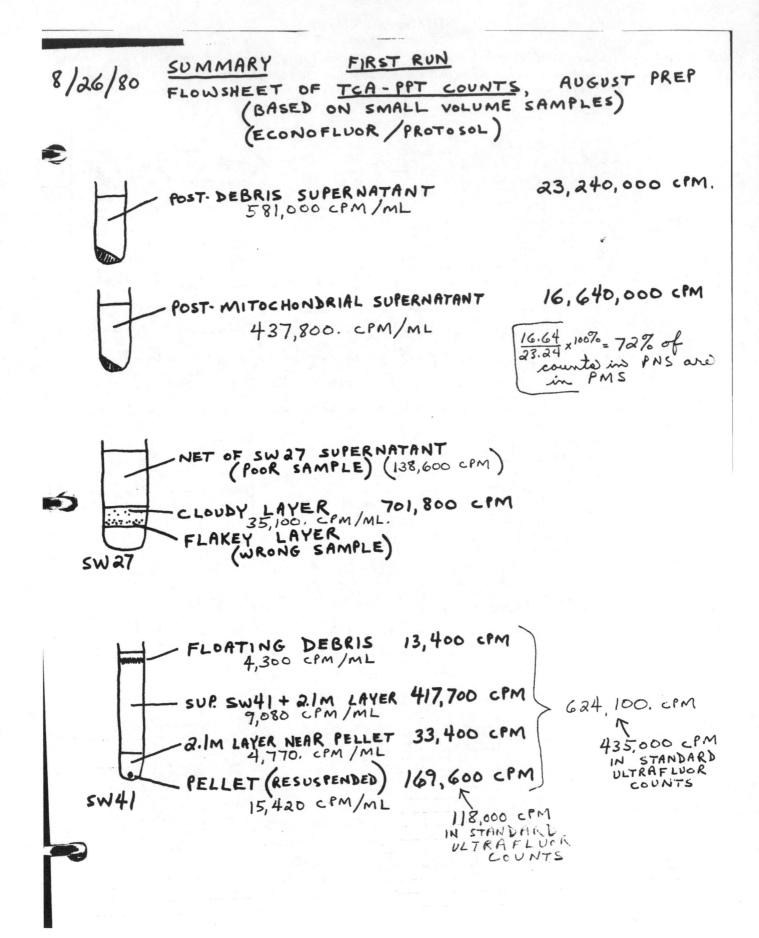

8/26/80

SUMMARY   FIRST RUN
FLOWSHEET OF TCA-PPT COUNTS,   AUGUST PREP
    (BASED ON SMALL VOLUME SAMPLES)
    (ECONOFLUOR/PROTOSOL)

POST-DEBRIS SUPERNATANT   23,240,000 CPM.
    581,000 CPM/ML

POST-MITOCHONDRIAL SUPERNATANT   16,640,000 CPM
    437,800. CPM/ML

$\frac{16.64}{23.24} \times 100\% = 72\%$ of counts in PNS are in PMS

NET OF SW27 SUPERNATANT
    (POOR SAMPLE) (138,600 CPM)

CLOUDY LAYER   701,800 CPM
    35,100. CPM/ML.
FLAKEY LAYER
    (WRONG SAMPLE)

SW27

FLOATING DEBRIS   13,400 CPM
    4,300 CPM/ML

SUP. SW41 + 2.1M LAYER   417,700 CPM
    9,080 CPM/ML   624,100. CPM

2.1M LAYER NEAR PELLET   33,400 CPM
    4,770. CPM/ML   435,000 CPM
                                        IN STANDARD
PELLET (RESUSPENDED)   169,600 CPM   ULTRAFLUOR
    15,420 CPM/ML   COUNTS

SW41
                                118,000 CPM
                                IN STANDARD
                                ULTRAFLUOR
                                COUNTS

10/29/80

First Puromycin Experiment

Mice were killed ~ 8:30 AM. Tumors from the following mice were used.

10/29/80
BOX 21   102 G8   one   good   All
    24   103 G9   two   good x2   tumors
    19   102 G8   one   good   were
    17   110 G2   ~~two one~~good   more pearly
    13   "5/1/80 #3" one   good   than
                                        hemorrhagic

About 39 grams of tumor was homogenized in usual manner.

PMS spin #1 at 12,000 RPM gave about 25 ml of pinkish turbid sup, over a whitish layer, then dark red pellet.

About 11 ml Sol A added to each tube for wash ⇒ pinkish clear sup after spin at 15,000 RPM x 15 min.

About 2 ml aliquant set aside - freezer.

Then ~2 ml of 30% NP40·Tris was added to ~50 ml sup. Mixed ~10 min at 4°C by turning upside down by hand.

Gradients made in SW41 tubes using 2ml 2.M and 1ml of 0.7 M sucrose (Sol C and B). Then about 8½ ml of sup added to each of 6 tubes (for sixth tube used Sol A to bring tube to volume).

No need for mineral oil.

SW41 at speed 40,000 RPM at 11:45 AM.

Drierite changed in Beckman.

Chapter 7

Erin: The Miracle Child

Erin was born at the Bethesda Naval Hospital in Maryland in January 1981. Glenda and I had joked somewhat nervously about what might happen if she were in labor just before or during the Super Bowl, but actually all went well that day. Glenda had to stay in the hospital an extra day because of a low-grade fever, which gave me an opportunity to speak again with the pediatrician who had briefly examined our baby. I told him that I was a bit of a nervous new father, and I was not highly trained in pediatrics, so I asked him please to re-examine our little girl one more time very carefully. That way, I would know that when I got her home, if she was cranky or had some other issue, I would be more certain that the root cause was not really a major problem. He laughed and agreed, and all was well.

We brought our baby back to our apartment on the third day after her birth, but she didn't take her breast feedings very eagerly and she slept quietly most of the time. Others commented how lucky we were to have a "good baby." When she was 10-days old I came home from work and found Glenda crying because the baby again had seemed not to take the breast feedings very well, and was fussy and crying. Over the course of that evening I took a look at the baby more with a doctor's eye than a father's eye, but I knew little about babies. I was certain that she had been very carefully examined, twice, about a week ago by the pediatrician. But by 10 pm I noted that her respiratory rate had increased and she started having "rib retractions," an early physical sign of difficult breathing. I told Glenda that I might be over-reacting, but I thought that there were objective signs of a respiratory problem, and I suggested that we take the baby to the emergency room.

When we arrived at the emergency room, the staff was responsible enough to take a look at Erin within just a minute or so, and they immediately felt that there was some sort of important respiratory problem. During the next sixty minutes, her respiratory problem worsened rapidly, and Erin was intubated and placed in the intensive care unit. The chest x-rays showed fluid in the tissues of both lungs that possibly was pneumonia, and the heart was enlarged. Erin's blood oxygen worsened during the night and she suffered a cardiac arrest, but after a few minutes of resuscitation her heart was beating again, and

her breathing continued to be supported by the machine. Stunned, Glenda and I sat in the waiting area throughout the night, trying to remain supportive of each other.

After another hour or so it was clear that Erin was getting much worse. Her kidney function had shut down, the fluid in her lungs now was very bad, and her blood oxygen levels were low even when she was being given 100% oxygen to breathe. The doctors and nurses worked very hard to keep her alive, but she was fading.

The resident doctor came and spoke to us about possible mental retardation as a result of all the insults she had endured, and asked whether we wanted the baby to be resuscitated if she had another cardiac arrest. Glenda and I insisted that the team make every effort to save her if that occurred, and we would take the risk of mental impairment.

Some time in the night, the hospital priest was called to baptize Erin *in extremis*. From that point on Erin seemed to stabilize, and she didn't have another cardiac arrest that night. I spoke to my boss and I was permitted to spend time at the hospital with Glenda and Erin during the next several days. Erin's kidneys started to work again, and her blood oxygen level, although terrible, was improved. Erin did not have pneumonia, but instead had severe congestive heart failure likely due to a congenital heart defect. Glenda pumped her breast milk so that a little could be put down the nasogastric tube. The special fats in breast milk are very important during the first month of life to allow proper brain development. I went back to work at the NIH seeing endocrinology patients in the clinic and trying to do research since I had to make a living, but Glenda spent day and night at the hospital. We had no idea what was going to happen next.

After three weeks, Erin remained stable, was able to breathe 30 % oxygen on her own power, but was no longer improving. The doctors had decided that she had a congenital cardiac defect of some kind, likely a "hole in the heart." To clarify the anatomy, the medical team proposed to do a cardiac catheterization to image where the cardiac hole or holes were, and then they proposed to do some sort of limited cardiac surgery to try to further stabilize Erin. While we waited with bated breath, they wheeled Erin to the catheterization lab, tried to squirt in just a little dye to image her heart, and, unexpectedly, she had another cardiac arrest. She was resuscitated and brought back to the intensive care unit with no information gained about her cardiac anatomy.

One of the doctors came to speak with me and said the new plan would be to proceed with a cardiac operation even though the cardiac anatomy was not yet clarified. He said that they would tie a knot around her "ductus," a special short blood vessel outside the heart that is open when babies are in the womb, but which normally closes just after birth. They thought that Erin's ductus was still open, and perhaps if they tied it closed then her cardiac condition would stabilize a bit more so that they could try to repeat the cardiac catheterization. I was concerned about this approach and I asked a couple of questions, although I was ready to support whatever the medical team thought would be best.

By that time they knew that I was a physician, and I was always very collaborative, although cognizant that I was a father first. My questions did make them think a little more, however, and they actually then decided that instead of surgery, they would transfer Erin to Children's National Medical Center in downtown Washington, D.C., where there was more expertise about such things. I was happy to agree with whatever they thought was best. Glenda rode in the ambulance with Erin to the other hospital, while I found a place to park our car.

Within a couple of days the cardiac catheterization had been completed successfully, and Erin was found to have four defects in her cardiovascular system. She had a large hole in her ventricular septum, a moderate hole in her atrial septum, a patent ductus, and a narrowing of the aorta called a coarctation. Blood from her left ventricle could not exit easily into the aorta, so it was crossing through the hole in the ventricular septum into the right ventricle and then pouring into the pulmonary artery, flooding her lungs. The patent ductus, although technically abnormal, was actually a fortuitous conduit in this setting, since it allowed some blood to be diverted away from the lungs. Thus it might have been a serious error to have tied the ductus off in this special case.

A brief comment is indicated as to why a few days after birth the expert pediatrician had not discovered the existence of these major cardiac defects during his physical examination. The doctor was competent, but the physiology

was hiding the defects from him. In the womb, the lungs have very high resistance to blood flow, as there is no reason why blood should go to the lungs to pick up oxygen if the baby is "under water" and is getting oxygen via the umbilical cord.

At birth, the physiology has to change, since the umbilical cord is cut and the lungs have to start receiving blood and taking in oxygen. It is a miracle that this change can happen so routinely and so effectively in minutes in most babies. In fact, the high resistance to blood flow in the lungs only falls gradually over about ten days. In Erin's case, the initially high resistance of blood flow to the lungs kept the lungs from being flooded with fluid for the first few days, and made the heart murmurs very quiet and difficult to hear. With each passing day, vascular resistance in the lungs fell a little more, blood started crossing in greater volume through the holes in the heart, and the lungs became more flooded. If we had not taken Erin to the the emergency room when we did, she would have rapidly spiraled downhill in just the next one or two hours, and would have died at home that night.

At Children's Hospital, the cardiac surgeon, Dr. Watson, told us that Erin was much too sick and tiny to have the internal heart defects corrected now. But he did recommend a major surgery to open up the narrow aorta, and put a band around the pulmonary artery, on the outside of the heart. The band would allow the minimum necessary blood flow into the lungs while restricting excessive flow. The fluid in the lungs would be absorbed gradually, over a few days, back into the bloodstream, and then oxygen could be absorbed more effectively by the lungs. This would be only a stop-gap measure, and additional major surgery in the future after Erin had gotten bigger and stronger would be required to repair the internal heart defects. This all sounded very reasonable, and we agreed to the operation. Clearly, there seemed to be no other option.

The operation went well, and Erin improved slowly in the intensive care unit thereafter. After a few more days she was breathing on her own and was moved out of the unit into a regular hospital room. Her nutritional status was poor, and she was much too weak to suckle. There are dangers to chronic use of nasogastric tubes, so another small operation was performed to place a gastrostomy tube for feeding. This small yellow-rubber tube passed through the skin of the abdomen and entered the stomach so that a syringe could be used to inject small amounts of liquid baby formula through the tube and directly into the stomach. Erin continued to require nasal oxygen, and after another month in the hospital the oxygen levels really didn't improve much. Finally, it was decided just to stop the oxygen support and let her blood gas levels run on the low side, and hope for the best. Erin in effect was surviving at the top of a very high mountain while the rest of her family was at sea level.

Erin had trouble keeping the formula in her stomach, and it was disheartening and frightening to have four or five hours of patiently given small feedings spit- up in three seconds. If Erin did not keep down calories, she would die. So we had to put only small volumes through the gastric tube at a time. These small frequent feedings meant that someone had to get up several times each night to put in a little more formula – and that job mostly fell to Mom. It was exhausting and never-ending work, and Glenda deserves to be recognized as a real hero for carrying on with this for two years. I should mention here that she resigned her full-time teaching position at Howard University to be a full-time mother to Erin.

Erin grew very slowly, and was always very small for her age because her heart was still inefficiently pumping. Her blood oxygen was low, and she was barely getting an excess of calories. We had to add a special oily liquid supplement of expensive long-chain triglycerides to her formula to have her remain in positive caloric balance. At first the insurance company denied payment for this special nutritional supplement because, "Nutritional programs are not reimbursed – we will not pay for obesity treatment or weight loss programs." Multiple letters failed to convince the company that we were desperately trying to get a critically ill one-year-old to gain weight, not have a teenager lose weight. After many weeks, the insurance company recognized their error, and began paying again.

At about age two, Erin attended an eating clinic at Georgetown University to learn how to take solid food by mouth, which comes normally to nearly all children, but not to very sick little patients who have always been fed using a G-tube. We could observe Erin via a one-way mirror during her eating training (which started with vanilla ice cream) so that we could learn the proper reinforcement techniques without disturbing the clinical environment. Then we practiced what we had learned directly with Erin. Finally, we were able to discontinue the G-tube at age 2½, and that was a happy day.

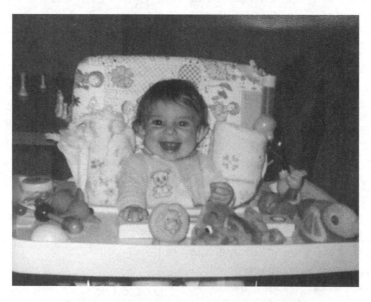

Erin with her Feeding Tube in Late 1981

Although very ill at the start, Erin was a joyful baby. You can see that we provided an enriched environment. Her dark yellow-brown gastrostomy tube extends to the right and connects to a white plastic syringe barrel hanging via tape and safety pin from the corner of her highchair. Only small volumes of formula could be placed in the syringe at frequent intervals or Erin would vomit, and lose all the valuable calories. I must have been working on a chess problem when Glenda took this picture.

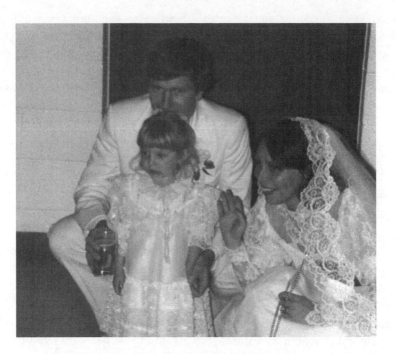

Erin as Flower Girl

*Erin was well enough in 1983, at age 34 months, to walk down the
aisle in my brother's wedding as flower girl.*

When Glenda put our tiny daughter in the folding seat of the grocery store shopping cart, she looked like a little six-month-old but she actually was approaching two years of age. One time in the super market, an elderly woman came up to Erin in the cart and said, "My, what a cute baby – goo, goo!" Erin promptly replied to the startled senior, "My name is Erin and my Mommy and I are going to get Cheerios, milk, bread and candy!" Erin loved to watch *Sesame Street*, and we constantly conversed with her and read to her, so she became very verbal. Somewhat belatedly, Erin was able to walk around when we clamped off her G-tube and tucked it in her pants. While our undersized Erin and her Mom were walking along a sidewalk looking in store windows one day, bystanders smiled as the tiny girl put her nose against the glass of one window, and then dropped their jaws when she exclaimed, "Wow, Mommy, I really like those two-toned Oxfords," the sartorial choice of Bert and Ernie, of course!

Erin's verbal precocity was manifest even as a four-year-old. One summer day she piled three or four items and boxes on her wagon to climb up to reach a small fruit on an ornamental tree in the yard. She tumbled onto the grass, of course, and ran crying into the house. Alarmed, Glenda tried to comfort her and find out what had occurred. When the sobbing subsided a bit, Glenda asked, "Erin, what happened?" to which Erin replied with a sniffle, "Mommy, I used bad judgment!"

When Erin was age 4, while we were in the Chicago area, she had another cardiac cath, and plans were made for the definitive surgical repair (as well as could be done) of her major cardiac defects. The afternoon before the hospital admission, Glenda, Erin, her new seven-month-old sister and I spent hours together in the Chicago Botanical Gardens, walking among the beautiful plants and flowers, seemingly oblivious to the challenge that lay ahead.

On that special morning in the Chicago Children's Hospital, April 11, 1985, Erin was cheerful and did not fully understand, of course, all that was about to happen. We rode on the elevator with her as she was being transported on a gurney to the floor where the surgeries were done. We kissed our little girl goodbye, and Glenda and I smiled and waved as the nurses wheeled Erin down the hall and through the swinging doors into the operating room. As soon as Erin disappeared through those doors, Glenda's brave mask dropped away and she collapsed into my arms in tears. Our daughter was about to undergo a severely traumatic and invasive procedure, and we might never see her alive again.

The surgical team, led by Drs. Idriss and Ilbawi, split Erin's sternum and removed most of her thymus. It was necessary to stop her heart and put her on a bypass machine to oxygenate and pump her blood for several hours while the heart was being opened and patched on the inside, and the aorta was widened. The surgeons used gortex patches to cover the holes in the atrial septum and the ventricular septum, and they removed the pulmonary band that had served its purpose for four years. The pulmonary artery also had to be widened using gortex.

During the long operation Erin's body temperature was lowered to reduce the metabolism and try to minimize tissue damage. Her core temperature was initially dropped to 22 degrees centigrade, and then held for hours at 25 degrees centigrade. After the internal heart patching was completed, blood was replaced in the closed heart, and an attempt was made to remove all air bubbles, since a small bubble that traveled to a brain artery would result in a damaging stroke. The heart was shocked back into action, the bypass pump was disconnected, and Erin was gradually warmed back up again. During the many hours of surgery Erin required dozens of units of blood, as had been expected, and we had lined up scores of volunteers from our churches (Glenda is Protestant and I am Catholic) to donate blood in the days leading up to the procedure. One staff member commented that their "fridge" had never been so full.

All that stitching in the septal areas made it possible that the heart's microscopic natural electrical conducting system might be damaged, and a permanent pacemaker might be a consequence if a stitch happened to have been placed in an unforgiving position.

We received reports from the operating room every couple of hours about progress. After many tense hours, we were allowed into the recovery room to take our first look at Erin post-op. She remained on the respirator with lots of IVs, tubes and wires, but her skin had good color, and the vital signs were good. The urine in the bag hanging by the foot of the bed was red, a sign of the hemolysis – the damage to red blood cells – that was caused by the hours on the bypass machine. I could see immediately on the cardiac monitor that there was a pacemaker spike before each beat. During the stitching an electrical heart block did occur, and a temporary external pacemaker had been placed with the wire exiting her sternal wound for the time being. It was hoped that normal electrical conduction might return if swelling in the septal areas improved in a few days.

In fact, about two days later while we were sitting with Erin after she had been extubated and was awake and alert, the beep-beep of the machine suddenly changed noticeably. I looked up at the monitor and saw that Erin's heart was now pacing itself, and the external pacemaker was no longer firing. At that moment I violated my self-imposed rule of never adjusting any of Erin's tubes, wires or IVs. It was such a triumphal moment when her cardiac conducting system started up again, meaning that no permanent pacemaker would be required, that I reached up and pressed the 'record button' on the monitor to run a paper strip of her heart beating on its own. That evening I put that ECG strip into her baby book at home.

Erin made a slow but steady recovery in the hospital. After several weeks, we proudly and gratefully brought her back to her own bed at home again. In a few months she would be able to return to preschool. Throughout her childhood she remained thin and petite, but she was very bright and, for the most part, very happy. She also was hardly ever sick, and we wondered if all of the blood transfusions received during her two big heart operations (at age one month and at age four years) might have had some sort of immunologically protective effect by exposing her to so many different proteins and viruses. I did have her tested for AIDS when she was in elementary school and, thankfully, she was negative.

All of the procedures for screening blood were still being worked out in the early 1980s, but luckily Erin escaped that virus.

Erin graduated from college with a B.A. degree with honors in 2003, and then went on to receive a B.S. degree in diagnostic imaging in 2006. She then married her college sweetheart and works as an x-ray technologist at a small hospital in Connecticut. It is somehow fitting that, having spent so much time in hospitals in her early years, she is now cheerfully and expertly serving many patients just as she had been served.

With Erin's definitive heart surgery completed in April, 1985, and then her successful recovery during the next weeks, I had a little time during 1985 to think about things like chess. As mentioned in a previous chapter, on June 1, 1985, I went to a small chess club on the north side of Chicago, signed up to join the U.S. Chess Federation, and played my first rated games.

Erin's Growth Charts

Erin was a seriously ill child, but she was bright and cheerful much of the time and seemed to get few respiratory infections – quite a bundle of contradictions.

The first growth chart shows her height (top curve) and weight (bottom curve) during her first 36 months. The first cardiac surgery was at about age 1 month, and that procedure, along with her g-tube, allowed her to survive. She limped along for the 3 years depicted below the 5th percentile in both height and weight. But she was growing, and she also was mentally fine. She only weighed 14½ pounds at age 1 year, so probably 99 out of 100 children were bigger.

The second growth chart covers the period from age 2 to 18 years. Her definitive heart surgery in Chicago occurred when she was 4 years and 3 months old. Although not all cardiac defects were addressed completely, the surgery was certainly a major success. She was able to continue to grow steadily, and showed a growth spurt at about 14 years. Her height eventually nearly caught up to the 50th percentile by age 18, but she remained quite thin through high school, with a weight at about the 10th percentile.

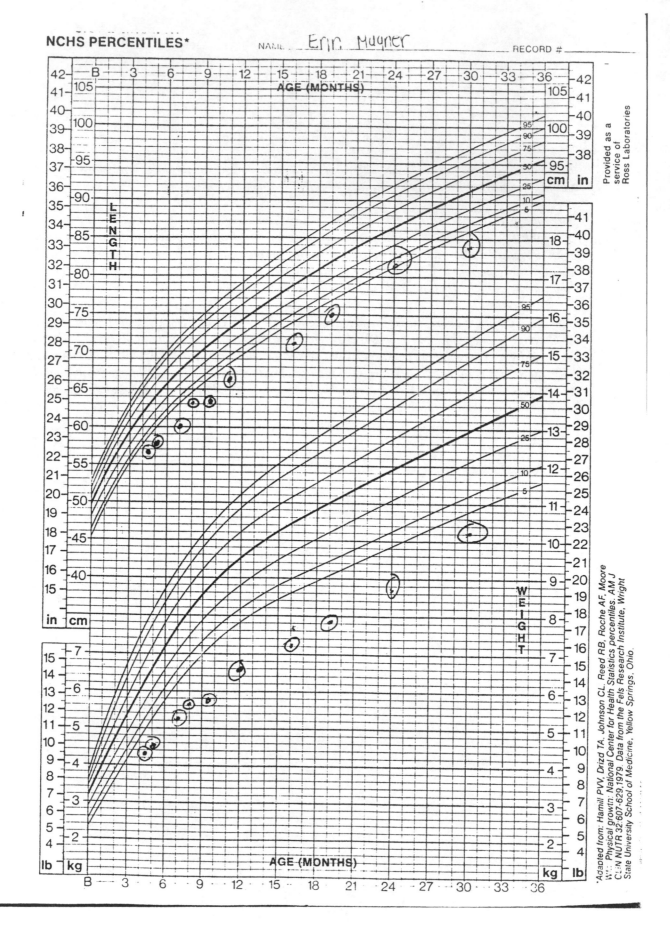

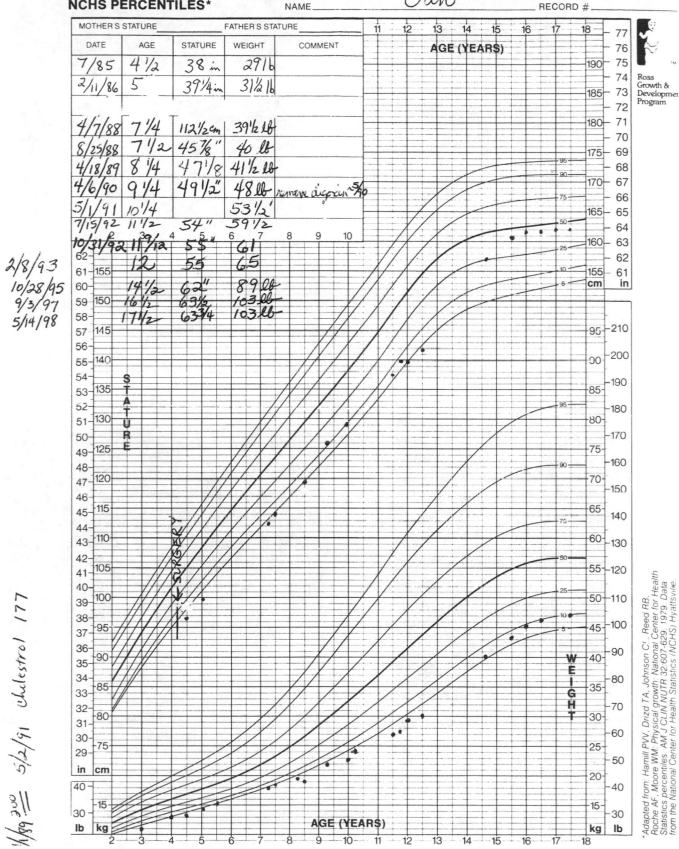

GIRLS: 2 TO 18 YEARS
PHYSICAL GROWTH
NCHS PERCENTILES*

NAME _Erin_   RECORD # _____

DATE	AGE	STATURE	WEIGHT	COMMENT
7/85	4½	38 in	29 lb	
2/11/86	5	39¼ in	31½ lb	
4/7/88	7¼	112½ cm	39½ lb	
8/25/88	7½	45⅞"	40 lb	
4/18/89	8¼	47⅛	41½ lb	
4/6/90	9¼	49½	48 lb	remove aspirin 5/90
5/1/91	10¼		53½'	
7/15/92	11½	54"	59½	
10/31/92	11 39/12	55"	61	
	12	55	65	
	14½	62"	89 lb	
	16½	63½	103 lb	
	17½	63¾	103 lb	

wt 31½
ht

2/8/93
10/28/95
9/3/97
5/14/98

1/89 300 5/2/91 cholesterol 177

SURGERY

*Adapted from: Hamill PVV, Drizd TA, Johnson CL, Reed RB, Roche AF, Moore WM: Physical growth: National Center for Health Statistics percentiles. AM J CLIN NUTR 32:607-629, 1979. Data from the National Center for Health Statistics (NCHS) Hyattsville.

Ross
Growth &
Development
Program

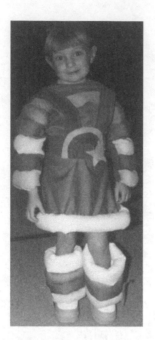

Erin at Halloween

Glenda was very creative during her construction of Erin's Halloween costume.

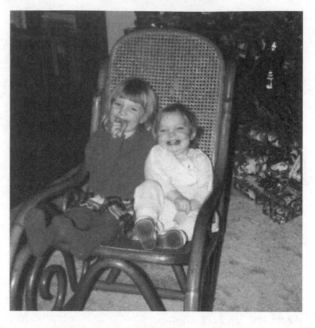

Erin and Carly Enjoy Christmas

Erin and her new baby sister, Carly, enjoy Christmas in 1985.

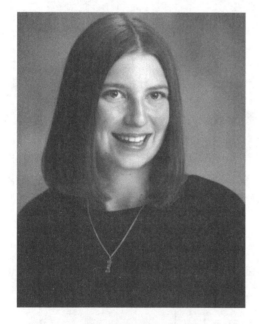

Erin Graduates From High School

Our sickly little baby grew in knowledge and grace, and graduated from high school in 1999.

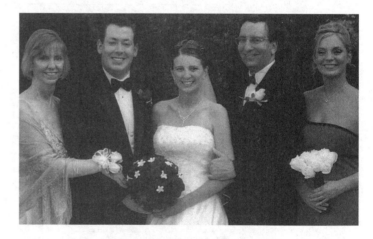

Erin Marries in 2006

Our first baby has grown and marries in July, 2006. From left to right are Glenda, my new son-in-law, Mike Moriarty, Erin, myself and Carly. It was a gorgeous and unforgettable wedding.

Chapter 8

Carly: My California Girl

Carly was born in September 1984. True to her nature about doing things her own way, she was born breech, as I explained in a prior chapter. So Erin is about three years older than Carly. But Carly was always bigger, more active, and more physically competent than her older sister, so you can imagine that that created some unusual dynamics in the family.

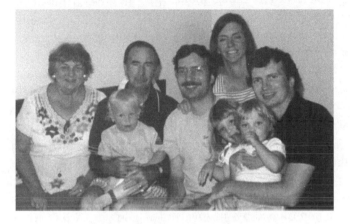

Families Gather in 1986

Three Magner families agreed to rendezvous in California in July, 1986 for fun and relaxation. Adults from left to right are Betty Magner, Louis Magner, Jim Magner, Glenda Pritchett, and Jeff Magner. Children from left to right are Jeffrey Patrick Magner, Erin Magner and Carly Magner.

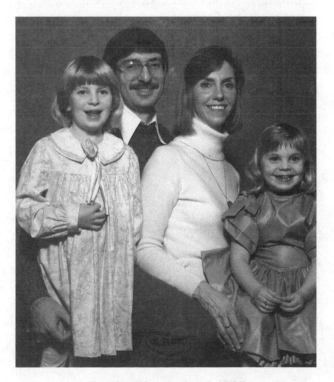

Family Photo about 1987

Erin, Jim, Glenda and Carly pose for a family photo.

Like Erin, Carly was very outgoing. She loved to sing and "perform," and she learned to play the piano as if she had been born to it. As a young elementary student she performed brilliantly several complex classical pieces at a spring piano concert, so I was dismayed that during the following summer months she decided that she would not practice the piano even one day! In September I thought that I would teach her a useful lesson about the importance of practice and continued effort. I sat her down at a piano and asked her to please play her classical pieces from that prior spring concert. The smug look dropped from my face when Carly effortlessly played them all nearly perfectly from memory, so I am not sure who learned the bigger lesson that afternoon. Parents should observe carefully and take to heart a real sense of wonder and awe as their children grow and develop. Human beings are truly amazing.

Carly made the transitions from Glencoe, Illinois, to Greenville, North Carolina to the New Haven, Connecticut area pretty smoothly, making new friends along the way. When she was about 16-years old she joined a group of high school students who were being trained by the local police to go into a bar and order a drink – if the student was not properly carded and was actually given the drink,the police waiting outside planned to move in and serve a citation. Although Carly was a fairly worldly teenager, she actually did not have at that time any experience ordering alcohol. The dozen or so students were assembled for an informal training session that included a mock-up of a bar area with bartender so that they could practice what they were supposed to say. The police instructor explained that the bar would have hard

liquor as well as beer in both bottles and draft. Carly was first at bat, so she somewhat self-consciously stepped up to the mock bartender, feigned a confident attitude, and in a loud voice announced, "I'd like a bottle of draft beer, please." After a second of stunned silence, the bartender and all of the police trainers roared with laughter. Blinking like a deer in the headlights and a little red-faced, Carly listened as they explained her error.

Carly was a superb student in high school, had major roles in several musicals, and sang with the Elm City Girls' Choir. She came to see me one afternoon with the thought that, yes, she could be admitted to many different colleges on the East Coast, but she had considered that the University of Southern California was a potentially interesting choice, since it had a close connection with Hollywood as well as offering top-notch academics. It was pretty expensive, however, and very far from home. "Dad," she asked, "If I were accepted to USC, would you let me go there?"

To no one's surprise, she was accepted, so our younger daughter now is a California girl, with a B.A. from USC. Carly is a Licensed Clinical Member of the California Association of Marriage and Family Therapists (CAMFT). Carly holds two masters degrees from Pepperdine University, an MA in Psychology and an MA in Clinical Psychology, with an Emphasis in Marriage and Family Therapy. She is a therapist at Laura's House, a domestic abuse treatment center. Most importantly, Carly fell in love and married Russell Ketchum, USC alum and southern California native. Russ leads a team of computer experts at Google. Though it is a little sad that we see much less of Carly now, we are thankful for the technological advances – email, cell phone, texting, Skype – that allow us to keep in close touch, almost daily. And of course, what matters most is that she is happy and is living a full and interesting life.

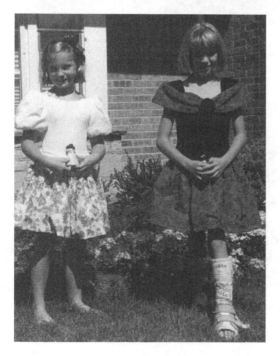

Carly and Erin on Easter Morning, 1991
Carly has grown quickly, and is 95th percentile in height and weight. Erin is small for her age due to her heart disease but is dressed elegantly for Easter, even if she still sports a cast due to the foot fracture sustained from turning cartwheels in the bedroom. She learned that she needed more space for those activities, so to the amazement of neighbors Erin turned many cartwheels and performed astounding acrobatics in the front yard while wearing her cast.

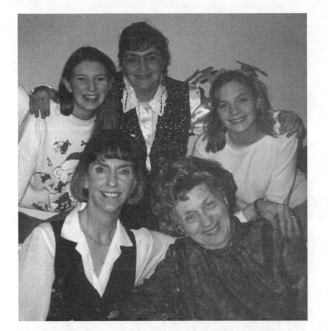

The Pritchett Side of the Family
*My wife's sister, Carol, is flanked by Erin and Carly
while Glenda sits beside her mother, Norma.*

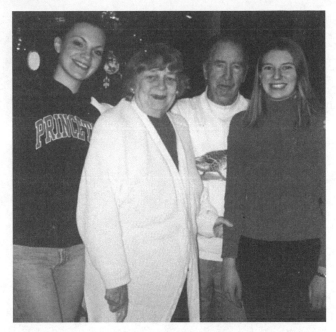

Visitors at Christmas
*Grandma and Grandpa Magner come to visit
in Woodbridge, CT.*

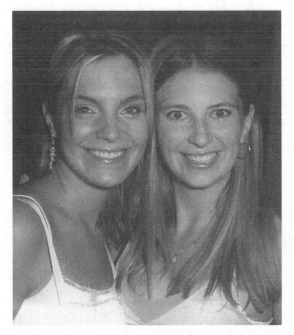

My Active Daughters
Carly and Erin enjoyed friends and fun in New Haven in the early 2000s.

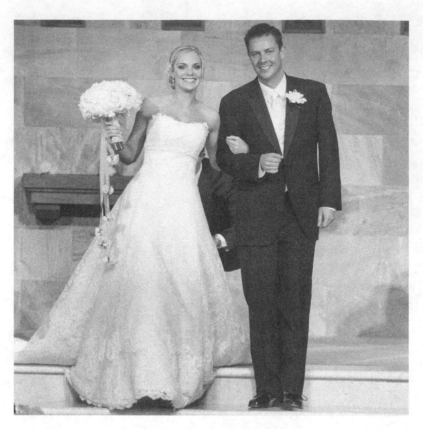

Carly and Russ at the Altar on Their Wedding Day: June 11, 2011
The happy couple, newly married! It was a beautiful wedding, and our family is so happy that my mother was able to attend and enjoy the festivities that June before her death in December, 2011. A new generation will carry on with love and life.

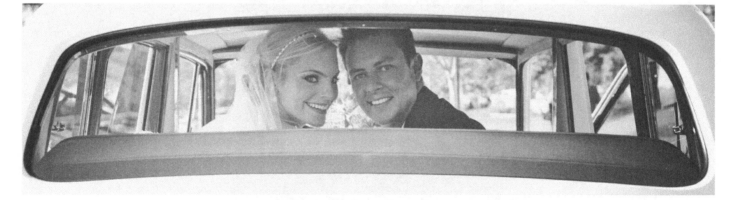

Carly and Russ Set Off to the Reception in Style!
After their wedding, Carly and Russ were transported in style to the reception.

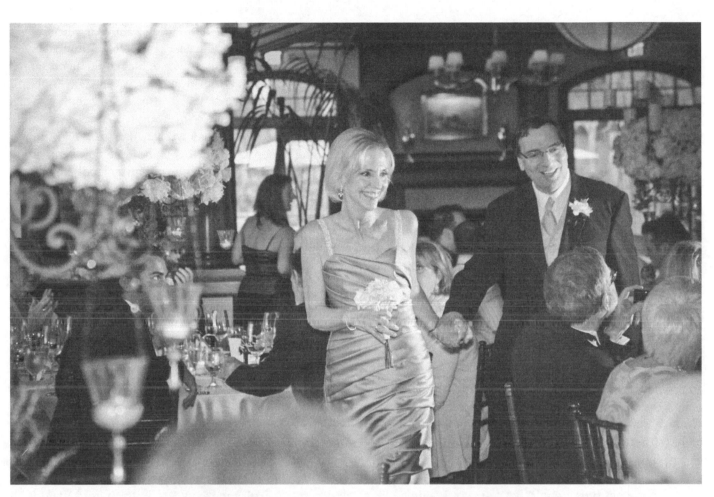

Glenda and I are Introduced at the Wedding Reception

Glenda and I made a traditional entrance at the start of the wedding reception. Glenda and Carly had worked on many details for the evening with the help of a wedding planner, and everything went almost perfectly, including a surprise appearance by members of the USC Marching Band that Glenda had arranged. During the weeks of preparations, Glenda would approach me with an idea about more flowers, a schedule alteration, arrange for the marching band, and so on – as Father of the Bride I quickly learned that my role was to smile and be supportive, and say "yes" to the ideas raised. As a surprise for Glenda, during the reception I made a little speech exalting her efforts and ideas, and introduced a song for Glenda that was fully appropriate: Roy Orbison's classic, "Anything You Want, You Got It!"

Chapter 9

Academia and My First Industry Job

In 1983 I had accepted the faculty position at Michael Reese Hospital, and it was great to be back in Chicago. It was exciting to set up my own research lab, and take on the clinical and administrative responsibilities of a young faculty member. I saw a wide variety of endocrine and general medicine patients and some were quite challenging.

A memorable case was a 53-year old male immigrant from Kiev who had been exposed to radiation during the accident at Chernobyl. This electrical engineer generally had been well, although he was a heavy smoker. He was operating electrical equipment indoors about 50 miles from Chernobyl when the accident occurred in April, 1986. He was told to continue working at his post; some type of radiation screening the next day showed, he said, that he had been exposed to "radioactive fallout." In December, 1986 he presented to the Kiev Research Institute of Endocrinology with a thyroid mass and enlarged cervical lymph nodes. A partial thyroidectomy and removal of larger nodes was performed, and the very brief translated pathology report stated that he had "low-differentiated microfollicular struma maligna of solid structure; cancer metastases." This pathology description was not standard and meant little to me except that the tumor probably was a more severe type of thyroid cancer, but what type I could not tell. Mr. I. said he then received several thousand rads of external radiation therapy to the neck, but one year later masses reappeared in his neck. Because he was thought to have been injured by the Chernobyl accident, and because his case was thought to be serious, he and his family were given special permission to move to the U.S. to seek medical care and, somehow, in April, 1989, he had come to see me!

My preliminary testing showed that he had extensive metastatic cancer, and his neck masses were so rock hard that when I tried to sample them with a needle I could not get out any cells for microscopic evaluation. In May, 1989 he had surgical completion of his thyroidectomy and some tumor debulking from the neck, and we then discovered on pathology examination that he had medullary thyroid cancer. This is a rare and sometimes aggressive form of thyroid cancer, and may not really have been related to any radiation exposure from Chernobyl. It was just bad luck.

During the next two years I tried to manage his slowly worsening condition as best I could. The tumor made a chemical marker called calcitonin that could be measured in the blood, and that level increased from 3,600 pg/mL (a very high abnormal level) after his surgery in May, 1989 to more than 9,000 pg/mL in April, 1991 as x-ray evidence of his tumor also worsened. This type of tumor does not respond well to chemotherapy or radiation therapy, so I employed conservative and supportive measures. My wife and I went to have dinner with him at his apartment, and spent the evening looking at his family photos and talking. He asked me to keep him from dying, but there was little that I could do. In November, 1991 he developed back pain and presented to the emergency room with low blood pressure, and he died soon thereafter. Although I could not keep him from dying, I was able to understand his diagnosis and his prognosis, and I had carefully explained those to him in 1989 so that he could live his life accordingly. I was able to manage small problems along the way, and assist with pain relief. These efforts, I think, made his life better than it otherwise would have been.

My boss, Dr. Arthur Schneider, had published an important body of work about the onset of thyroid cancer in adults who had received thymus irradiation as young children. He had good contacts with thyroid experts in Japan, and from time to time a Japanese scientist would come to Michael Reese Hospital to work in his laboratory for a year. Because I had set up my lab and had obtained a federal grant, Arthur helped me arrange for a young Japanese physician-scientist to come work with me.

Yoshi Miura and his wife found a small apartment in Hyde Park, and soon Yoshi enthusiastically began experiments. He was skilled and hard working, and contributed valuable data to our efforts. We published several papers together, along with other colleagues as co-authors. Yoshi and I were pleased to present an abstract of some of the work at the 8th International Congress of Endocrinology in Kyoto in 1988. I had the opportunity during that week in Japan to see many interesting sights. I booked a tour of China during the next three weeks, and brought home a lot of stories to share with my wife, who graciously allowed me to go exploring while she cared for our children at home. Interestingly, after seeing some sights in Hong

Kong, I stood in line to catch my flight to Guilin in southern China and found that a senior scientist I had known fairly well at NIH, Dr. Saul W. Rosen, who years before had been Bruce Weintraub's mentor, had also joined this small ten-person tour. We arrived at the the primitive Guilin airport at dusk, and just a few bare lightbulbs were hanging in the very spartan and empty terminal. There seemed to be some confusion among the immigration officials about what to do with this plane-load of people, and we stood in line outside the terminal with the other 30 passengers for about an hour waiting to have our passports stamped. Suddenly we were all waved through the entry point with no inspections and were allowed to board a bus to the hotel. Struck by the lack of rigorous entry control (this was in 1988, and our group was very obviously made up of only middle class tourists and businessmen), Saul laughed and quipped, "If something is not worth doing, it's not worth doing right!"

In addition to Yoshi, I also recruited a trainee from South Africa to join our team at Michael Reese Hospital. Victor Perkel was experienced in internal medicine and was seeking endocrinology training in the U.S. I struggled a bit with the forms related to his green card and the hospital's sponsorship of his entry into the country. I was troubled by one line on the form that stated that the work position would have to be a permanent position. I knew that endocrine fellows only stayed at an institution for a couple of years, or possibly three years, and then usually moved elsewhere. But then I saw in the fine print that the federal definition of a permanent position was one that was anticipated to last at least 36 months. This gave me a new perspective on the true meaning of permanence, so I completed all of the necessary paperwork, and soon thereafter Victor and his family arrived. After he had been living in Chicago for a week or two, I asked him if he was having any difficulty adjusting to the city.

"Everything is going pretty smoothly, except I'm a bit bothered by the robots," he replied.

"The robots?" I asked.

"Yes, the robots," he repeated.

I asked more emphatically, "The robots?"

Perceiving my confusion, he paused and shook his head. "Sorry. I mean the traffic signals. We call them robots."

It turned out that it was not only the robots that confused him. The next day he related to me a somewhat embarrassing situation that had just happened. He had never been to a McDonald's fast food restaurant, since the company did not do business in South Africa. Confident in his ability to purchase food successfully at a local McDonald's, he patiently stood in a short line all the while watching the actions of the other customers very carefully so that he would be certain to place his order correctly. Finally reaching the counter, he smiled and ordered a Big Mac, a small Coke and some chips.

"Chips? We don't have chips, sir," came the reply.

Rendered speechless for a few seconds, he stammered, "But I just saw two other fellows order chips!"

After another moment or two of confusion, it became clear to the clerk that he meant to order French fries. Soon Victor sat down to his lunch triumphantly, having had only one small glitch during the process.

Victor was smart and a hard worker, and we published several papers together. In addition to Yoshi and Victor, a series of skilled technicians assisted me in my laboratory, although I had only one technician at a time as a result of budget restrictions. To get additional "boots on the ground," during many of the summers I accepted a bright college student to join my team in the lab for a few weeks. The hospital paid them a small stipend, and I tried to give each student some one-on-one time, although they probably learned the most from my technician. I think that each student over the years had a valuable research experience, and if they made any reasonable contribution to the work, I always included them as co-authors on the next paper, which they very much appreciated. I was chagrined one summer when I accepted a very bright young co-ed to join my lab for a few weeks, but a month before her scheduled time she called me and explained sheepishly that she would have to back out of the job.

"I have just won an all expenses paid study trip to Switzerland for this summer," she explained.

"Wow," I replied, and I expressed my sincere congratulations. But then I added, actually just in jest, "But if you stop to reconsider for a moment, wouldn't you rather work in my lab in Chicago doing fascinating biochemistry rather than traveling here and there in Switzerland?"

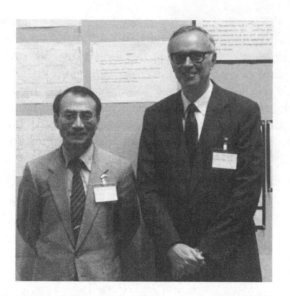

A Japanese Colleague with Dr. Arthur Schneider in Kyoto, 1988
My boss at Michael Reese Hospital for nine years was Dr. Arthur Schneider, an astute scientist, a superb clinician, and a perfect gentleman.

She was silent for a moment, so then I added, "And consider that Chicago is actually exactly like Switzerland. Only flatter." Now realizing that I was just teasing her, we both had a good laugh together.

In addition to interviewing college students for the summer positions, I also interviewed individually each year about 20 medical students who were applying to be interns in the hospital's internal medicine training program. I really enjoyed meeting these bright applicants, and I was quite interested to see what they were doing with their lives. One of my particular points of interest was to analyze the chronology of what they had listed on their applications so that I could understand what they had done year by year since high school – a period of eight years for these applicants. Sometimes a little probing would disclose that they had traveled in Europe for one year, or worked on an archeological dig. During one interview with a muscular young man, I was having difficulty understanding what he had done for one twelve-month period where there seemed to be a gap in his CV. He hemmed and hawed a bit, and I still had no clarity after a minute or two.

"So just tell me," I continued with a mildly stern tone. "Is that the year that you were in jail?"

His wide eyed expression instantly told me, somewhat to my horror, that I must have struck a nerve.

"But let me explain right now, doctor," he blurted, "that it was not really my fault!"

We finished the rest of the interview in a fairly routine manner, but I'm sure he walked out wondering what amazing investigative techniques had been employed by the hospital to discover his secret. I had only been joking, of course, when I had mentioned jail.

Because I was so busy with patients, teaching and research during my years at Michael Reese Hospital, I had little time for chess. I had joined the USCF in 1985 and I played a few games at that time. I played in several small tournaments during late-1991 and early-1992. I suffered several losses and my rating declined. I had no time for study of chess and in 1992 a new nine-year gap in my chess- playing career was just beginning. I had other priorities in my life.

I was having difficulty getting my National Institutes of Health scientific grant renewed, so my small research laboratory at Michael Reese Hospital was operating with a very limited budget. I was busy seeing endocrinology and general medicine patients, and I had a hectic and happy family life. Dr. Schneider, my immediate boss, was a skilled scientist and physician, and was just about the best possible boss. But Michael Reese Hospital was starting to have financial difficulties. In 1992, I decided to look for a more promising job outside of Chicago. I interviewed at a hospital in Honolulu, but this would have been a purely clinical job with little opportunity for research, and when the realtor drove me around to look at small houses, the prices were astronomically high. (Of course, a few years later the prices fell substantially.)

Steve Usala, an old friend from the University of Chicago who was then an endocrinologist on the faculty at East Carolina University in Greenville, North Carolina, invited me to give a lecture and look at a faculty position there. The medical school buildings and laboratories, and also the hospital buildings, were relatively new, the people were nice, the salary and benefits were acceptable, and I was offered lab space and a paid lab technician to help me for twelve months. North Carolina was a lot warmer than Chicago, and the houses were affordable. So I talked it over with my family, and took the job. We sold our house in Glencoe, Illinois for a profit, and before we had to move out I sent Glenda down to pick out a house.

She described her favorite house on the phone (remember, I had lots of patients in clinics in Chicago, so I could not just take off anytime I wanted), and with my long-distance approval she bought it. We also bought a new minivan to provide good service for the family. A few weeks later, in early August, 1992, we loaded up the car and headed south.

Having decided to drive straight through from Chicago to Greenville, Glenda and I taking turns, we found ourselves in western North Carolina in the early morning hours. The girls had slept, of course, and were now wide-eyed and hungry, on the look-out for a place to stop for breakfast. A likely spot appeared up ahead – Waffle House – not an establishment with which we were familiar but one which no doubt would fit the bill of the moment: breakfast and coffee. Once inside, we noticed a unique informality and familiarity among the wait staff and customers. After having been addressed numerous times as "Sweetie," "Honey" and "Sugar," Carly turned to us with a puzzled look – "Why does everybody act like they already know us?" Texan Glenda grinned and answered, "That's the South, Honey."

When we pulled into the driveway I was pleased with Glenda's choice. She had picked out a four-bedroom colonial in a nice neighborhood about four miles from the medical school. Glenda had found some nearby teaching opportunities, and my daughters were quite positive about the move, so all was well.

But one problem with Greenville, North Carolina was that there were few active chess groups for miles, and my job and family kept me very busy. I played a few games against my Astral computer between 1992 and 1997, but I played in no tournaments.

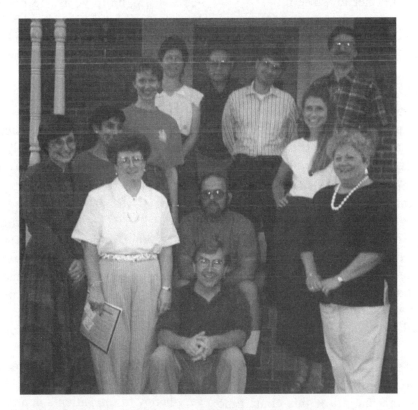

Endocrinology Colleagues from East Carolina University
I worked at East Carolina University in Greenville from 1992 until 1997, and made good friends there. Dr. Gene Furth, at center back, was an endocrinologist and the Chairman of Medicine who recruited me to the position. I am in the plaid shirt in the back, and next to me is my long-time friend from the University of Chicago who had relocated to Greenville before me, Dr. Steve Usala. Dr. David Snyder is wearing the scrubs, and seated in front is our Chief of Endocrinology, Dr. Kirk Ways. Our talented fellows, Dr. Radha Reddy and Dr. Fiona Cook, and other staff also attended this backyard outing. As budget cuts and other issues punished our Division in 1996, the other physicians left one by one, leaving me the only endocrinologist in the Division. With regret, I decided to leave academia in 1997 and tested the waters in the pharmaceutical industry.

I enjoyed the clinical work, even though I was seeing many more patients than I had at Michael Reese Hospital. The endocrine clinic had many patients with type 2diabetes, and there also was a wide variety of other types of patients. The in-hospital consultations were always interesting, and service as an attending physician on the General Medicine Ward was particularly challenging, since many of the patients were quite ill. The students, interns, residents and fellows provided an opportunity for teaching, and lots of lively discussions. I wrote several book chapters, and published articles with colleagues about the useful education of diabetes patients about their disease, diet and medications. I also published interesting clinical cases, including a woman who had lost pituitary function after a severe hemorrhage when she delivered a baby, a woman who lost certain white blood cells temporarily when given a thyroid medication, and another woman who I discovered was allergic to the blue dye in one of her pills (a problem easily corrected by switching her to white pills).

Most important to me was my scientific research, and I published several interesting papers during the mid-1990s, including a few making use of *in situ* hybridization to assess the upregulation of certain enzymes in pituitary cells that were synthesizing the hormone TSH. But I still had trouble getting substantial grant support.

A "slow-rolling crisis" began in early 1995 when our new Chairman of Medicine, Dr. W., insisted that faculty should reduce time spent doing research and writing book chapters, and instead should have more clinic hours to try to bring in more revenue. As a sensible and responsible faculty member, this was fully understandable to me. After all, the University was paying my salary. I dutifully complied by adding more clinic hours, more months of inpatient consultations, and I doubled my General Medicine Ward time to two months annually.

The four endocrine physicians who worked in my department were not so sure that all of this clinic time was really appropriate for academicians, but we all basically pitched in and did more clinical work. We felt, however, that our key roles should be teaching and research, along with a sensible amount of clinical work to help pay the bills for the medical school. We couldn't help it if the insurance reimbursements for endocrinologists were relatively low. Students, interns, residents and fellows, who accompanied us as we saw patients, still needed to learn how to take care of patients with endocrine diseases.

I loved a joke that circulated in our department at that time that seemed quite apropos. There once was a remote monastery of monks whose goal was to pray three times daily for the salvation of the world, help the poor a little if they could, and teach young boys how to become monks. The monks took pride in being very self-sufficient, so they tended small gardens and eked out a living as best they could. One day, a bright monk came to the Superior with the idea that if the monks sold some of the wine they made each year, there would be more funds available to make life more efficient for the community. Even the poor could be helped a little more. The Superior approved the sale of wine, and over the next years the monastery sold more and more wine. Soon it became a booming business. But a new Superior became concerned as costs of business rose, and more and more wine had to be sold to support the infrastructure. The Superior asked the monks to pray less each day and and teach less each day, and instead spend more time making wine. After a few more years, he reached a crucial decision. In order to meet the new quotas for the next year's wine deliveries, the praying and teaching would have to stop completely!

Over the next year or so, during 1995 and 1996, my four partners all took other opportunities elsewhere. I was left alone with the work of five endocrinologists, though I obviously could not multiply my efforts that many times. I worked hard but many patients simply had to seek care elsewhere.

I decided that I could still find a way do scientific research, but probably not in a traditional role at an academic institution. Although I had just been granted tenure as a professor, Glenda and I came to the decision that I would leave academia and join a large pharmaceutical company. It is hard for me to fully express in writing the sadness I felt as I planned to end my academic career. I loved interacting with students and trainees, and I immensely enjoyed the privilege of running my own small scientific research laboratory. I also was very happy to see patients in an academic setting — but I just could not envision myself focused nearly entirely on seeing patients. The freezers in my laboratory were full of valuable (at least to me) probes and antibodies and plasma samples that could provide novel scientific insights in endocrinology for many years – but now they would all be discarded. The federal government had supported my scientific efforts for years, and I had reciprocated by publishing scores of scientific papers and book chapters. I had done everything right, and although I had never had the attitude that the government owed me a grant, I do admit that I felt somewhat betrayed. Federal grant funding was so tight that I simply could not continue my work.

I flew up to Connecticut in late-1996 to interview for a posting at the West Haven facility of Bayer Corporation. I had no idea how things worked in a big drug company. I was polite and just kept repeating at each interview that I was a well- trained internist and endocrinologist who knew some biochemistry and was very interested in science, and I was ready to make the change from academia to industry. They liked me, and on the second visit a few weeks later they offered me the job of Associate Director, which was an acceptable position, but with a fairly low level of managerial responsibility. I knew that I had to learn the ropes. I was to start in February, 1997.

Sadly, I wrote out my letter of resignation to my chairman at East Carolina University, where I had hoped to work until I retired. I was astonished by his reaction, since he was incredulous that I was about to quit my job. I was more incredulous that he had not realized that I was serious about needing a reasonable opportunity to do research, and not wanting even more clinic time. I had told him calmly at several prior meetings that if he insisted on assigning me more and more clinic time, I would have to strongly consider leaving the university. Since I would still have a wife and children in Greenville for a few months in 1997, I offered to return to volunteer to give several scheduled endocrinology lectures to the medical students, as there was literally no one else to give them. He accepted this proposal, and it was really no trouble for me to give three or four lectures in March and April since I would be back in town on occasion to see my family.

After my children's school year ended in June, my family joined me in Connecticut. The Endocrine Group at Bayer had a bit of a momentary crisis that they intended me to solve my first week. My new boss at Bayer was an older gentleman, and he had been doing the medical monitoring of the patient laboratory data and patient adverse event data in two large Phase 3 studies of patients with type 2 diabetes, but this was a big task for him on top of his other many responsibilities. One study was testing a Bayer oral product, Precose (acarbose), in a novel combination with the oral drug metformin. The second study was testing acarbose in combination with injectable insulin.

The basic idea was that these studies should prove that the standard drug, such as metformin alone, for example, would lower blood glucose pretty well, but the blood glucose would be even more improved if metformin were combined with Precose. The young physician who had been doing the medical monitoring of these two ongoing studies had left the company rather unexpectedly for a personal reason, and Bayer really needed a physician to be able to step in to pick up these duties – so that turned out to be a good break for me.

Several people on the team there were very helpful to me, since I was so inexperienced about drug development. I just learned quickly on the job with their help, and every week I learned more and more new things just by rolling up my sleeves and doing things. It was in a way like doing a medical internship but while sitting in a chair in front of a computer most of the time. I felt strange not being "on call" and there really were no emergencies. I came to work at about 8 am and left at about 5 pm five days per week, although there were a few busier periods.

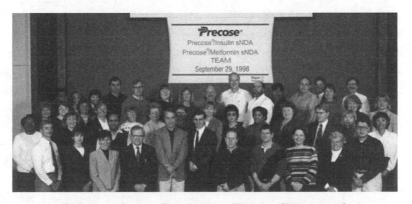

Celebrating a Success at Bayer Corporation
Having joined Bayer in February, 1997, with no pharmaceutical company experience, I pitched in to manage two large Phase 3 studies and worked with a skilled team to get FDA approval for two new indications for our drug for diabetes, Precose. These successes were a big relief to me in my new environment. I am in the back row at the right with the mustache.

The patients in the clinical studies were scattered at many hospitals and clinics in many cities across the United States, and there were physicians at each center who were actually responsible for day to day issues that might arise with a patient. I was more the record keeper at that point. The doctors at each center entered data on their "case report forms" week by week, and when all of the patients in a study had passed a pre-defined clinic visit, the database of a study was "locked," and large tables of data became available for me and my colleagues (statisticians, drug safety experts, etc.) to analyze. A large formal study report document had to be written for each of the two studies, and as the main physician analyzing the medical results, I played a large role in that. Both studies were successful, showing that the Precose made a meaningful contribution to patient care when added either to metformin or to insulin. We then worked with the expert external physicians who had participated in these studies to prepare scientific abstracts for presentation at medical meetings, and wrote up the medical papers for full publication. The two papers subsequently were published in the journal *Diabetes Care* in 1998. We also wrote up lots of paperwork to submit to the Food and Drug Administration and to other regulatory agencies in many countries in order to have the official prescribing information updated about Bayer's drug. I learned many lessons about all of these complex processes, and the day-to-day experience was invaluable.

I had never begun seeing patients directly myself in the New Haven area when I moved there in 1997. Initially I had declined the opportunity to have a half-day clinic once a week at a local hospital because I was afraid that I was so inexperienced at my drug company job that I didn't want to divert my attention;

I was intent on focusing on my new job to be sure that I didn't mess anything up. In 1998, after successes with the two diabetes studies, their publication, and successes with the FDA and other regulatory bodies, I received a nice promotion, which gave me more responsibilities. By mid-1999, however, I had a number of additional accomplishments under my belt, and just as I was beginning to consider taking on some clinic responsibilities I received another pleasant surprise – I was promoted again, this time to a more global position.

Recall that Bayer's main headquarters are in Germany, and it is a large and well- established global company. In my new role with global responsibilities in endocrinology I would still be living and working primarily in the New Haven area, but I would travel more and be involved in all phases of drug development from basic science efforts, through preclinical development, clinical development and post-registration studies. It is beyond the scope of this book to explain all of this, but the relevant point was that with more international travel, sometimes on short notice, I felt uncomfortable having a scheduled clinic with patients waiting.

I might have to cancel the clinic with only a few days notice if an important trip or meeting came up. I felt that such cancellations would not be fair to the patients who had signed up to see me, and it might even be medically dangerous for them. So at first in 1997 I didn't have a clinic in New Haven because I feared I might mess up my job, and then later by 1999 I couldn't have a clinic because I had been promoted for doing my job very well. Life is funny.

I was busier than ever, and I traveled the globe. I continued to work with Precose, the marketed product, but now I also worked on early drug candidates being considered for use someday by patients with type 2 diabetes. I also worked on projects related to osteoarthritis and osteoporosis. I became involved with early clinical studies of a Viagra-like drug for male sexual dysfunction, and I wrote the clinical study protocol for the Phase 2 dose-finding study for this drug, which eventually became marketed as Levitra.

Over several years our team became very knowledgeable about sexual dysfunction of many types, and we met regularly with top physicians who were studying these areas. I was amused one time when I was stopped by a lady with a clipboard at a shopping mall. She asked me to fill out a questionnaire constructed by a group wanting to raise awareness of the serious problem of sexual harassment. I only filled out their form to question # 3, which asked "Do you ever talk about sex at work?" I just handed the questionnaire back to the nice lady, since I knew then that my score on their questionnaire was going to skew their results completely!

By the summer of 2001 I was settled enough with my job and family to play in a chess tournament again. The annual Bradley Open near Hartford, Connecticut would be my new coming-out party.

Chapter 10

A New Job At Genzyme In Cambridge

During the summer of 2003 I changed jobs. Bayer had run into a number of financial and other difficulties, and although I really enjoyed working at Bayer, I decided to accept an opportunity at Genzyme Corporation in Cambridge, Massachusetts. Genzyme was a smaller company than Bayer and had a more entrepreneurial culture. The endocrine drug, Thyrogen®, at Genzyme was recombinant human thyroid-stimulating hormone (rhTSH), which was on the market for use in patients with thyroid cancer. I had extensive knowledge about TSH from my past academic career, so this was a very comfortable fit for me. I started as Senior Director of Clinical Research, but then was soon promoted to Vice President of Clinical Research, with focus on the endocrinology area.

In mid-2003 I stepped into the middle of an ongoing Clinical Development project that needed my attention. For a number of years Genzyme had generously provided free Thyrogen to a number of doctors for thyroid cancer patients who had need of the drug for certain special

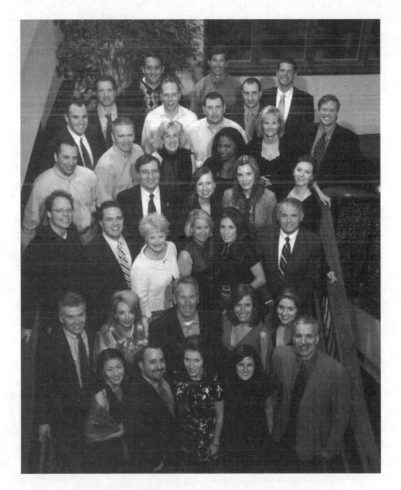

Working with a New Team at Genzyme

In 2003 I moved from Bayer to Genzyme Corporation, Cambridge, Massachusetts. I am near the center of this photo wearing the dark blazer with dark necktie, surrounded by my new very talented and very friendly colleagues. My academic research from 1980 until 1997 had focused on the biochemistry and cell biology of thyroid-stimulating hormone. I now had the opportunity at Genzyme to apply those years of experience to assist with further clinical development of a marketed drug for thyroid cancer, the recombinant human form of TSH. My extensive prior scientific career in the TSH field along with my new knowledge about global drug development acquired at Bayer made me essentially the perfect clinician-scientist for this position at Genzyme.

medical conditions. This was a program that was set up by Genzyme in conjunction with the FDA, and was a so-called Compassionate Use Program. Many of the patients had seriously advanced thyroid cancer that had spread to their lungs or bones, while other patients lacked the ability to make sufficient TSH in their own pituitary glands so required the injections of rhTSH for certain treatments or testing to be effective. Other patients had a history of serious clinical depression or other medical illnesses that would put them at risk if they stopped their routine daily thyroxine medication as part of an old regimen to raise their blood levels of TSH, so those patients could be more safely managed using the injections of rhTSH. Doctors had completed paperwork requesting the Thyrogen be shipped for these special patients, and in many cases the Genzyme Medical Director had approved the shipment.

The project underway in 2003 was a formal clinical research protocol, approved by regulators and institutional research boards, to engage those doctors who had participated in the Compassionate Use Program in many cities. The doctors were to complete case forms based on the records of patients who had received the Thyrogen. Doctors would record on the forms various blood test and nuclear medicine scan results, and other results, that would allow Genzyme to compile a summary of the experiences of these very ill patients. Genzyme hoped that if the data showed substantial patient benefit as well as safety then a regulatory dossier could be prepared and sent to FDA to seek favorable package insert language changes for Thyrogen. This would broaden the range of patients who would be eligible for Thyrogen use.

The case report forms were completed by the doctors for about 115 patients. Genzyme study monitors traveled to the various clinics around the USA in which the patients had been treated to provide assistance to investigators if conflicting or ambiguous information seemed to be entered for a patient. Data on the case report forms were entered into a central computer database in Massachusetts. Then the Genzyme data managers and statisticians went to work to generate tables and listings — summaries of key clinical parameters in tables, as well as detailed computer printouts showing in an organized way every data point captured for every patient. This huge electronic package then was delivered to me to perform a detailed medical analysis focused primarily on the efficacy of Thyrogen in these patients, while a Genzyme doctor in pharmacovigilance used the same package to perform an analysis of the clinical safety of Thyrogen use in these patients. Then our small team wrote up a formal Clinical Study Report, an internal confidential company document that is also supplied routinely to the FDA, to record our analyses and conclusions.

The data seemed to be favorable for Thyrogen, and over the next several months our team proceeded with the next big step to attempt to get a favorable Thyrogen label change. We completed the extensive paperwork required to file a dossier with the FDA. A day before the dossier was trucked to the FDA in Rockville, Maryland we took a photo of Paul Gelep, business and program management expert at Genzyme and long-time expert on Thyrogen, as he held some of the volumes of documents. That was in 2004, but now such dossier submissions are done electronically. This was a lot of work, and our team was extremely hopeful about the review by FDA, but after preliminary review the FDA told Genzyme that although the data were promising this had been a retrospective collection, and FDA decided that a prospective randomized trial would be required before any label change for Thyrogen could be allowed. This was a disappointment, of course, but to salvage some good from this worthwhile scientific effort we proceeded with publication of the clinical data: Robbins R, Driedger A, Magner J and the Thyrogen Compassionate Use Investigator Group. Recombinant human TSH-assisted radioiodine therapy for patients with metastatic cancer who could not elevate endogenous TSH or be withdrawn from thyroxine. Thyroid 2006; 16 (11): 1121-1130. I should mention that Genzyme remains interested currently in finding a way to obtain the official label language that would allow broader use of Thyrogen in patients with distant metastases of their cancers, but we are still working on that.

Regarding other aspects of my job, many routine duties required attention. Annual reports were written for regulators (Thyrogen was already registered in major countries), and I worked with our internal Genzyme Regulatory team to obtain new registrations for our product in multiple small countries. One episode that illustrated the triumph of enthusiasm over experience was obtaining a

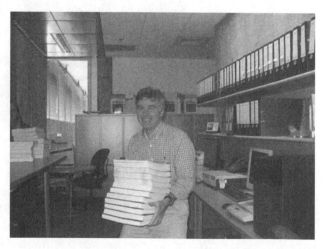

Paul Gelep, who has worked at Genzyme with Thyrogen for decades, weighs the team's efforts.

label update of Thyrogen in Switzerland, a country that has a unique drug registration process. The Genzyme office there e-mailed me directly saying that they needed me to look over their Thyrogen dossier – which they had compiled by cutting and pasting pieces of other existing Thyrogen dossiers.

The problem was that the Swiss needed a very rapid turnaround of my comments within just two days, and then the dossier would be formally submitted to the government. I felt that the dossier was unclear in many places in large part due to the inexact cutting and pasting, a naturally messy process. So for many hours I just rolled up my sleeves and did my best to rewrite and reorganize many pages of the clinical sections. For improved clarity I invented new headings of document sections to present a much more logical flow of ideas. Pleased with my efforts after a huge amount of work, I sent the large document back to the Swiss, who promptly submitted the package to their government. Several months later I learned that the Thyrogen label had been approved in Switzerland, and I was very pleased with myself since I felt that I had made a major contribution to improving the quality of the submission. All was well.

The humorous end of the story is that several years later our main Regulatory Department at Genzyme Headquarters in Massachusetts collected that Swiss dossier and several others from Europe to prepare a consolidated report of some kind. The sections of the documents did not match up, of course, because I had moved many parts around in the interest of clarity and accuracy, not respecting usual section boundaries in such official documents. An executive from our Regulatory Department reviewed those documents and then approached me, and she asked if it was true that at the last minute I had rewritten nearly the entire clinical dossier for Switzerland. I proudly said that I had. She laughed and confided that her team had decided that I had been quite creative in my efforts! She informed me that it was not allowed to just make up new headings for the sections of regulatory dossiers, and my work was very unconventional, although scientifically perfect and very well written, and had clearly gotten the job done. We both had a good laugh, since I might have caused an implosion of the whole effort, but it was clear to me that my extensive re-write had made a confused and unintelligible document at once fully clear to the poor Swiss government doctor (who was not likely a thyroid cancer expert) who had to read and understand that dossier to vote on approval. I suspect that the government doctor much appreciated my making the document easily understandable, and he then gave a well-informed, positive decision for our company!

Other parts of my job also kept me very busy. For several years our team worked on a possible application of a low dose of rhTSH with oral radioiodine to treat benign

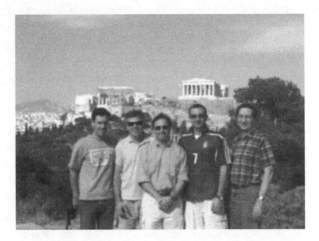

Part of the USA Thyrogen Team takes a break during a meeting in Athens.
From the left: Marcelo Cheresky, Paul Gelep, Peter Cooke, Mark Allyn, James Magner.

multinodular goiter. The project involved writing and executing several clinical protocols, and we published three medical articles about our results. Currently, this is still a work in progress.

Another Clinical Development project involved developing a plan to seek registration of Thyrogen for use in thyroid cancer patients in mainland China. That country is potentially a huge commercial market for many sorts of products, including drugs related to management of thyroid cancer. I had many teleconferences with my Chinese Genzyme and Sanofi colleagues, and I made trips to China to speak with nuclear medicine physicians, surgeons and a few endocrinologists from different cities in that huge country. Our team designed two clinical studies that potentially might be required for registration, and those extensive documents were translated into Chinese and submitted to the SFDA. But this is also a work in progress at this time.

I also worked for several years to achieve registration of Thyrogen in Japan, and made multiple trips there. I spoke slowly using very clear power point slides as I presented to the Japanese government health authority, KIKO – the committee members all wore headphones so that they could hear a simultaneous translation as I spoke. Genzyme achieved government approval of the diagnostic indication of Thyrogen in Japan, and then later the remnant ablation indication, so our team is very proud of this work.

The remnant ablation indication for Thyrogen had been achieved first in Europe in 2005 based on a global study that actually was ongoing and in the last stages when I joined Genzyme in 2003. So in late-2003 I was handed a huge package of tables and listings of the study data, and I wrote up the medical efficacy portions of the internal report, the Clinical Study Report, explaining the positive results of the study in great detail. I then helped write up the medical portions of the massive regulatory dossier filed in Europe, and months later argued our case in London before the relevant committee of the European Medicines Agency (EMA), the CHMP. I had met several weeks before that meeting with the European Thyrogen Rapporteur in Dublin to explain our case, and he was generally supportive. A rapporteur is the point of key medical contact between a pharmaceutical company and the EMA. But during my presentation to the CHMP in London several committee members raised some difficult issues – I stood at the podium and quickly provided some unrehearsed but logical and convincing responses, and then I was asked to leave the room. A vote was taken and Genzyme won over the committee, so I was greatly relieved. The pivotal clinical study that supported this approval was written up with the external investigators and published as Pacini et al. in 2006.

Although the EMA granted the new remnant ablation approval in 2005, the FDA wanted more follow-up data on the patients seen in the pivotal study. Our rapid design and execution of another clinical study to get that additional required data is described in the appendix along with the resulting publication of that follow-up study. FDA approval of Thyrogen for the new indication occurred in 2007, and was cause for displaying a celebratory banner in the lobby of Genzyme's Cambridge headquarters.

In 2010 Genyzme faced a new kind of crisis. The manufacture of biotechnology drugs is highly complex since they are products of living organisms. Complexity can lead to problems, and a variety of manufacturing issues appeared in 2010 that led to a drug shortage of Thyrogen and several of Genzyme's key products. We were confident that all issues could be resolved within two years and we would be right back on track. Of course, because product availability was an issue, company revenues fell as did the company stock price. Company management, then led by the charismatic Henri Termeer, was approached by Sanofi, a huge, powerful company that was in search of a growth platform. Sanofi wanted to buy Genzyme, but Termeer refused. His argument was that Genzyme's problems and low stock price were very temporary – but those, of course, were the very reasons that Sanofi wanted to acquire Genzyme! Carl Icahn also got involved in the next series of dramatic events. In the end, Sanofi executed a hostile takeover of Genzyme and took possession in 2011. This was a stunning turn of events for Genzyme employees, and during the next months we spent a lot of time getting used to new software systems and processes. Fortunately for Genzyme, Sanofi had no intent of buying and then dismembering the company. Instead, Sanofi wanted to purchase a highly functioning independent-minded

biotechnology company, and Sanofi wanted most Genzyme people to stay and continue doing exactly what they had been doing, and maintain a high performance. Someone described it as Sanofi having purchased an expensive, shiny, high-performance sports car, and they did not want it to get scratched!

With the takeover by Sanofi, a number of Genzyme employees chose of their own accord to depart. Most relevant to my work as the Thyrogen Clinical Development doctor was the departure of all three physicians who had been dedicated full-time to Thyrogen Medical Affairs (two in Europe and one in the USA departed). Since 2003 I had primarily worked on Clinical Development tasks, but I had occasionally helped with Medical Affairs tasks in the USA and even overseas. Top management approached me in November, 2011 and requested that I continue full-time in Clinical Development, but they wanted me also to pick up full medical responsibility for Thyrogen Medical Affairs globally. As Thyrogen was marketed in 65 countries, taking on both Clinical Development as well as Medical Affairs for Thyrogen would be a big task, but I agreed. There was actually no one else to do this. There were Genzyme Medical Affairs personnel stationed in many countries around the world, but these physicians worked in Medical Affairs for all of Genzyme's products – they spent at most 10% of their time on Thyrogen issues, so they were not that well-versed in the latest in thyroid cancer research and science.

A point of explanation is that Clinical Development tasks involve such duties as writing company-sponsored clinical protocols, executing the clinical studies, analyzing the results, and writing the Clinical Study Reports. One also advises management about the strength of the data and the unmet medical need, and whether the big effort of trying to get a product label update based on the new clinical data is reasonable. If given the green light, the Clinical Development doctor then works with a team to prepare the large regulatory dossier that would be needed, make explanatory power point slides, and present to and interact with the regulatory authorities to achieve the product label update. This doctor also writes required reports for regulators, and answers ad hoc regulatory inquiries about medical issues. A different doctor, in Pharmacovigilance, is an expert on safety and all of those regulations, but works closely with the Clinical Development doctor on the above tasks. The Clinical Development doctor also works with the basic scientists who are trying to develop new products using animals, and also he looks at in-licensing opportunities from other companies that might be purchased to be new products. Thus, Clinical Development for a globally marketed product in a company of Genzyme's size pre-2011 is a full-time job.

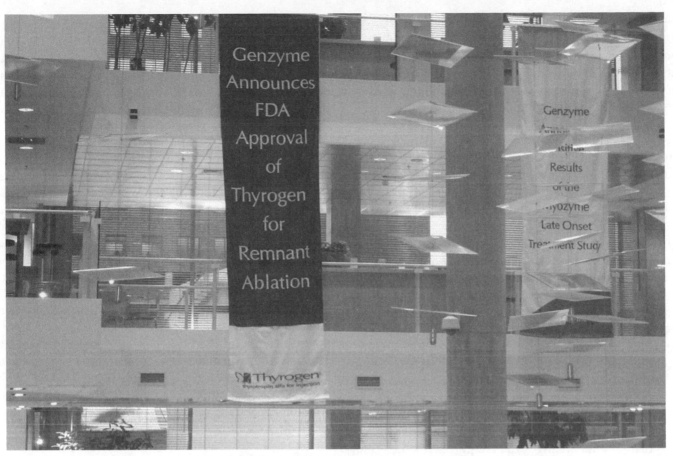

A Banner Hangs in the Genzyme Lobby to Celebrate our Success with Thyrogen.
In 2007 the success of our Thyrogen team in getting the remnant ablation indication in the USA was celebrated at Genzyme headquarters with a banner, some champagne and some speeches.

In contrast, a Medical Affairs doctor answers questions from prescribing doctors, and is allowed if asked to speak "off-label" to address a question, whereas Sales is not permitted to speak "off-label" in many countries, including the USA. The Medical Affairs doctor is a resource to the Medical Information Department, which is contacted daily by doctors with questions. Medical Affairs also advises Marketing as that group designs new advertising brochures or prepares new power point slides for company-paid physician speakers. All such Marketing materials have to be "on-label" and are steered through a complex series of approval steps conducted within a Promotions Review Board (PRB). The Medical Affairs doctor also prepares medical updates for the Sales Teams, and commonly attends Sales Meetings several times each year to interact closely with Sales personnel to answer their questions and provide other training. Medical Affairs also supervises the activities of skilled professionals known as Medical Science Liaisons – these persons are often graduates of pharmacy schools, and are allowed to answer "off-label" questions as they visit prescribing physicians in their offices or at medical conferences. The Medical Affairs doctor also helps shape the publication strategy for the product, and entertains doctors' questions about

Investigator-Sponsored Studies (ISS) that they have an interest in performing at their local university. These study proposals originate with the external doctors and might be prospective clinical studies, registries, retrospective studies, or even basic science studies. The Medical Affairs doctor also reviews applications for grants for Independent Medical Education programs (such as grand rounds programs at hospitals). There are complex systems of software for managing all of these tasks in a way that is auditable by regulators in view of the need to be compliant with many regulations and to be transparent if payments are being made to doctors who are acting as speakers, advisors, consultants, or investigators. And all of the above activities need to be budgeted for, and then the budget must be managed. Nothing is simple, and everything must be carefully documented.

In view of the above two job descriptions, I had a busy work life in late-2011, 2012 and 2013. I was fortunate fairly quickly to put in place a European Medical Affairs Director for Thyrogen, Dr. Ana Crespo, who was able to perform many Medical Affairs duties in that region, which includes some Middle East countries. Then in mid-2013 I brought on board a skilled endocrinologist, Dr. Richard

Weiss, to be the USA Medical Affairs Director. For Asia (including Australia) and Latin America I relied on close cooperation with the excellent regional Medical Affairs personnel we have based in those areas, and who keep up very well with thyroid cancer issues even though Thyrogen is only one of their many product responsibilities.

An interesting Thyrogen project unfolded over several years that happened to be a perfect blend of Medical Affairs and Clinical Development tasks – since I wore both hats things worked extremely smoothly. This section is a little technical, but medically-inclined readers will appreciate this. Patients with thyroid cancer often have a total thyroidectomy performed, and in many cases then receive oral radioiodine treatment (remnant ablation), but the recommended amount of radioiodine to use for the ablation procedure has varied over the decades. During my endocrine fellowship that started in 1980 and for years afterward I often chose to use 29.9 mCi 131-I for that procedure in routine patients because the nuclear safety regulations in the USA allowed for that amount to be given as an outpatient. A few years later larger amounts of radioiodine were recommended for routine patients, such as 100 mCi, and in later years in the USA that amount was made legal for outpatients in many states. But a randomized prospective trial really was required to determine scientifically whether 30 mCi or 100 mCi was the correct amount to use on a routine basis. A Genzyme Medical Affairs physician based in England starting in 2005, Dr. Mike Holmes, was instrumental in working with some UK physicians in the early stages of this enterprise. Genzyme provided funding and Thyrogen to support a large Investigator-Sponsored Study in the UK that was a four-arm randomized trial of thyroid remnant ablation. The four regimens tested were Thyrogen plus 30 mCi, versus Thyrogen plus 100 mCi, versus thyroid hormone withdrawal plus 30 mCi, versus thyroid hormone withdrawal plus 100 mCi. This trial of 438 thyroid cancer patients showed beautifully that all four methods of thyroid remnant ablation were equally effective, yet patients who received only 30 mCi could be discharged sooner from the hospital and had fewer adverse events, while patients who received Thyrogen (versus thyroid hormone withdrawal) had a better quality of life. This wonderful UK study actually was done in parallel with a very similar and equally well done large prospective clinical study in France that enrolled 752 patients, and that provided the same excellent results. Both studies were published in the same issue of the *New England Journal of Medicine* in May, 2012. The first authors were Ujjal Mallick for the UK study, and Martin Schlumberger for the French study. With publication of these important papers, I served on a team at Genzyme to quickly write up a regulatory dossier to get improved Thyrogen label language in Europe and also in

USA, and we succeeded in both regions. Subsequently scores of other countries have updated their Thyrogen product labels as they followed the EMA or FDA lead after careful review of the necessary applications. This combination of ISS data published in a prestigious journal leading to regulatory action has been rare in the past, but things just worked out perfectly for us this time.

On another occasion a few years ago I had traveled to London to rendezvous with a German expert, Dr. Markus Luster, to argue before the CHMP to allow patents with higher risk thyroid cancer to receive Thyrogen. I proposed that Thyrogen use should be allowed for all patients with a history of differentiated thyroid cancer and who have been thyroidectomized, except for those who have distant metastases. This would make Thyrogen legal for greater than 90% of patients with differentiated thyroid cancer. In brief, the CHMP agreed, but required that the Thyrogen label could be changed immediately as long as at a later time Genzyme fulfilled two post-approval commitments. The first requirement was provision of data about so-called T3 patients that were a subgroup being studied in the Mallick et al. study mentioned above. That data requirement would be easy to fulfill. The second post-approval commitment was for Genzyme to provide data on patients with even more advanced thyroid cancer, so-called T4 patients. A problem, however, was that no T4 patients were being included in the Mallick *et al.* and the Schlumberger *et al.* studies that were then enrolling. In the appendix of this book I explain in a legend how we worked out a mechanism to provide the required data on T4 patients. All required data were provided to EMA successfully. We then published the data as shown in the appendix, the Bartenstein et al. study of 2014.

As you have seen in this book, since 1980 I have been closely involved in basic science studies and also clinical studies of the pituitary hormone TSH. It was wonderfully fortuitous to have during my career the ability to work on very biochemically oriented TSH work, as well as projects that directly affected patients in clinics and hospitals. When I was working in academics I saw patients personally in clinics and hospitals. I diagnosed diseases in individual patients, wrote prescriptions or organized surgery or nuclear medicine treatments for them, and often saw my individual patients regain health. It was very rewarding work, and I likely helped several thousand individual patients over a number of years. But working in the biotechnology / pharmaceutical industry in the later part of my career was actually an expansion of those efforts. Although I spent much time sitting in front of computers, my work in industry probably affected for the better not just thousands of patients, but actually more than a million patients around the world. It was a wonderful privilege to have been so engaged.

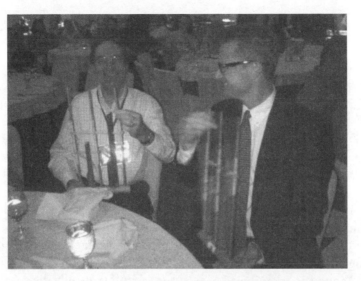

Jim Magner and Mike Schneider make some music.
At the opening banquet of an Asia and Oceania Thyroid Association meeting in Bali my colleague Mike Schneider and I learned to play a traditional Balinese musical instrument that could sound a single note. We could only make a tune when joined by many other such instruments each playing a different single note. The banqueters' group effort, when directed magnificently by our host, was actually very successful for first-timers.

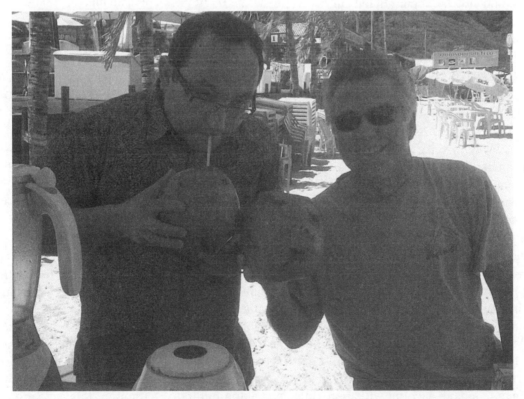

Cyril Calles and Paul Gelep
Cyril Calles and Paul Gelep relax on a beach in Brazil during a break from a meeting about Thyrogen.

Chapter 11

Plan to Play More Chess Someday by Saving for Retirement

Although we all are leading busy lives these days, it would be nice to plan to play more chess in retirement. This will only be possible, however, if we have saved properly to allow that free time. I have inserted this chapter because if any of this material helps you to become financially more secure, that may be of more benefit to your future chess activities than learning seventeen variant lines of the Queen's Gambit Declined.

Money is very important in our modern culture. But accumulating money was never the top goal in my life, and probably should not be for anyone. After all, I chose to become an endocrinologist, among the lowest paid of the medical specialties. Money is important because we must buy things from others that we do not produce ourselves – milk, bread, hamburgers, lightbulbs, gasoline, etc. The prices of these things tend naturally to rise over time, and we have to plan for that. We must provide not only for ourselves, but for our families. And we must plan to continue to pay for things when we can no longer work. Money should not be accumulated, in my view, as an end in itself. Money instead should be viewed as a valuable tool that must be used wisely to satisfy essential needs and help one to achieve important goals, and money must be saved carefully so as to be available when we might need it. Very importantly, money can be used to help others.

There is no magical way to make a lot of money, although I suppose that a small number of people win a substantial lottery every year. The painful truth, but one that must be fully recognized and internalized, is that the most important way to accumulate money is to be paid by someone (or by yourself if you own a business) for doing a useful job, and then one must spend a lot less money each month than one makes. Saving a high percentage of one's salary is key. And then that saved money must be wisely allocated among several reasonable investments so that the money can grow over time. Many of you know "The Rule of 72." One's account if untouched will double in value in the number of years equal to 72 divided by the annual rate of gain. Thus, not allowing for any taxes, one's money in a bank account will approximately double in 10 years if one is being paid an interest rate of 7.2% annually. An important detail is that as money accumulates there actually is more and more money available to double, so this compounding effect can be substantial over many years.

There is an old story about a chessplayer in the Middle East two centuries ago. He provided entertaining conversation and recreation for a powerful king, and sometimes played chess with him. One day as the two sat together in conversation, the chessplayer asked the king to be paid for his service for the coming year in grains of wheat that could be counted out on the chess board. The king called in his financial minister and a written contract was agreed and signed. The king felt a little badly because instead of paying his advisor 100 gold coins during the year, he would only be required to pay grains of wheat counted out on the 64 squares. There was to be a single grain of wheat on the first square, and that was the salary for the first day. Then there was to be double that amount of wheat on the next square as payment for the second day. On day three the payment would double again, and that would cost the king 4 grains of wheat that day. The cost would be 8 grains the next day.

Of course, readers who are mathematically inclined will recognize that by about square 40 or 45 the king will be required to pay all the wheat in storage in his entire kingdom! And after only 5 or 10 more days the king would owe all the wheat in the world. If this had been a real story, it would probably have ended with the execution of the brash chessplayer by the angry tyrant, which should serve as a lesson to any of you about to enter into salary negotiations. But the real point of the story is the immense power of compounding an amount by a constant fractional percentage.

Having made the widely known points that saving and investing sensibly are the true keys to accumulating wealth, there are many other important tidbits to mention. One must study hard, work hard, and make the proper connections so as to optimize one's earning potential. An entertaining and very readable account along those lines has been given to us by Benjamin Franklin in his autobiography. Although this selection might sound formidable since Franklin did so much during his life, his autobiography is actually a slim paperback volume that can be purchased for about $10 new. He wrote the first part and then was interrupted, so he completed the last part in old age (actually, many scholars believe that the book was not actually finished).

The somewhat old-fashioned language takes only ten pages or so to get used to, and the authenticity is well worth this minor inconvenience. Frugality is but one of many topics that are addressed. He was willing to leave home, and travel to new places. Expertise at reading and writing was vital. He was willing to serve on committees and do other unpopular jobs of that kind, since he actually then could have a direct hand in shaping outcomes of important or relevant questions. Notable was Franklin's skill at being in the right place so as to be the obvious choice when some task had to be done for a fee, such as printing up paperwork for the legislature. His personal reflections on trying to be a good person, and his record keeping regarding his ability to refrain from committing small sins are delightful accounts. Many educators would assert that this is one book that every American should read (or anyone of any nationality, really), and it can be read in just a few days, or during a couple of airplane rides. This book is listed among my key reading suggestions in an appendix given later.

Recently I received an annual summary from the Social Security Administration – nearly every American adult gets one of these summaries – and I looked a little more carefully at my record of annual earnings in the document. (Note that for some years in the past the record shows the "earnings base" on which certain taxes had been collected, rather than the true total earnings.) Yes, there on the list was $224 during 1967, the money I had earned at that fast-food summer job. A part-time job during college provided earnings of $606. Earnings in later years were listed as well.

I was fortunate to have generous and supportive parents who paid for most of my education, although I also received small scholarships and took out a few small loans. I had about $10,000 in debt when I graduated from medical school, much less than many students have today, and I was able to pay that debt back within the first ten years of my working life. During 1977, my six months of internship in San Antonio from July through December provided earnings of $5,485. Glenda, who had educational loans as well, had a part-time job at that time, and made less than $1,000, I think. The costs of rent and groceries were less then than today, of course. During 1978, when I was in internship and residency training, my annual earnings were $12,032. In spite of these small earnings, we easily aligned our spending so that we were always saving a little. When the Dodge Charger died in 1979, Glenda and I picked out a new Chevy and, with the help of a small car loan, we had no difficulty buying the car.

During my three years as a fellow at NIH (1980-1983) my salary increased to about $30,000 to $35,000 annually, and Glenda and I actually felt pretty well-off. We went out to eat more, and took a few short weekend trips. Of course, Erin was very sick then. Our apartment building management announced that they were going to sell the apartments as condos, and we either had to buy or move. So in 1981 we purchased a small house in Wheaton, Maryland. Interest rates were very high then, and our mortgage rate was about 12%. In 1983 I took the new job at Michael Reese Hospital in Chicago, and we sold the Wheaton house for a small loss, but we were happy and excited to move on to a new opportunity. We actually had saved a few thousand dollars by that time. Both Glenda and I bought additional life insurance since Erin would need substantial resources should we not be around to provide for her. We also maintained our car well so that we could keep it running as long as possible.

As a new Assistant Professor of Medicine at Michael Reese Hospital in 1983 my salary was a little more than my NIH salary. Glenda and I found a small 1600- square foot house in Glencoe, Illinois that was empty and seemed like a good opportunity for us. Glencoe is an upscale community north of Chicago that has excellent schools, and one could easily ride the Chicago & Northwestern train to Chicago each day. The house had been lived in by three elderly siblings, a brother and two sisters, who over the years did little repair or upkeep. When the last sister died, she willed the house to the Salvation Army, and that group promptly sent a truck to remove all the appliances from the kitchen to be sold at their thrift store. The Salvation Army is a superb charity, but the organization is not well suited for dealing in real estate. The house stood empty for a year or so, and high weeds grew in the yard, which irked all of the neighbors. We heard that a number of offers had been made on the house, but the Salvation Army committee had a business meeting only once per week, and the proposed deal often did not get on the agenda for several weeks, causing the interested party to withdraw the offer. I judged the house to be structurally sound, but it needed serious cosmetic attention – all the carpeting ripped out, floors refinished, lots of painting, and a major upgrade of the kitchen.

Thinking that this house was a good deal, I mentioned to our realtor that we might offer a bit more than the asking price, but she strongly suggested that we offer exactly the asking price, as opening up a negotiation-by-committee might just delay the process. Sure enough, our bid was accepted. We lived in a Holiday Inn with Erin, now a two-year-old, for several weeks while a contractor made the house livable. Before long we moved into our refurbished little house on Old Elm Lane, and the neighbors all were supremely happy to see us! Ironically, we learned several years later that a couple, with whom we became good friends, had made an offer on the same house that summer – but without the invaluable advice of our real estate agent.

By December, 1984 I looked into several Dreyfus mutual stock and bond funds to improve the investment mix for our savings. Over the next eight years, we followed our same careful spending and saving practices, while enjoying a full family life. Financially speaking, we had never been better. When it was time in 1992 to move from Glencoe, Illinois to Greenville, North Carolina, the real estate situation in the United States had improved dramatically as compared to 1981. Property prices had appreciated and interest rates were lower. We sold the Glencoe house for a nice profit, and we purchased a larger and nicer house in North Carolina for less than our Glencoe sales price, so we knew that we would have extra funds to work with. The new house was a two-storey colonial in the Brook Valley neighborhood of Greenville. It needed a new furnace, air conditioning system and a new roof, so the owner was happy to talk to us. There is quite a story to this house, and the whole situation seemed like another real estate opportunity for us.

Reverend "X" and his wife owned the Greenville house. He was a prominent televangelist in the region and collected lots of money mailed to him by earnest but misled viewers. He spent the money on a lavish lifestyle that included the large house in Greenville, along with expensive power boats and other luxuries.

He was investigated for fraud and used his TV program to attack his detractors. He was indicted and stood trial, and during that period he collected signatures and ran for mayor of the city. As part of his campaign, he put up a large billboard on which his photo was superimposed with a large figure of Jesus behind him, implying that the Lord supported his candidacy 100%! He also went on a national news magazine program to make the argument that his boats and luxuries were his reward for doing the Lord's work.

Unfortunately for the preacher, he lost the election, was convicted of a crime, and sent to jail. His wife decided to sell the house and downsize. She also wanted to sell us the huge grand piano in the living room for "only another $10,000," but we declined that generous offer. The wife was thrilled to sell the house, we were quite happy with our purchase, and we may even have helped pay a bill or two for an attorney! Yes, indeed, the Lord works in mysterious ways.

By 1992, I was an Associate Professor, and my salary was then incrementally up another notch, but was not very high. We continued to save and invest. Our two girls were doing well, so Glenda took on some part-time teaching jobs, and that helped build our savings.

In 1997, when we moved from Greenville, North Carolina to Connecticut, we sold the Greenville house for a profit with the help of Bayer Corporation of West Haven, Connecticut, which was my new employer. Relative to North Carolina, real estate prices in Connecticut were significantly higher. We found a suitable house in a suburb of New Haven with good schools and a reasonable commute by car. The house had a somewhat sad story, since the family was near bankruptcy. We worked out a fair deal that helped out that family, and it was a good opportunity for my family as well. I moved in first in February, as I had already started working for Bayer, and when the school year ended in North Carolina, Glenda and the girls joined me in June, 1997.

I worked six and a half years at Bayer, and I learned a tremendous amount about global drug development. But when that company began having a number of difficulties, most notably the voluntary withdrawal from the market of its profitable cholesterol-fighting drug, Baycol, I kept my ears open for another opportunity. In 2003 I started working at Genzyme Corp. in Cambridge, Massachusetts, where I rented a small apartment and came home on most weekends. Glenda and my girls remained in Connecticut. After all, I wanted to make sure that this job move was a good fit for me. In time, I was promoted to Vice President of Clinical Research, and my responsibilities were related mostly to projects in Endocrinology. The real excitement for me at Genzyme was that I got to apply my many years of research work on TSH to one of Genzyme's marketed products, recombinant human TSH (Thyrogen).

Soon my girls were older and away from home. But Glenda was very happy with her job in Connecticut, so we have continued what may seem to some to be an odd arrangement, with me home only on weekends. In 2003 the housing market in Boston seemed very pricey, so I decided just to wait awhile before buying. I was dumbfounded in 2004 and 2005 as house prices continued to rise in the Boston area. For several years the prices had risen much faster than wages, so I knew that this was a very peculiar and unsustainable situation. I looked at some expensive real estate in Cambridge and, just as an experiment, I spoke to my bank. To my great surprise, they offered to loan me a very large amount of money to make the purchase. I knew that this was crazy, and I deduced that many banks must be lending lots of money very loosely. I turned down the loan, continued to rent my apartment, and worried what was going to happen when this housing price "house of cards" eventually collapsed.

In mid-2007 I was so concerned about the threat to all property values, and to the U.S. financial system, that I started selling nearly all of my stocks, and I completed that task by October, 2007. I mentioned my concerns to several pretty smart business people at work, but they were sanguine. I was going to be giving up potential gains just to hold a few treasury funds and bank accounts in dollars. I knew that something bad was going to happen, but I had no idea when. In only another year, the unsustainable housing price madness started to unravel. But I had preserved my capital, and could then invest after the big downturn. This financial story holds another lesson that can be well appreciated by chessplayers. Basically, if you are having a pretty good game, the key thing is to avoid a big mistake. It might be better not to make that speculative attack, for example. Just play a steady solid game, keep an eye on the clock, and watch carefully to be sure that you don't leave a rook hanging. Avoiding a mistake can be as important as finding a creative path forward.

Chapter 12

Ancestors and Grandma Metzger

Many people are too busy today in the United States to find out much about their ancestors, or to reflect very often on the challenges they faced and overcame. Recent generations of one's ancestors can provide insight, however, into why one was born in a particular state and city, and why the family is involved in certain businesses, organizations, religious communities or activities. I suspect that none of my ancestors ever played a single game of chess. But they had busy lives trying to provide for their families, and I would love to find an old diary explaining how they balanced all of their responsibilities. Perhaps some of the sections in this book are intended for my great-grandchildren as my explanation to them about finding balance in life. We each have many problems and responsibilities, but also worthwhile interests in other activities, like chess. Readers understandably will have little interest in my ancestors, so I will keep this brief. But many readers will have ancestors with similar stories, and these may resonate. Besides, readers should be encouraged by my story to speak with their older relatives and try to find out some of the family stories before these are lost to the grave. Readers will also note that I have many gaps in what I know about ancestors, so younger readers should start soon to gather information from their older relatives.

In 1787 a man named Thomas Magner was born near Cahir, Ireland. He married Mary O'Neal, who bore him six children. Due to the terrible famine in Ireland, one son of Thomas named John, who had been born in Clare, County Tipperary in 1819, traveled to New York City in 1847, and he then encouraged his parents to move to the U.S. Thomas, Mary and their surviving children traveled to Portland, Maine, which had a large Irish community. Thomas died there in 1857, but his wife lived on into old age, and died in Portland in 1881. John apparently felt no need to hang back by the Atlantic coast, but instead was encouraged to seek new opportunities along the western frontier, which in those days was Ohio. In April, 1851, John married a young Irish woman, Bridget Begley, in Cincinnati. Their first son, Thomas, was born in January, 1852, and he was my great-grandfather. In 1857 the young family took a boat down river to the Mississippi, and then up to Keokuk, Iowa, and later traveled through Quincy, Illinois to the little town of Camp Point, where new railroads were being built. I

believe that he worked on the railroads during the Civil War. In 1864 the family moved to Clayton, Illinois, where Bridget died in 1906. Although aged 87, John moved to Jacksonville, Illinois, where some of his children lived. John died there in 1910.

Thomas married Anna Elizabeth Rossiter in 1878, and later that year they established a family home in Jacksonville, Illinois. Thomas, like his father, worked for the railroads, although after a time he was working more as a manager. He held the title of "Road Master" for the Wabash Railroad, and specified which rail cars were to make up various trains to optimize the commercial returns, and he also made some of the train schedules. Thomas apparently was well-liked and skilled, and a railroad switching area near Kinderhook, Illinois still bears a sign that reads "Magner Junction."

Thomas died in 1932, but Anna lived in the home with two adult daughters who never married. When Anna was about 85-years old, she went down the steps to check on the furnace and fell, breaking a hip. That was generally the kiss of death for an elderly person at that time, but the two daughters cared for her very well at home, getting her up and about in a wheelchair. I can remember meeting her when I was 3 or 4 years old. Anna turned 100 years old in 1955 and that was a rather unusual accomplishment in those days, so she received a nice write-up in the newspaper and President Eisenhower sent her a birthday card. Anna died a few months later.

Thomas and Anna had a son, James, born in 1882, and he was my grandfather. James married Rose Etta McHatton in 1910. James worked in a hardware store, and Rose Etta worked in a nearby general store, often selling bolts of cloth to ladies to make dresses. James eventually had a long career at the local post office near their home, and he was the supervisor of the office when he retired. My father, Louis, born in 1925, was one of their seven children. Rose Etta attended mass every day while her sons served in World War II. She died in 1955 when I was only four-years old, actually just a few months after Anna had died, so I have only a few faint memories of Rose Etta. My grandfather lived until 1967, but because Jacksonville was 70 miles east of my boyhood home, I only saw him a few times a year. He was a kind, smart

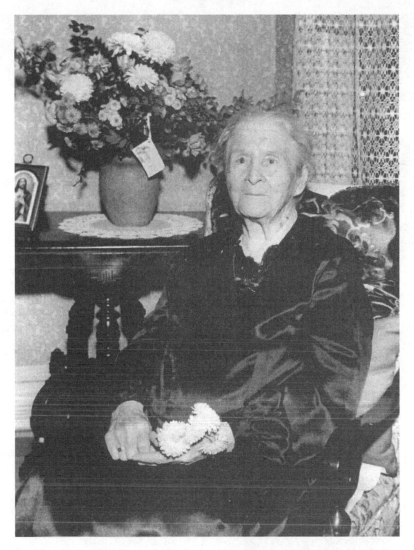

Great Grandma Anna Magner aged 100

I remember meeting Anna. She was lovingly cared for by family for more than 15 years after breaking a hip, and she enjoyed the notoriety of turning 100, which was decidedly uncommon in 1955.

man with white hair and rimless spectacles. Regarding my ancestry on my mother's side, I know that John J. Metzger, one of my great-grandfathers, was born in 1842 in Kuenzelsau, Wuerttemberg, Germany. At age 3 he was brought by his parents, Martin and Margaret, to New Orleans (1846), and the family then settled temporarily in Brownsville, Texas, but they found conditions there unsafe. Martin moved the family to Iowa, and then to Edwardsville, Illinois where he worked at farming until his death in 1853. The widow immediately brought most of her ten children to Quincy, and John, the youngest of this large brood, after a time joined the volunteer fire department. He was elected chief by a popular vote in 1872, and he was reappointed to that position over many years by several mayors of Quincy.

John attended some school, and then over six years learned the harness maker's trade with Banard & Lockwood. During this period, in November, 1865, he married Elizabeth Keuter. Having saved some money, he then opened his own small harness shop on Hampshire Street. The business grew, and he sold out his stock after two years. He then moved his family to York Street and operated several businesses there from 1869 until 1885. In that year he partnered with Christopher Ward to found a pork packing enterprise, Metzger & Ward, and later expanded these operations by partnering with Henry Behrensmeyer. In 1891 John sold his share of that business to his partner, and began his own new company, the Metzger Pork Packing Company, which was highly successful.

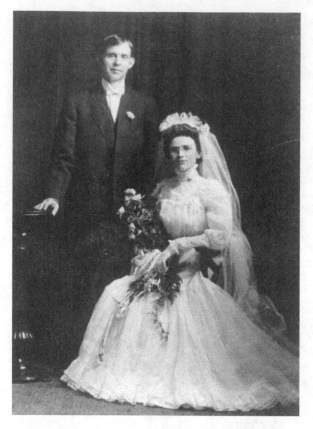

James Magner marries Rose Etta McHatton
The wedding took place in Jacksonville, Illinois, June 28, 1910.

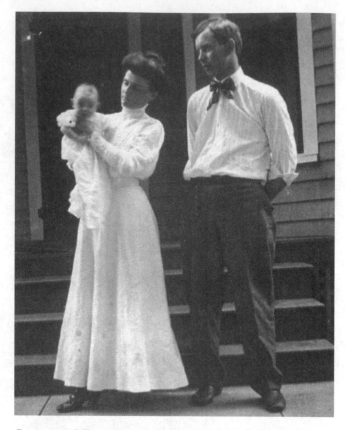

James and Rose Etta Magner with their first child, 1912
James and Rose Etta with their daughter, Frances, in front of their home in Jacksonville, Illinois.

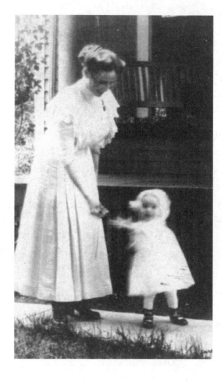

Rose Etta Magner plays with Frances in 1913
Rose Etta clearly was thrilled to be a young mother. She eventually had seven children although one died as an infant from a staph infection of the severed relic of the umbilical cord. My father was the youngest living child. All of the children were educated and became relatively successful in life. The four boys served proudly in World War II in distant posts, and all survived the war.

John and Elizabeth had nine children, although only four daughters and a son survived into adulthood. Their youngest son, born on March 11, 1889, was Arthur, who was my grandfather. Arthur attended elementary school, and then worked in a family-run grocery and confectionary shop that was adjacent to the family home on York Street. The family owned some good "black-dirt bottomland" along the Mississippi, which they farmed, and as a youngster Arthur loved to float rafts among the trees during the regular floods. He was good with tools, and learned to make wooden molds used at the local iron works as part of the process of making cast-iron kitchen stoves.

The Metzger family was a fairly prosperous one in Quincy, and they purchased one of the first automobiles in town. As the mechanically-inclined youngest boy in the family, Arthur kept the contraption running – oil can, wrenches and spare tires at the ready – and he had the job of hauling his four sisters here and there around the town, which he greatly enjoyed. In one of the early cars, the gas tank was under the dashboard. When the car was driven up the steep hill near the river the gravity-draining tank would not feed the gasoline properly, so the engine would stall. So Grandpa always just drove the car up that hill in reverse. In the early 1920s, Arthur and a friend were walking down the street and saw two attractive young ladies walking ahead of them. The boys flipped a coin to see which girl each would ask out – and a few years later each boy ended up marrying that girl. Arthur married Loretta Steinbrecher on May 17, 1922. They lived first in extra rooms at the Metzger family home, although when my mother, Elizabeth, was born on April 27, 1926, other arrangements were soon implemented. Loretta caused a bit of a scandal during the 1920s when she became one of the first women in the town to have her traditional long hair cut short in the new fashion. After a lot of tongue wagging for a time, Arthur's sisters and many of their female friends one by one had their hair cut short too!

The Wabash Railroad station in Quincy was across the street from the little grocery store (actually more of an ice cream store) that was owned by the Metzger family. During the prohibition days, the family quickly realized that there was more money to be made by selling whiskey to thirsty travelers than they could make selling ice cream. At the instigation of my grandfather's mother, rye and other necessary ingredients were grown on the family farm, and the distillation and bottling also was done there. My grandfather then sold drinks or bottles of whiskey out of the ice cream store to the train passengers, and many travelers who made that same trip regularly were repeat customers.

Things went well enough until the Great Depression hit. The Metzger family had invested years before in several acres of land along Lind Street, and a small well-built two-room shack dating back to about 1850 stood on that property. Arthur was handy with tools, and with help he built-out the shack into four rooms to create a simple house. He, Loretta and my mother moved to this refurbished house in May, 1933, thereby saving rent payments. But times were hard. Grandpa, who had worked in the grocery business in the past, had a job making wooden casting molds for a cast-iron stove company, and he also converted a station wagon into a popcorn wagon, and he cruised the parks on the nicer evenings.

He had learned well an important insight into human nature. Even during very tough times, many people feel that they still deserve to spend a small amount for a little entertainment or recreation. When many people each spent a few pennies for popcorn, it helped pay the bills. Grandpa put up for sale a beloved but ageing model-T, and was chagrinned when the man who wanted to try it out by driving it around the block never returned with the car. That was another lesson about human nature. Grandma Metzger pinched pennies and learned to make do. She grew vegetables in the yard, and one fall stewed a crop of tomatoes and preserved them in dozens of jars to use over the winter. She stored the jars in the cool cellar. A few weeks later she retrieved a jar, set it on her kitchen counter, and as she unscrewed the lid the contents suddenly exploded with great force, splattering red tomato all over the walls and ceiling of her white kitchen. Grandpa carefully examined the other jars, and noted bubbles of gas in all of them, so he gingerly carried them, as if they were nitroglycerine, one by one up the stairs and out into the furthest part of the back yard. Although she was quite young at the time, my mother still has an indelible memory of the glee she felt as her parents allowed her to throw stones at those jars, eventually exploding them all harmlessly outside.

The Depression years had a long-lasting effect on Grandma Metzger, and she always remained very frugal. Treats for my brother and me often were pie crust edgings sprinkled with cinnamon and sugar, or a little icing spread on white crackers. At Christmas our tradition was never to spend money on wrapping paper or bows, but just to put the few gifts in brown paper bags – it was still great fun to open the bags and see what was inside! One problem for us as youngsters was that some gifts were very practical, such as new socks or underwear, so we had to be patient as we worked through those sorts until we got to the toy or book or game. Also, Grandma never wanted to pay postage to send a gift to her sister, Helen, in California – nor did Helen. So each year they exchanged Christmas cards in the mail, and each enclosed a check for $20. The practice only began to strike me as odd when I was about 10 years old and I realized that it would have been simpler for each not to write a check. But by my mid-teen years I realized that the symbolic nature of having the physical check and setting it out on the dining room table was what was important to both Grandma and Aunt Helen. Many of the ladies of that era were toughened by the rough economic times in the 1930s. For the rest of their lives they would clean, sweep and work until they dropped, saving money as they applied their own sweat and effort to whatever task was at hand. Grandma used an old wringer washer in the basement and never agreed to buy a more modern washer, even though by the 1970s she easily could have afforded it. She walked up and down the steps and hung the laundry outside to dry. A sad footnote to the wash story is that when she was about 78-years old she missed a step on the stairs and fell onto the concrete basement floor, breaking her hip. She lived alone, and although she was in great pain, she crawled up the basement stairs, and then managed to stand and take steps on her broken hip as she made her way to her bathroom to wash up a bit, since she knew she would need to go to the ER. She also changed her dress, and called for a taxi to come pick her up at her front door and take her to the hospital. We learned later that at first the ER physician couldn't believe that her hip could be broken, since she had walked on it in great agony. But the x-rays confirmed the fracture, and immediate surgery was required to place a pin. Within a week or so Grandma was up and walking again in spite of pain, since she was absolutely determined to maintain her independence.

Another relative in my family, Aunt Ruth, who was Grandma's sister-in-law, was another tough German lady. When her husband, Jack, died, a small line appeared in the newspaper about the funeral arrangements, and this notice must have been seen by an unscrupulous salesman. Ruth was home one afternoon when an unexpected knock came on the front door. A salesman explained to Ruth that the gold-embossed bible that Jack had ordered last month had arrived, and he was personally delivering it for him, although $30 was due on delivery. Without missing a beat, Ruth calmly replied that this was surprising since Jack had not mentioned this purchase to her, but that Jack would be home from work by 5:30, and he was welcome to come back then and speak to him about it. The salesman made a quick retreat, and never returned.

Grandpa Metzger also was frugal and tough. My brother and I often listened as Grandpa explained about his old radio, or sat with him in the front seat of his Chevy parked in the garage, or learned to build and fly kites. Grandpa showed us how to make a perfectly satisfactory glue from flour and water for use on the kites. We first chose two lumber-yard-derived strong wooden sticks of appropriate lengths (for example, one stick about five feet long and the other about four feet long) and used a fine knife to notch the ends of the sticks in a direction parallel to the face of the kite. The shorter of the two sticks became the horizontal member, and was tied at right angles to the longer stick about three-quarters of the way toward the top of this vertical member. A string was run circumferentially tightly from end to end of the sticks through the notches, and the assembly was placed flat on the kitchen table on some colored light-weight wrapping paper with the full length of the horizontal stick touching the paper.

Glue could be used to connect overlapped pieces of paper if a single piece wasn't already large enough. Scissors were used to trim the excess paper, but we left about three-quarters-inch of paper beyond the diamond defined by the circumferential string. After snipping the paper here and there strategically to allow proper folding, the edges of the paper just beyond the string were coated with glue using a finger, and were folded over the string to attach the paper to the kite framework. A length of string was used to connect the two ends of the horizontal stick while slightly bending that stick, thereby giving a somewhat rounded shield shape to the front surface of the kite. Two holes then were punched carefully in the paper (quickly surrounded by small pieces of tape to prevent tearing) directly over the vertical stick. One hole was a few inches above the horizontal stick, and the second hole a few inches above the bottom end of the vertical stick – the exact placement of all of these elements was part of the art of the craft. A length of string about 1½ times the distance between the two holes was gently placed through the top hole in the paper and tied to the vertical stick, then the other end of this piece of string was placed through the bottom hole in the paper and tied to the vertical stick, creating the belly-band.

The kite was placed on its back, a single finger was placed under the belly-band, and the band was extended toward one end of the horizontal stick – a small loop of string was tied with a knot in the belly-band at that point, and served as the site of the attachment of the flight string. A small tail made from a strip of light cotton cloth, perhaps 12 inches long to start, was tied to the

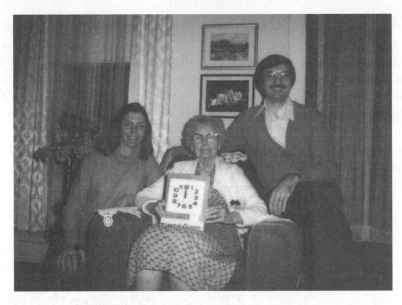

Glenda and I Visit Grandma Metzger

Glenda and I occasionally got to visit Grandma Metzger in Quincy, IL before her death in 1984. Shaped by her experience as a make-do mother during the Depression, Grandma Metzger had a practical and no frills approach to life, and successfully met many challenges during her 84 years. A gift of a new clock with large easily visible numbers satisfied her perfectly.

bottom of the vertical stick using a six-inch length of string. Depending on the wind, the tail might need to be longer to provide greater ballast. The kites always flew great!

Many other memories are tied to the old house on Lind Street. My brother and I built "tents" in the living room using blankets, and when we stayed overnight I sometimes slept on the living room couch and would listen in the dark to the old wind-up clock before I fell asleep – the tick-tock seemed so loud during the still of the night, yet one hardly noticed it during the daytime. One of my earliest memories in the house apparently stemmed from events on October 4, 1957, when I was six. Late that evening I was playfully skipping and singing as I ran from room to room. I was startled when my parents and grandparents, who were intently watching the 10 pm news in the living room, shouted at me, "Quiet! Quiet! This is important!" I was never a boisterous child, so this unexpected rebuke made a memorable impression. Although I did not understand what was happening, I could sense their fear and concern about something. That was very much out of character in our family, and this made a strange impression. Years later I recognized that they must have been watching the first news report that the Russians had launched Sputnik. The ability of the Russians to fly a satellite over our heads was dramatic proof that the Russians also had the intercontinental ballistic missiles that could deliver nuclear bombs as well. Americans today may not fully appreciate the genuine shock and fear that Sputnik aroused in the U.S. among ordinary citizens.

Grandpa had angina. Nitroglycerine pills helped, but sometimes he would need a shot of whiskey first thing in the morning to get going. When angina put him in the hospital for 3 or 4 days at a time, Grandma would smuggle in the shot of whiskey for him each day, and he recovered. One night in March, 1965, he had a very bad spell, and we all went to see him that evening at home in his bed. During the night he was taken to the emergency room, but died shortly after being admitted to the hospital. The wake and funeral were very impressionable experiences for me at age 13.

I found out years later that Grandpa had kept a loaded pistol in the house – it was a very old gun with a mother-of-pearl handle. He apparently had wanted to have it under the counter years before when he was working in the store selling whiskey to strangers who were just traveling through town, and he decided to keep it at home thereafter. After Grandpa died, Grandma took the pistol to the police station to see if they could unload it for her, since she wanted to keep the gun but not the bullet. The police found that the bullet had corroded into place, so it was a good thing that no one had ever tried to fire the gun. After some oil soaks and other tricks, the police got the bullet out, and dutifully returned the pistol to Grandma. In time, Grandma developed snow-white hair and became nearly blind, but still shuffled around in her house with a little help from "meals on wheels." She survived a breast cancer operation, and took tamoxifen orally to hold the tumor at bay. This worked for several years, but one time when I visited her in early 1984, she pointed out to me large rock-hard lymph nodes on both sides of her neck. By that time I was an experienced physician, and I knew well exactly what those lymph nodes meant.

Grandma asked me, "Is this the cancer coming back?"

"Yes, Grandma, it is the cancer. But you should still have some time left." While never wanting to rob a patient of hope, I always was very honest with all of my patients, and also with my relatives.

Grandma Metzger lived on at the Lind Street house until she died of cancer in October 1984, a couple of weeks after telling her by phone about the birth of our second daughter. We gave Carly the middle name Marie, which was Grandma Metzger's middle name, and Grandma was very pleased to hear it.

During the 1970s and 1980s Grandma was challenged by the noise and traffic in the college neighborhood, especially when a new student cafeteria was built right next door. It was the late-night loud wedding receptions held there that bothered her the most. If during the night students threw beer cans over the fence into her yard, the next morning Grandma would walk the fence-line and toss each can back onto the other side. In spite of noise and other neighborhood distractions, Grandma was committed to staying in her own little home that had so many memories. I hope that I can do the same someday.

Chapter 13

Texas Hold'em Poker

Curious About Games

Since boyhood I have enjoyed games, and I liked chess, but I did not learn to play Texas Hold'em poker until 2007 when I was 56 years old. I had seen No-limit Texas Hold'em briefly in 2006 as I flipped up or down TV channels, and I was intrigued by the graphic presented next to each hand being played showing the percent likelihood of winning. This percentage changed as a given poker hand progressed. Clearly there was a lot of luck in this game, but also there were some mathematics and strategy of some kind, since not uncommonly a player with very poor cards could win the pot by deception and bluffing. It was also clear that deception was vital to manage to win the largest amount of chips possible when a player happened to have a very good hand, since an opponent's chips could not be taken from him unless he himself voluntary put them out in the center of the table to be stolen! My initial impression in 2006 based on the TV shows was that the game was about one-half luck and one-half skill. Since I am not a gambler, I did not look further into the game until a fortuitous event occurred the next year.

A Funny Thing Happened...

Monday, July 23, 2007 was to be our 30th wedding anniversary. Glenda and I have an interesting marital arrangement that has worked fine, in part because our adult children are grown and independent. I live part-time in Cambridge, Massachusetts while Glenda lives in our home in Connecticut where she teaches English at Quinnipiac University. Glenda told me that when I drove home that weekend I should be prepared because, of course, we would be doing something a bit special in honor of our anniversary. She volunteered that she was going to be taking me on a surprise trip for two days. But the destination was a secret!

I arrived home on Friday, July 20 and was told that we were leaving by car in the morning. Off we went that Saturday with me, perplexed but amused, in the passenger seat. As we headed from New Haven toward New York City I speculated aloud that New York was the destination. Glenda just laughed, and as we crossed the George Washington Bridge into New Jersey it became clear that was not the case.

"If we're going to Florida," I quipped, "then this is going to take a while!"

It turned out that we were headed to Atlantic City because Glenda had purchased concert tickets for that evening to hear Josh Groban, one of my favorite performers. We enjoyed a lovely anniversary dinner and a great show.

The next morning after breakfast we decided to walk around in the casinos for an hour before starting our drive back to Connecticut. This was a unique experience for us since we did not frequent casinos. I was vaguely aware that the House had the odds in their favor, and in games like roulette the House consistently won about 5% of all money bet. I suspected that the unpublicized margin on slot machines likely was even a little higher than that. It was a fool's errand to gamble in casinos.

We happened to walk by a large poker room set behind some glass windows. She had sat with me a time or two as we had puzzled over the game on TV. Although I was tentative, Glenda encouraged me: "You are smart and great at chess. You could learn to play poker."

I should comment that I believe that this may have been the first time in recorded human history that a wife has steered her husband by the arm into a poker room, and insisted that he learn to play poker!

So I bought $100 in chips at the cage, and sat down somewhat tentatively at what I was told was their least expensive game, a Limit Hold'em table. My all male opponents and the dealer were quite friendly and helpful as I learned about small blinds and big blinds, and how the game worked. I now realize that the players probably were salivating as they watched a truly novice player wander in with his chips and sit down at their table! Probably because the game was Limit, I surmise now that I was somewhat protected from their predation—with reasonable, basic play I could not really lose money too quickly. In fact, I caught on in minutes, and started to win a hand now and then. Glenda watched through the glass. After about 90 minutes I still retained about half my chips, which was probably a bit of a miracle. I cashed in my remaining chips, and chalked up the $50 loss as an expense for my first and quite memorable poker lesson. It was fun! But even at this novice stage I recognized that Limit was an entirely different game than the No-limit games I had watched on cable TV. There seemed to be much more luck and less true strategic maneuvering possible in Limit, which was a natural consequence of the betting restrictions operating in the Limit game.

Learning A Little More About Poker

I certainly had no interest in gambling, but I resolved that in the coming months I would try to learn a little more about poker. I discovered that there were No-limit Hold'em games, which I speculated should contain more strategy, at casinos located nearer our home. It happens that due to my work away from Connecticut I frequently had to drive west from Boston to New Haven, and then back again. Located about mid-way, and just a little aside from the most direct route, are two major casinos in Connecticut with poker rooms: Foxwoods, and Mohegan Sun. It was not a high priority for me, but I thought it might be interesting to learn more.

I participated at first in the convenient low-stakes No-limit cash games (convenient because one can show up and depart any time one wishes). One could buy-in for only a relatively small amount of money to gain experience. Because I was making a stop for an hour while driving home or back to work, the convenience was very helpful. It seemed that some of the cash game players were highly skilled and very experienced, whereas others had intermediate skill, and some were quite inexperienced like me. This was quite a mix of diverse players. I quickly learned that some cash game players are not brainy strategists, but instead are often inveterate gamblers who play their hands in rather unorthodox and high-risk ways. They take this strategy because they have come to a casino to spend their hard-earned money, and they want to take chances, even big and somewhat illogical chances, to win money. If they lose their chips these gamblers do not view this as a major problem, apparently—they just take out their wallets and buy more chips. But if such a player gets lucky, a careful and logical player can lose money to them in the short-run. I did tend to lose small amounts during those months—more poker lessons.

I next tried inexpensive tournaments (rather than cash games) at Foxwoods and Mohegan Sun, and also at Rockingham Park in New Hampshire. This type of No-limit Hold'em structure was much more sensible for me in view of my interest in the strategic principles of the game. It was less convenient, since a tournament starts at a scheduled hour, and then continues for many hours. But the strategy of play is somewhat different than in cash games, since one's tournament chips are very precious and, in most tournament structures, cannot be replaced. One cannot take many high-risk gambles and just get more replacement chips at any time (some tournaments do have a re-buy option near the start of the tournament, but only in early levels). Thus, one needs pretty consistently to make logical and strategic moves. Ill-considered gambles will almost always result in disaster. With experience I got pretty good at tournament play, and my estimate at that

time back in about 2008 was that in tournaments with typical Saturday players, success at winning a cash prize is perhaps based 25% on luck and 75% on skill. I supposed that truly World-class players could win games using 90% skill, but I was still not really certain that the impact of chance could be made that low. There is more about the estimation of the luck factor later in this story when I talk about the reality and importance of the high variance in poker results, and how the standard deviation of earnings almost always compares to the mean of earnings.

Concerning luck in poker, a fellow player once told me that it was not so important to be lucky, but to avoid being unlucky! In other words, after careful and very skilled strategic plotting, even if one traps an unsuspecting player, the victim may win the hand in the end by an improbable chance event that can cripple you. This is called a bad beat. A typical such example is to entice a good player to make big early bets with his pocket jacks when you are holding pocket kings, which gives the opponent a pre-flop chance of eventual success during the hand of only about 20%–yet one of the two remaining jacks in the deck may subsequently show up and ruin you. And that happens one in five match ups of that type!

At this point let me interject that during the rest of this chapter an elementary understanding of the game of No-limit Hold'em is presumed, since it is not my goal in this book to teach about poker. Instead, I want to share a few thoughts about poker that may resonate with other players.

The Importance of Supplementing Subjective Assessments with Quantitation

In 2008 I also bought a couple of books about No-limit Texas Hold'em and got more indoctrinated into the mathematics and the intermediate-level strategies. Precise odds calculations were complicated and cumbersome, and clearly could not be done in detail while playing at the table. But with a little more reading I soon discovered a number of quite useful "rules of thumb" for almost instantly doing very simple approximate calculations mentally. One of these short-cuts is the "Rule of Four:" One first simply counts (based on one's two hole cards and the three cards showing in the flop on the table) the number of outs (the very good cards potentially to come that would improve one's hand significantly). Then with two cards still to come at that point in the poker hand, the probability in percent of hitting at least one of those valuable cards is approximately four times the number of outs. (With one card to come it is half that.) For example, if one holds two spades, and the flop contains two spades, then one of the two remaining cards to come will need to be a spade to create the spade flush, a powerful hand that often wins against a more average hand. As there are four spades showing, then of the 13 spades in the deck there are 9 spades unaccounted for. Now some spades could be in the hands of your opponents, which could be a very serious problem, especially if an opponent has two spades with one card of a higher rank than yours! But for this example, with two cards to come and 9 spades that are outs to importantly improve your hand, the probability is roughly 9 x 4 = 36% that one of the two remaining cards to be dealt will allow you to hit a flush. This quantitative knowledge allows you to properly think quickly about the specific confrontation you are currently in, and influences the size of your remaining bets. The calculation grounds your thinking before you consider other objective and subjective assessments of the situation.

In fact, the correct strategy in this situation actually will depend on a lot more than just the basic math and the number 36%. The current context of the hand, for instance, is of supreme importance. At one extreme is the case of all bets being small so far with the hand occurring early in a big tournament with five players still participating in the hand. One could certainly consider wagering a small fraction of one's remaining chips to bet on the 36% chance of success if other factors (several to be mentioned soon) are appropriate. At the other extreme, imagine that this hand instead is occurring very late in a tournament with only three players remaining in the entire tournament, with all three in this hand. Suppose that you and an opponent have many of the remaining chips (say 20% and 65% of the remaining chips, respectively) while the short-stack player has nearly as many chips as you do, and he is all-in for about 15% of the chips in play. Suppose also that the big-stack opponent is also all-in with his 65% of the chips in play. In this context, one needs to take a breath and consider the pay-out ladder of the prize money. Your hole cards of, say, the 9 and 10 of spades might already be beaten by either or both of your opponents, although in general it is not very likely that either of your opponents will also have two spades. The conservative play in that case near the end of the tournament would be to not risk your precious chips, but instead to fold your pretty good potential flush, and let the big-stack potentially knock the small-stack out of the tournament in third place, leaving you a guaranteed second place prize. There is usually a big step up from third place money to second place money. You would hope then to take on the victorious big-stack in subsequent hands during heads up play. The point is that the same 36% chance of improving your hand actually has vastly different implications for what might be the correct play in different contexts.

I had mentioned above that numerous other factors must also be quickly weighed while sitting at the table. Such factors include the ranges of hands you believe that each of your opponents might be betting with at that specific stage of the tournament, in view of the types of hands that they have previously played and shown publicly at the conclusion of prior hands.

Alternatively, rather than an all-in situation as described in the above example, if the betting has been smaller with potential for future bets in the hand, one must consider one's position at the table relative to the opponents. That is to say, in what order must players reveal if they are going to bet and how much? This is actually a vital consideration, since a player that acts last in the hand usually has a substantial advantage over his opponents – the player that acts last is able to process the most available information before he must act. The player that acts last is also able better to control the pot size, which helps to mitigate risk if he has only a moderately good hand. Most hands play worse out of position (when you need to bet before your opponent), although some types of hands play somewhat better out of position than do others.

Another vital skill is bet sizing. Only with proper bet sizing can one truly optimize one's earnings. A novice might reasonably ask why bet on any hand that has less than 50% chance of winning? Understanding the quantitative answer to that question is vitally important in order to make a long-term profit in poker. This has to do with something called pot odds, which is the ratio of the current pot size to the required or proposed bet. When confronted with a decision about whether to call a bet, for example, one mathematical factor to consider is the comparison of two numbers: (A) the current pot odds, compared to (B) the current odds of winning the pot by hitting one of the outs needed. The calculation of (A) is straightforward since current pot odds are simply the ratio of the current pot size to the size of the required bet. If the pot has $10 and the required bet is $1 then the pot odds are 10:1, or, in other words, if you bet you must put in 10% of the pot. Calculation of (B) is bit more complex, since you must know what outs will improve your hand sufficiently to allow you likely to win the pot, and consider how many unaccounted cards are available that might contain those outs. That "Rule of Four" is the shortcut method that helps to do an approximate calculation of (B) fairly quickly after a flop. When seeking a flush with two cards to come, for example, as explained above, one might have a chance of 36% of making the flush. To make the purely mathematically-based decision, compare (A) to (B): since 36% is larger than 10%, it makes sense based on the arithmetic to call a $1 bet (with a $10 pot) if you have a 36% chance of hitting your flush. Notice that if the bettor had bet a larger amount than $1, this would have made it more expensive for you to call, making your pot odds less favorable. So if the bettor had put in $10 instead of $1, then your required bet of $10 into a now $20 pot would give you pot odds of 50%, which is larger than your odds of winning (36%), making a call mathematically unfavorable for you. Note, however, that quickly doing the math is only part of the story in poker, since if by recent experience you think that the specific person betting likely is bluffing, you might choose to ignore the mathematical disadvantage and make the call anyway.

Thus, bet sizing is important not just when facing a decision about whether to call a bet, but also when you are the initial bettor and you wish to make a large enough bet to make the pot odds unfavorable for your opponent.

The idea of pot odds has been further enhanced to create the concept of implied pot odds. Implied pot odds allow a player to justify a bet at a current point in the hand (currently with insufficient pot odds) if the natures of the hand and of the players are such that as the hand continues to play out it is very likely that the opponent can be enticed to put quite a few more chips into the pot in a likely losing effort if certain outs actually do appear. Most dramatic is when a player can be enticed to lose all of his chips in one hand. The unfortunate player will be "felted" – after he has just lost all his chips there is nothing remaining in front of him but the table's green felt! Please consult a good poker book to get quantitative examples of calculation of implied pot odds. But in my present style of play I routinely just assess implied pot odds subjectively, and they are important.

Bet sizing also affects decisions when you have a very good hand and you want to gain some value from an opponent. With a very good hand, if you bet too large your opponent might fold and you will not win more chips from him, whereas if you make a smaller bet, the opponent might put in more chips not realizing that he is already beaten. In that case, the bettor is making a so-called value bet. The precise size of the bet to make depends on many objective and subjective factors – you must choose a bet size that the opponent will actually call. Frequently the value bet is somewhat smaller than the current pot, but in unusual cases in which the pattern of play suggests that the opponent believes that he has a winning hand, then a larger value bet could be tried.

Another situation is when you have a losing hand but you want to bluff, so a big bet could be made – but you potentially might lose a lot of chips. A related concept of a deceptive tactic is the over-bet. If you have an almost certainly winning hand, you could make a large bet just to make it appear that you are making a large bluff while holding a weak hand – but then your opponent might fold, and you will get less value than if you had made a smaller bet!

Proper bet sizing allows for ultimately losing hands to lose the minimum practical amount, and proper bet sizing also can optimize gains for winning hands.

Subjective Elements

I had mentioned that numerous other factors must also be quickly weighed while sitting at the table, such as what ranges of hands you believe that each of your opponents might be playing. You must also assess whether your individual opponents generally are tight or loose, and also whether they tend to be timid or aggressive. Have they shown any bluffs, or do you think that they are bluffing a lot? The type of player who has the combination of characteristics of being tight-aggressive can be a quite dangerous opponent. A nick-name for one type of player is a "rock." They are often older players who are betting with their retirement money, often are neatly dressed, have their hair combed, wear a retired military hat, and they keep their chips in neat stacks. If such a player rarely comes into a pot, but now is making a big bet, it is often best to fold even if you have pocket jacks. Of course, such a player might change up his style once in a while to play a hand very loosely. In contrast, a consistently loose-aggressive player makes big bets with weak hands and often wins those confrontations unopposed. This can be quite profitable for him in the short run, and the nick-name for this sort of player is a "maniac." Yet when handled intelligently, the loose-aggressive opponent over time will give away his chips to more sophisticated opponents.

A very important concept relates to how players tend to be loose or tight in different situations, and how you can take advantage of this change in the behavior of opponents. An extreme example might be a 60 year-old middle-class mathematics professor who generally plays very tightly. Early in a tournament, when he makes a significant bet, he usually has a very good hand, so you can most often fold. Vital is to recognize that if he loses many of his chips during the day, then when he is short stacked he will feel the need – probably justified – that he must begin to play more loosely. He will play with weaker hands. So early in a tournament, you should fold your pocket jacks to him, but later in a tournament, when he is short stacked, if he makes a big bet you should call or raise. A note of caution is that if you yourself choose first to go all in against an opponent, you should pause and first think about that player's recent hands won and lost, and also be certain to check the size of his chip stack. If you go all in against a player who is doing fairly well at the game in recent hours, and who now has an average-sized chip stack, then he may fold to your all in bet so as to avoid an unnecessary risk. Alternatively, if the opponent has many chips, or very few chips, your all in bet is more likely to get called, making things risky for you. In those two chip stack situations the player feels very comfortable and wants to call or, alternatively, the player feels very desperate and feels he must call. A highly confident big stack or a desperate short stack who calls can sometimes beat your A,K with 4,5, for example, so take care. That has happened to me.

Expert poker players try to find so-called "tells" in their opponents. A tell is a behavioral signal given off by a player unknowingly when he is bluffing, or, alternatively, when he has a strong hand. A player might change his breathing, put chips into the pot with a different hand motion, have a more visible pulse in his neck, nod his head, or do some other little behavior that is unique to him in that poker situation. Because players must often show what cards they actually were holding at the end of winning hands, watching a player carefully over a few hours might reveal his tell. As these sorts of signals became more widely known by players in past years, the deception in the game rose to new levels. More players began wearing sunglasses to hide their eyes. Players sometimes would act out a false tell that they knew would be picked up by an opponent and misinterpreted! I have performed false tells many times myself, even though I am only a player with an intermediate level of experience and skill.

Thus, whether it is interpreting a poker tell as true or acted, guessing whether a player is bluffing and what cards he holds, and so on, the mind game in poker is very important. One thinks about what the other player is thinking, and one also thinks about what he may be thinking that you are thinking! Among cognitive scientists this is called recursion, and this very sophisticated process likely developed in early humans over more than a million years. The evolution of recursion had much to do with social interactions within Stone Age groups of humans living in small groups. In small groups vital issues included who had what social status, who would get a good share of food, and who would get sex with whom. These sorts of social concerns and associated deceptions likely were part of what drove the amazingly rapid increase in human brain size, and later the development of more sophisticated languages and social structures. From a natural selection point of view, males had an incentive to have sex with several females, and to prevent to some extent other competing males from having sex with their female partners. (Note that among humans there is more often pair bonding than the alternative strategy of formation of groups of females guarded by a male, as is seen in lions, horses, gorillas and many other mammalian species. The human pair bonding strategy reduced violence between males, improved the survival of males, and promoted social stability. Such benefits of pair bonding improved the survival of the entire small group, as compared with that of other small groups that were competing for resources.) But a female needed to have sex with males with good traits and also insure social support for herself and her children. A clever female often had a back-up male to support her without the knowledge of her usual sexual partners. Over thousands of years human females gradually lost the public physical signals, common in some other primates, that show their maximal periods of fertility, and losing these physical signs helped obscure paternity. A strong dominant male human would believe that any child of his sexual partner was his. Note that after a strong young male lion takes over a group of females from an elderly weakening male, the young male routinely kills all the existing cubs so that all cubs raised will be his own. That gruesomely effective male strategy had a cost to the species too high for the small groups of primitive humans who in many cases were barely getting enough to eat to survive and reproduce in their environments.

When a poker player has the weak hand 2,3 but an ace appears on the flop, that player may sometimes bet to pretend that he has an ace. But his opponent (who perhaps holds pocket kings) knows that such a shifty player may bet to make this pretense to cause him to fold a very good hand. Yet, the betting player knows that his opponent will know that he will sometimes represent having an ace when he does not. Such recursion can proceed to many levels of thinking. Cognitive scientist Michael C. Corballis wrote a book in 2011, *The Recursive Mind: The Origins of Human Language, Thought, and Civilization*, in which he discussed different "orders" of thinking competence and sophistication. He noted that many mammalian species have a zero-order theory of mind. Anthropologist Russell H. Tuttle has also written on this topic in his 2014 book, *Apes and Human Evolution.* Non-human animals have varying abilities to perceive, feel, know and, in a real sense, think to some degree. But only humans have a recursive first-order theory of mind, with the ability to perceive, feel, know and think what others are perceiving, feeling, knowing and thinking. Dr. Tuttle illustrated this unique human phenomenon of recursion by quoting the character Prince Geoffrey in James Goldman's play, *The Lion In Winter*, as Geoffrey discussed with the Queen the action of King Henry toward his sons: "I know. You know I know. I know you know I know. We know Henry knows, and Henry knows we know it. We're a knowledgeable family."

The Cadillac Of Poker

There is no room in this chapter to discuss about a dozen other very important assessments often required to play one's best. And all of these assessments must be done on-the-fly while actually playing in a unique and constantly changing mix of players, hands and contexts. Most of the assessments are quite subjective. Thus, No-limit Texas

Hold'em poker is said to be not a card game played by people, but instead a people game played by persons who hold cards.

The famous poker champion Doyle Brunson calls No-limit Texas Hold'em the Cadillac of poker because in his view it is the supreme test for a poker player, as compared with other varieties of poker commonly played. It is a game that takes only an hour to learn, but a lifetime to perfect.

Beginners make lots of mistakes when they play No-limit Texas Hold'em. They play too many hands, and they bluff too much. They fail to adjust their starting range of acceptable hands as a table gets fewer players. They often can't quickly do simple calculations of probability. They do not properly consider position, and they do not properly assess opponents, in part because they may not be paying careful attention during hands in which they are not participating. They misjudge the context of actions, and context is extremely important. They cannot minimize losses or maximize gains because they fail to size bets optimally. And they have trouble reading what cards an individual opponent likely may have in view of the opponent's current and past actions. The more one practices, however, the better one can get.

Chess Or Poker?

In 2011 I published my first book, *Chess Juggler*, so many readers already know that I enjoy chess. Now that I play both chess and poker, I suspect that some readers might wonder what I think about a number of excellent chess players who in recent years have been investing more time learning about and playing poker. Ylon Schwartz, for example, is a chess master from Brooklyn, NY who is now a professional poker player. He had a peak USCF chess rating of 2408, and in poker he won a major cash prize ($3.7 million) when he took fourth place in the WSOP $10,000 NLH main event in Las Vegas in 2008. I looked him up on Wikipedia recently, and he shared there some general observations. He believes that many of the skills needed to succeed in chess are useful in poker, and that the memory skills needed in chess are also used in poker when one retains details of betting patterns of opponents in poker. He believes that analogous thinking is required when playing certain chess strategies or assessing how to bet when one has a good poker hand but does not want the opponent to fold. Schwartz also thinks that geometrical relationships between pieces on a chess board may be considered in some ways analogous to geometries simulating the cards plus chip stacks of fellow poker players. I personally find little real overlap in having skill in chess and having skill in poker other than just the basic obvious needs in both games to be smart, well-practiced, attentive, logical, calm, and determined to win. One also

needs stamina to continue to play at a high level for hours in a long chess or poker tournament with only short breaks. That stamina factor is said to give younger players an edge against older players, although the older players tend to feel that their experience actually gives them the edge!

One statement made in Schwartz's article that I clearly agree with, and which has been made elsewhere, is that chess is a game of complete information, in contrast to poker. That makes a big difference about potential exhaustive analyses, such as by computer, of chess versus poker. It is common knowledge that strong computers will be able routinely to defeat even the best human chess players. This is accomplished technically in many cases by brute force computing of millions of options. But there is so much subjectivity and nuance in poker that it will be a huge challenge ever to invent a computer that will consistently beat top human poker players. I guess time will tell.

As an aside, let me recount that years ago one of my friends asked me if I was depressed about my chess career, since good computers could consistently beat me. In other words, if technology had surpassed humans in chess, why do humans even bother with chess anymore? Of course, I enjoy chess as a game – it is fun to play! I'm not focused on the prize or trophy that I might be awarded. So I responded to my friend that it was the activity of playing chess itself that attracted me to it, the fact that I enjoyed it. I then countered his question with another question. So why do people still insist on punishing themselves with the rigor of training for a marathon run, and then making that grueling run, when technology can now transport that same person in an automobile over the same distance in a fraction of the time? The answer, of course, relates to the love of running, and the sense of accomplishment by the development of the skill and stamina required to perform well.

Alexander Grischuk, who is among the world's top 10 chess players, has begun playing poker. Other excellent chess players who now play a lot of poker include Almira Skripchenko, who is said to be among the world's top 50 chess players, and who by 2014 had poker earnings exceeding $250,000. Another is a Polish chess Grandmaster, Radoslaw Jedynak, who is sometimes known as "Radoom." He lives and plays in Warsaw, and he earns money on the computer by playing in many poker games on-line simultaneously. Simon Ansell from London is a chess International Master who has played a lot of poker in recent years. Simon attained the status of Supernova Elite in 2009 in the PokerStars rating system.

Some of these players faced off in the first major combined poker and chess tournament held on the Isle of Man in October, 2014, hosted by PokerStars. The cost for entry was 220 pounds. The approximately 73 players were first paired up in a series of chess games, and victories in those games were important to determine how many chips each would be allowed to start playing with in the subsequent poker tournament!

A chess and poker player who is a spokesperson (her title is Mind Sports Ambassador) for PokerStars and who has been closely associated with the Isle of Man tournament is FIDE Grandmaster Jennifer Shahade. She is a two-time American Women's Chess Champion, and the editor of Chess Life Online. She has written about the similarities and differences between chess and poker, and has lectured about this at Massachusetts Institute of Technology ("Poker Lessons from Chess," January 30, 2013) and at a TED talk in Baltimore in January, 2014. She has some interesting ideas, and I will paraphrase some of her opinions. One of her observations is that decision trees are longer and more complex in chess than in poker. A key skill in both games, she believes, is to know when to play quickly, and when it is time to take a lot of time to calculate and reflect very carefully. Because both games have practical time limits, one needs to use time wisely and choose correctly between limited and longer analyses. She raises the question: when should one calculate as opposed to when should one just evaluate and then act? She also points out that during a chess game, when it is your move you should largely focus on tactics (the short-term issues), whereas when it is your opponent's move you can take a broader view of the board and the game and use that time to focus on long-term strategy. Analogously, in poker, when playing a hand one must think tactically (and a bit strategically), but when not in a hand one can reflect more on long-term strategy. During that time you can consider adjusting your opening range of hands for the current table, recheck chip stack sizes of all opponents and imagine good spots that may come up, and consider which opponents you might want to isolate or avoid in marginal situations. For example, you will be prepared to act rapidly if you get a fair hand like pocket tens, since you will have watched for an opportunity to isolate and play against a small-stack while being willing to fold against a large-stack.

Shahade has pointed out another useful generalization about chess and poker: one can play well for hours, but then one mistake can ruin everything. One must avoid blunders. It takes discipline to recognize that it might be better to do very little for a period rather than make a fatal error.

Luck Versus Skill In Poker

There is no need to have a long debate about the importance of luck versus skill in chess. Winning a clear majority in a series of chess games is more than 99% based on skill.

True, a chess opponent may fortuitously make an oversight, but so may you! In a series of 100 chess games between two specific persons, the majority of the chess games will almost certainly be won by the person who has the most chess skill. This is comparable to having two basketball players take free throw shots – after each has made a hundred attempts, it is trivial and highly accurate to determine that a player who made 89% of his free throws is more skilled at shooting free throws than the other player who made only 66%. Uncertainty could arise, however, if the two success rates were 89% and 86%, of course, so the degree of variability and reproducibility of actions also is a consideration if the scores are close – statistically speaking this refers to the standard deviations of two mean values, and to the coefficients of variation.

Poker is a bit different, since luck and skill are both clearly involved, but how can one measure their relative contributions? It is necessary to talk about variance in poker, which is a superficially simple topic although the details can be complex.

Earlier I had mentioned how during a single confrontation the eventual win rate of a high pocket pair versus a lower pocket pair is about 80% after all the cards have come out in Texas Hold'em poker. That is wonderful for the player with the high pair, but there is a problem. If one plays poker for 10 hours, with about 30 hands played per hour, then over that day's course of about 300 hands a player may likely have had a high pocket pair against a lower pocket pair several times. How has he fared? Since his probability of winning one heads up encounter is 0.8, his chance of winning two encounters is 0.8 x 0.8 = 0.64, and his chance of winning four such encounters is below 50%; winning four times has a probability of only 0.8 x 0.8 x 0.8 x 0.8 = 0.41. The caveat is that four repetitions of a type of event can allow for a lot of variance to influence the overall result, very unlike the example above about two basketball players each attempting 100 free throws. Thus, a reasonably lucky player could win all four heads up confrontations with his high pair, but if he were particularly unlucky he might lose three of the four confrontations to the player with the lower pair – he could even lose all four confrontations to the lower pair! We would like to be a bit more quantitative about that risk, however.

In addition, during 10 hours of poker there are many different types of confrontations that each could happen several times, and each type has its own descriptive probabilities for outcomes. Such types include flush draws, straight draws, and several others, with a very common type being the classic poker race between two players: a pocket pair versus two higher cards, such as 9,9 versus K,Q. The pocket pair has a small advantage over the two over-cards by about 53% to 47%, but those precise probabilities depend on whether the over-cards are suited, and are close in rank so as to enhance straight possibilities. If over a 10 hour period a detailed list of poker hands played and their outcomes was kept, one could apply some algebra to determine a summation statistic for that day describing what a player's theoretical rate of winning hands should have been as well as his actual rate of achieved hand wins – one could then compare the expected versus the observed rates of winning those hands. Without getting highly mathematical, let me say at this point that for even top poker pros, their actual performance often will differ substantially from what should have theoretically happened – variance has a very big impact on poker outcomes over short periods. But how short are those periods? What length of time would make more clear the influence of skill versus variance? It turns out that even over the course of a year of poker games, variance can still be a big influence on how much a poker player is winning. We can get a bit more quantitative in this chapter, but let me say that the influence of variance in poker is subjectively many times higher than that seen for good basketball players shooting free throws. So there is real skill in poker, but natural variance plays a big role in the win record for any player over a year or so. Of course, the longer the period of observation, the lower the influence of variance is on the assessment of a player's performance. But shockingly, we are talking about assessing years rather than months of results to achieve some realistic assessment of true poker skill.

Poker players know that over a day or two they sometimes run good and sometimes run bad. But let's see if we can get a bit more quantitative (I want to credit the mathisfun.com web site for portions of the simple examples I am using here). A convenient measure of performance for cash game players is the amount of cash won or lost at the end of each day of play – that is much more practical than a detailed record of every hand. The amount of cash won or lost on five consecutive days provides a so-called distribution of winnings, although that is quite a small sample. It happens that our player of interest is either very good or very lucky, and he has won money on each of the five days. His observed winnings are $600, $470, $170, $430 and $300, and his mean amount won per day is $394. To get the variance, subtract the mean from each day's winnings, which gives positive and negative numbers. Then square each of the differences to make them all positive numbers, add them, and divide by the number of samples to determine the average. The variance is $[(206)^2 + (76)^2 + (-224)^2 + (36)^2 + (-94)^2] / 5 = \$21,704$.

It is great news that we now have the formally-defined variance, but what does it really mean? Is there a standard way to interpret the variance? Conveniently, the variance is the square of the so-called standard deviation, a widely used and well understood tool for assessing data that are in a normal distribution. So in this case, the standard deviation is the square root of $21,704, which is approximately $147. In a normal distribution of data, one can use the standard deviation to assess each of the individual data points to determine if a result is far out of what the usual pattern might dictate. In a normal distribution, 68% of the data points fall within one standard deviation from the mean, while 95% of the data points fall within two standard deviations of the mean. Use of standard deviation allows an assessment of the volatility of the results seen.

Another useful statistic is the coefficient of variation (COV), which is formally calculated for a distribution of results by dividing the standard deviation by the mean. In this case the COV is $147 / $394 = 0.373, and notice that there is no $ in front of the COV. Because dollars are being divided by dollars, the units cancel out, so the COV is a dimensionless number. That is an advantage of use of the COV, since a standard deviation must always be viewed in terms of a mean with consideration of units, whereas the COV is dimensionless and can be used more easily when comparing data from different sources or with different units.

But returning to the string of cash wins for our player, with a known mean and known standard deviation for that distribution, one can think of the mean of $394 as the current best estimate of the true win rate, whereas the standard deviation of $147 is a measure of the luck factor over time. For this player and for this small distribution of results, it seems that skill is much more important for his outcomes than luck. But in the real world of poker players, the story is actually different. Analyses of players' results not presented here show that over 300 hands in a day of poker, or even over 3,000 hands in ten days of poker, the standard deviation of the results is much larger than the mean. It is not until one surpasses more than 10,000 hands of poker, or about 33 days of poker, that the standard deviation in some cases becomes smaller than the mean. And many non-professional players do not play 33 days of poker in an entire year!

Another very useful objective statistical tool that helps to assess the patterns in such data is the confidence interval, and interested readers should look into that concept. One finds when looking at representative data that, for most players, perhaps 50,000 hands or more are really required for an accurate assessment of a player's probable skill at poker, versus the effects of luck.

A cruel mathematical truth about such gradually accumulating data that roughly fall in a normal distribution is that, as data are collected over time, variance tends to approach its true value much more quickly than does the mean, which can take a long time to converge toward truth. For poker, this means that the variability in poker results will be apparent to a specific player early on, but the true skill-based performance of a player cannot really be known until a long time has passed. I guess that if one is truly terrible at poker, and has no drive to improve by carefully studying the actual principles, one should hope to be "fortunate" and lose consistently in the first six months! One could thereby have early confirmation of one's deficits, and quit poker as soon as possible!

Perspective In Poker

The good advice many players hear is that it is all one long session. There is no point trying to play each day so as to end the day with at least a small profit. That just cannot happen in poker because the variance is too large. It is the intrinsic nature of the game to have such variability. The meaning of the statement that it is all one long session is that one cannot take too seriously one's results from a weekend of play – one needs to judge one's play over a couple of years. A vital positive result of realizing the nature of poker, with its high variance, is that if one is having a losing day, one then knows that there is no point going on tilt and making big gambles to try to catch back up to one's average play, since that very likely will just cost more money. Instead, one needs to make a good decision about each individual hand over many days, weeks and months – then let the results over a long time speak for themselves.

Poker is one of the few sports in which a very skilled player can actually go for a fairly long period with a losing streak. The variance in poker actually makes it very difficult for an individual player to judge his own skill, and it is also difficult to assess the true weaknesses in one's game. Learning from what happened a day ago commonly may be misleading. Instead, one needs to understand well the many fundamental points required to play poker with skill. These concepts include objective elements, such as the mathematics of poker probabilities, adjusting starting hands, the importance of position, proper bet sizing, etc., along with dozens of subjective elements, some mentioned in this chapter. Practice is important for improving at poker, just as if one is learning to play the piano, but poker is different than some activities since one cannot really efficiently and easily learn the vital fine points of poker merely by playing. Early in your career you must learn from books or a coach the objective and subjective elements that are vital for success in poker by understanding the nature of the game. Only then does practice play a role as you gain experience consistently applying those generally winning techniques. Even if you lose during a day or a week of play, if you have made the correct decisions but lost anyway, you need to understand that this is the variance in the game. But confirming that your decisions have been largely correct by discussing hands with a skilled colleague is important because you may not at first recognize some sub-optimal actions that you have taken.

In many ways poker is much more like real life than is chess. Although during a game of chess a player may be genuinely surprised by a turn of events, in reality chess is a much more purely analytical game than is poker. All the chess information is there fully visible to be analyzed. In poker, by contrast, one never knows what is going to come up next, and vital information during individual hands also is unavailable. In poker, like in real life, preparation and knowledge of fundamental principles are important for success, but many more subjective skills are also required. In both poker and life, one must be watchful and cautious, but one must also be flexible, inventive and prepared to take reasonable risks when an attractive opportunity seems to be at hand. And then one must be courageous, make a decision and take action, but then live with equanimity with the consequences. One needs to avoid big mistakes, but numerous small mistakes are normal. In both poker and life, one must be determined to win, and continue fairly consistently to make good decisions every day.

Chapter 14

Religion: Free Will, God and the Meaning of Life

Although professional scientists generally avoid writing anything about religion or God, I think I should. Writing about this topic has many traps, of course, and can cause many misunderstandings. But most people feel a strong urge to better understand their place in the world, they wonder about how the universe came to be, and whether there is really any ultimate purpose. One thing is very certain: the universe is very complicated and actually is a very strange place. I write this chapter to explain my thinking about the ultimate meaning of human life and my religious views, and to show how my thinking evolved over time. Many readers with strong scientific backgrounds may have struggled with such questions, and I am happy to share briefly my religious journey (which is still a work in progress) to see if any of it might be of benefit to others.

I want to give a brief outline of my progress, and then share some additional thoughts.

- My childhood was spent with family within a religious tradition in small-town America (in my case Roman Catholicism, with regular church attendance).

- Excellent elementary and high school education (Catholic schools) provided a solid foundation in Old Testament and New Testament content, Catholic doctrine, and some discussion of the world's many religions. High school religion classes included broad reading (such as the Jewish philosopher Martin Buber's influential book, *I and Thou*). I was introduced to and very impressed by Søren Kierkegaard's concept of the necessity of a "leap of faith." I was exposed to the works of Thomas Aquinas and his "proofs of God." I never at any time in my life had a literal interpretation of biblical or religious writings.

- I had solid biology and chemistry education from the age of 14 on, and I had a detailed understanding as a teenager of natural selection and Darwinian evolution. I had first-hand knowledge of geology and fossil collecting as a teenager. Starting at age 12, I pursued extensive reading in astronomy, biology, biochemistry, cosmology, physics, math, special and general relativity, and quantum mechanics.

- At ages 18 to 22 I was very concerned that humans probably did lack free will. It seemed that human action was totally shaped by "nature and nurture" (genetics and environment), but I hoped that a good argument for the existence of free will would emerge. I had a strong belief in the "unity of truth": that scientific truth and religious truth must in the end be fully compatible, even though there appeared to be many contradictions.

- During the college years (ages 18 to 22) I pursued an aggressive formal program of broad education in science and mathematics, with an emphasis on biology, biochemistry and chemistry. I also attended university classes in biblical redaction criticism (Old Testament and New Testament) at the University of Illinois. The science and biblical classes were supplemented with extensive independent reading.

- At age 22 I read Arthur Stanley Eddington's book chapter "The Decline of Determinism," and I have been thereafter fully convinced that quantum mechanics allows "plenty of room" for the existence of free will. In this period I also read about Kurt Gödel, but I did not then fully grasp the significance of his work.

- During the medical school years (ages 22-26) I attended a class on New Testament issues at the divinity school at the University of Chicago. I studied medical ethics in some depth during medical school with Dr. Mark Siegler, an expert in the field. A key ethical concept learned during that period that I made extensive use of during the rest of my medical career was the consideration of what might be "ordinary" versus "extraordinary" medical management in different patients in different clinical settings and situations. I remained active in Catholicism throughout my years in college and medical school, and throughout the rest of my life.

- In 1977, at age 26, I married a Protestant who is very engaged in her religious community. We have had a happy marriage, and we have raised two daughters through countless small and large crises in a happy, Christian home. Both daughters are practicing Christians.

- By about age 35 I was very impressed with many books by the philosopher Mortimer Adler, and especially by his book, *How To Think About God*. (Adler was not a religious person at the time he wrote that book, and he noted in the subtitle that it actually is a book for pagans! Adler later converted to Roman Catholicism, a process that he describes in his second autobiography.)

- By 1988 (age 37) I was convinced intuitively that science did not have all the answers, but I was very cautious about reasoning based on religion or "revelation." One potentially can go far astray into confusion and superstition if one takes small steps away from science. As reflected in the essay that I published in *The Scientist* in 1988 (see appendix) I felt that one should not be intellectually lazy and just take a leap of faith without first struggling with rational and scientific approaches to the problem of humankind's ultimate meaning. It is true, I thought, that one needs as a final step to make a leap of faith, but one should be determined to make full use of reason to make the leap as small as possible!

- By 2000 (age 49) I had learned more about the attempts in the early 20th century of Bertrand Russell and colleagues to formalize rigorously complex systems of thought. I also had learned more about Kurt Gödel's proof that no complex rigorous system of thought could be made entirely self-consistent – there always would be a very large (probably infinite) number of genuinely true statements that could not be proven to be true within even highly complex formalized systems of reasoning, including mathematics. Sophisticated science is a formal rigorous system of thought, but there necessarily are an infinite number of truths that science can never prove. Science is vitally important, but science cannot have all the answers! This collapse of Russell-like programs to pursue all truth by pure rational means opens a small crack to allow one to make legitimately a first assumption of a "greater truth" to contribute to, provide vital context, and substantially influence the use of rational arguments. I expressed this concept in the book review placed on-line in 2013 (see appendix) as I commented on the philosophical shortcomings of Krauss in his book, *A Universe From Nothing*.

- In 2014 I first read Martin Gardner's book (the 1999 updated edition), *The Whys Of A Philosophical Scrivener*. This is a remarkable book written by a towering scientific intellect who also has a strong background in philosophy. The book has critics, of course. But Gardner explains why he believes in free will, and why he is not an atheist. I should mention that Gardner comments on Aquinas and also on Mortimer Adler, but Gardner finds that pure rationality has many shortcomings when it comes to thinking about the big questions in life. In the end, Gardner uses rational means, of course, but he also condones a substantial leap of faith as being both necessary and legitimate as one assesses whether human life has any ultimate meaning. He is genuinely hopeful about the human condition, although with some humor he admits that the atheists have all the best arguments!

Einstein: It Is A Very Mysterious World

Having presented an outline above of my intellectual journey (still in progress, please recall) regarding the ultimate meaning of life and the significance of religion, I next wanted to present a variety of related anecdotes and ideas that I have found interesting through the years.

As a teenager I was impressed by an anecdote about the young Albert Einstein. It was said that when he was 4 or 5 years old he was given a compass to play with. The movement of the needle was astonishing to him – something strong and invisible was moving the needle so that it always pointed north no matter how he walked about the house. Einstein recalled that this was his first realization that there had to be "something behind things, something deeply hidden." He had already grasped that the world was large and complex, but after playing with the compass he realized that the world was actually profoundly more complex and more mysterious than it appeared.

With the rise of quantum mechanics in the early 20th century, the world became not only more mysterious, but seemingly extremely strange. Einstein was uncomfortable with the bizarre world of quantum mechanics, in which chance seemed to rule supreme, and he complained that, "You believe in God playing dice." The biologist J. B. S. Haldane once remarked, "The world is not only stranger than we imagine, it is stranger than we CAN imagine." Now in the 21st century, after the discovery of the substantial gravitational influence of apparent "Dark Matter," and the confirmation of the existence of an abundant amount of "Dark Energy" that is causing the entire universe to accelerate its expansion, it remains clear that our universe is very, very strange, indeed.

Einstein was not a proponent of organized religion, but he had an elegant mystical sense. Max Jammer published this quotation from him: "I'm not an atheist, and I don't think I can call myself a pantheist. We are in the position of a little child entering a huge library filled with books in many languages. The child knows someone must have written those books. It does not know how. It does not understand the languages in which they are written. The child dimly suspects a mysterious order in the arrangement of the books but doesn't know what it is. That, it seems to me, is the attitude of even the most intelligent human being toward God. We see the universe marvelously arranged and obeying certain laws but only dimly understand these laws…."

The Quotable Einstein, Princeton University Press, presents additional passages of interest:

"My religion consists of a humble admiration of the illimitable superior spirit who reveals himself in the slight details we are able to perceive with our frail and feeble minds. That deeply emotional conviction of the presence of a superior reasoning power, which is revealed in the incomprehensible universe, forms my idea of God."

"Thus I came…to a deep religiosity which, however, reached an abrupt end at the age of 12. Through the reading of popular scientific books I soon reached a conviction that much in the stories of the Bible could not be true…Suspicion against every kind of authority grew out of this experience…an attitude which has never left me."

"Science without religion is lame, religion without science is blind."

And the following is my favorite:

"There are two ways to live: you can live as if nothing is a miracle, or you can live as if everything is a miracle."

Deism in Colonial America

Some would categorize Einstein's comments above as expressing a type of Deism. Many of America's founding fathers were very interested in science, participated in some form of organized religion as a perceived and expected cultural commitment, but also often tended toward a type of Deism. The argument in support of a Divine Creator / Designer based on the elegance of the design of living things was popular at that time, as espoused by Reverend Paley and his story about finding a watch and knowing that there existed a designer. We

have known since Darwin, however, that natural selection itself operates to produce the appearance of careful design as selection gradually aligns a species to its environmental niche. So biological design by the Almighty no longer holds much weight in the 21st century, but one wonders still about the apparent design within physics and the inanimate world. The following quote by Thomas Jefferson captures his thinking about design in both the living and the non-living:

"I hold (without appeal to revelation) that when we take a view of the universe, in its parts, general or particular, it is impossible for the human mind not to perceive and feel a conviction of design, consummate skill, and indefinite power in every atom of its composition. The movements of the heavenly bodies, so exactly held in their course by the balance of centrifugal and centripetal forces; the structure of the Earth itself, with its distribution of lands, waters and atmosphere; animal and vegetable bodies, examined in all their minutest particles; insects, mere atoms of life, yet as perfectly organized as man or mammoth; the mineral substances, their generation and uses, it is impossible, I say, for the human mind not to believe, that there is in all this, design, cause and effect, up to an ultimate cause, a Fabricator of all things from matter and motion, their Preserver and Regulator, while permitted to exist in their present forms, and their regeneration into new and other forms. We see, too, evident proofs of the necessity of a superintending power, to maintain the universe in its course and order."

All forms of Deism may not encompass the notion of a God who can be prayed to for assistance, or who will preserve life beyond the grave. George Washington, Ethan Allen, and Benjamin Franklin were hopeful about the goodness of Providence and the existence of an afterlife. Thomas Paine in *The Age of Reason* and other writings expressed many thoughts consistent with a sort of Deism. And Paine also seemed hopeful about an afterlife:

"I consider myself in the hands of my Creator, and that he will dispose of me after this life consistently with His justice and goodness. I leave all these matters to Him, as my Creator and friend, and I hold it to be presumption in man to make an article of faith as to what the Creator will do with us hereafter."

As a bit of an aside, I want to raise another point about colonial America and whether prayer has efficacy, or whether God performs "miracles." Washington believed in the efficacy of prayer. I really do not know what to believe about such questions, but let me share three bizarre occurrences during the Revolutionary War that seem so outlandish to me that I just do not know what to make of them.

The first strange series of events occurred when Washington had taken up position with a large part of his army on Brooklyn Heights during the defense of New York City in late-August, 1776. Numerous British warships with large numbers of troops were present in the harbor, and 20,000 British troops were landed on Long Island under General Howe to make their way toward Washington's position. Washington in effect had his back against the East River. As the situation progressed during daytime, Washington called for more and more colonial troops to be brought from Manhattan Island across the river in small boats to reinforce his defenses on Brooklyn Heights. If the British could send ships up the East River, however, Washington's army would be surrounded there with no hope of victory or retreat— the American Revolution might have ended that week. Fortuitously, a strong north wind prevented any infiltration of British ships into the East River behind Washington's position. Not the world's most experienced general, Washington began to realize during the late afternoon that his position was hopeless, and that he must retreat to save his army. The small boats then were used all night to move many of the men, cannon and arms from Brooklyn Heights back to Manhattan. Astonishingly, this was done in silence and in such order that the experienced British force did not realize that this was happening over many hours. But as the sun was about to rise many colonial troops still needed evacuation, and they were by then a much smaller and helpless group than hours before. Amazingly for August, just before sunrise an intensely thick fog hugged the ground and persisted well into the morning. According to historian David McCullough in his essay, "What the Fog Wrought," a man standing only a few yards away could not be seen. During the persistent fog the remainder of Washington's troops and their arms were silently rowed back to Manhattan (except for several very large cannon). When the fog rose later that morning, Howe was astonished to see that the entire colonial army and all of their arms had completely vanished! Military historians today marvel at this improbable series of events.

A second fortuitous episode occurred when Washington's cold and starving troops, up to 12,000 men, were encamped for the winter at Valley Forge. There was no prospect of resupply and desperation forced Washington to order nets to be deployed into the river to see if any fish might be obtained. A huge haul of fish was caught, so large that locals reported that nothing like it had ever been seen in the area. The army ate well and gradually recovered. Sounding almost biblical, I again do not know what to make of this event except that it is intriguing, and it must have had a remarkable impact on the minds of Washington and his men. Pulitzer Prize-winning author John McPhee has researched this and related stories, and he found a variety of conflicting accounts. The fish were apparently shad (*Alosa sapidissima*), which were known to be commercially important in the area and which sometimes ran in large schools when spawning in the early spring. Sources suggested that possibly multiple large catches occurred in 1778 to save the army. McPhee has humorously referred to shad as America's "founding fish."

Throughout the war Washington had fought and retreated, then fought again and retreated again. He knew that he must at all costs preserve the army even if he could win very few battles. Finally, Washington moved decisively in September, 1781 with the hope that the French fleet would appear at the correct time and place to allow a battle to be won. A long-term plan of this sort had been discussed previously with French commanders, but there was no certainty if or exactly when Admiral de Grasse might sail his fleet north from the Caribbean. Washington fully committed himself. He marched his Continental Army of more than 8,000 troops and French forces of more than 7,000 troops toward Yorktown, where the southern British army under General Lord Cornwallis, with about 6,000 troops, had camped intentionally along the coast in view of the overwhelming command of the sea by the British for resupply of food and arms. In spite of poor means of communication between American land forces and the French fleet, the French fleet appeared off the coast at just the right time and Washington then continued his march toward Yorktown. Cornwallis had been expecting relief by sea by General Clinton headquartered in New York City. The next inexplicable error by Cornwallis was his decision to concentrate his troops more closely, sensible in a way but at the cost of abandoning vital forward positions that were immediately taken by the Americans without opposition, allowing the Americans to dominate the battlefield. The French and Americans then inched forward, making use of a highly effective night attack to seize by force additional forward positions. As the siege continued into mid-October, the noose tightened and Cornwallis was forced to surrender his entire army. This stunning development essentially ended the war with victory improbably going to the Americans. Again I know not what to make of this remarkable ending that would have strained the credulity of any modern movie audience had it been fiction. But I have no doubt that these events profoundly affected the minds of the founding fathers as they proceeded in the next years to establish the new nation.

I should say that as my many European colleagues finish reading the above paragraphs they may now be wondering if I have been smoking something. But I felt that these stories were just too good to be left out of this chapter.

Gödel and an Infinite Number of Unprovable but Genuine Truths

Turning back now to more rational topics, I want to briefly discuss the work of the Austrian logician, Kurt Gödel. For this discussion I rely heavily on a version of the book *Gödel's Proof* by Ernest Nagel and James Newman that was edited and republished in 2001 by Pulitzer Prize-winning author, Douglas Hofstadter. Hofstadter is a professor of Computer Science and Cognitive Science at Indiana University.

This story begins in the early 20th century when prominent mathematicians such as David Hilbert sought to develop complex formal systems in which rock-solid empirical proofs could be demonstrated for mathematical topics. Key among such logicians were Bertrand Russell and Alfred North Whitehead, who wrote a sophisticated massive three-volume work, *Principia Mathematica*, which appeared in 1910 to 1913. Russell and Whitehead believed that they had developed a system based on pure logic that would ground mathematics on a firm foundation for all time. In the late 20th and early 21st centuries, such a manner of purely rational thinking is admired by those who feel that science and rationality have all the answers, and anything that is not purely scientific and purely rational is bunk.

Some years after the appearance of *Principia Mathematica*, Kurt Gödel began to have some doubts about this approach. He found a way to turn the logic symbols used in the long proofs within the book into numbers, and he found ways to use the numbers to rigorously calculate the equivalent of the proofs. But a problem appeared. *Principia Mathematica* was about numbers, and Gödel had accurately turned the content of the book into informative numbers that could be intelligently manipulated. Thus, the formulas in *Principia Mathematica* were actually just saying things about each other, and in some cases they apparently were just saying things about themselves. This raised in Gödel's mind the potential existence within *Principia Mathematica* of the sorts of classic self-referential paradoxes known for many years, such as "This statement is false." Russell and Whitehead had intended for all time to set aside circular reasoning by using a rigorous logical system, yet Gödel could show that there were many strange consequences within a closed logical system. Gödel in effect could rigorously derive formulas that said, "This formula is unprovable by the rules of *Principia Mathematica*." Next, Gödel demonstrated that there were true formulas that could not be proven using the rules of the closed logical system. Finally, he then showed that his method applied to any system that tried to accomplish the exalted goals of *Principia Mathematica*. Gödel forever destroyed the ambitions of those who believed that mathematical reasoning can be captured in the rigidity of axiomatic systems. Gödel's publication in 1931 negated *Principia Mathematica* and raised serious questions about the meaning of mathematical truth – and more generally, what is the meaning of truth at all?

In sum, there does not exist any purely rational system of thought in which every postulate can be straightforwardly proved as true or false. Every system of reasoning must have at its base one or more unprovable assumptions. And within any purely rational system of reasoning, there are many genuinely true statements that cannot be proven to be true. If a statement properly formulated within a rational system is both genuinely true, but undecidable within that system, then necessarily the system is incomplete. Within the book by Nagel and Newman as edited by Hofstadter, a key section is entitled "The Heart of Gödel's Argument," which takes the reader through the logic in a step-by-step manner.

The implications of Gödel's incompleteness theorem are far-reaching. First, there are many genuine truths that are unprovable. Another implication relates to the prospect of artificial intelligence. Sophisticated computers currently operate by fixed rules of inference of formalized axiomatic procedure. Even though procedures may be improved for future machines, still no future operating system will be complete and able to handle all problems. The formal operating procedures will always be, necessarily, incomplete. Although some scientists may currently think in the 21ˢᵗ century that sophisticated artificial intelligence is only a few years away, it seems now more likely, in view of Gödel, that the human brain makes use of rules of operation that are hugely more sophisticated than any current computer. Hofstadter warns against mysticism, but writes, "The theorem does indicate that the structure and the power of the human mind are far more complex and subtle than any non-living machine yet envisaged."

In view of Gödel, rational science cannot have all the answers. As a professional scientist I still believe that it is entirely proper and highly desirable to stick as closely as possible to rational science. But rational science, even in the realm of mathematics, is necessarily incomplete and cannot properly describe many genuine truths.

By 2013 I had reached this stage in my intellectual journey, and that is why I composed in 2013 the review of Krauss' book (see appendix) in the manner chosen. But in January, 2014 I stumbled upon Martin Gardner's engaging but controversial book, which I will briefly discuss.

The Ghost in the Machine

The universe turns out to be highly mathematical. It is as if a sophisticated mathematician had written out thousands of equations on a long scroll and then stepped back and clapped his hands. By some magic the particles and energies described in the equations instantly "came to life." As one author has described it, the universe "began to fly." An electron having a specific location and properties is simply the collapse of a wave function -- a product of pure mathematics. How is this possible? It is an analogous situation to the production of qualia -- mental experiences – by the chemicals and electrical events in our brains.

The closing paragraph of *The Matter Myth* by Davies and Gribben reflects on this mystery, and I paraphrase it here:

"Descartes founded the image of the human mind as a sort of nebulous substance that exists independently of the body. Much later, in the 1930s, Gilbert Ryle derided this dualism in a pithy reference to the mind part as 'the ghost in the machine.' Ryle articulated his criticism during the triumphal phase of materialism and mechanism. The 'machine' he referred to was the human body and the human brain, themselves just parts of the larger cosmic machine. But already, when he coined that pithy expression, the new physics was at work, undermining the world view on which Ryle's philosophy was based…. We can see that Ryle was right to dismiss the notion of the ghost in the machine --- not because there is no ghost, but because there is no machine."

Martin Gardner's Book

I will refrain from saying too much here about Martin Gardner's book, *The Whys Of A Philosophical Scrivener*. Of note, the book was first published in 1983, but then Gardner revised and updated the book in a 1999 edition, so be sure to read the latest. The book is amusing and profound, and thoroughly entertaining. The reviews show that scientific readers both love and hate it. If I understand Gardner's work history correctly, he wrote a Mathematical Games column for *Scientific American* for many years, but then to the great disappointment of thousands he asked to stop writing this column in 1981 so that he could fully apply himself in his old age to a special project. It seems clear to me, based on the obvious care and love with which he crafted *The Whys Of A Philosophical Scrivener*, that the special project was the production of that book. His extensive updating of the 1999 edition with many humorous notes demonstrate that this project was very important to him personally.

Some of the chapters of Gardner's book include the following:

"Goodness: Why I Am Not an Ethical Relativist"

"Free Will: Why I Am Not a Determinist or Haphazardist"

"The Proofs: Why I Do Not Believe God's Existence Can Be Demonstrated"

"Faith: Why I Am Not an Atheist"

"Prayer: Why I Do Not Think It Foolish"

"Immortality: Why I Do Not Think It Impossible"

"Surprise: Why I Cannot Take the World for Granted"

In view of the above selection of chapter titles, readers who know me can understand why I was enchanted. I recommend that you take a look at it.

Chapter 15

Closing Thoughts

Anecdotes can be entertaining, but also instructive and helpful. My hope is that a thoughtful reader might glean practical advice from my ramblings that will prove useful in many areas of life. A more detailed listing of specific points of advice, which I have updated from time to time and shared with students over the years, is attached as an Appendix. I also hope that this book might support and reassure readers who face difficult problems – readers who possibly are having very basic philosophical/existential questions because of disappointments, job changes, illness, suffering and setbacks of many kinds. Sometimes these challenges can be overcome. Be tenacious! Learn, plan, prepare and execute! Work hard! Do your best to prevail!

But sometimes the challenges cannot be overcome. Keep in mind that failure can be instructive and, dare I say, fulfilling in the sense that a bold and sensible solution may have been implemented, seemed at first to be working, then appeared to provide additional promise after further tweaks, but fell short, unfortunately, in the end. Such battles command our attention and test our imagination and stamina. We had better believe that the effort is valuable even if failure is the result because, in the end, all of us and our families will "fail" in a very fundamental existential sense. What is the proper mental frame with which to approach this sobering prospect?

It is very important for the modern thinking person to fully internalize that the universe is vast and complex, and the Earth is very old (4.5 billion years). As individuals, our time on this planet is extremely brief. The books I cite in my reading list in Appendix B are very highly recommended, and several of them will help readers fully grasp these ideas. It is one thing to know these facts, but it is another to completely internalize them. Scientists through the centuries have held a range of religious views, often shaped by their times and cultures. Isaac Newton (1642-1727), regarded by many as a true genius and one of the greatest scientists of all time, lived during an era when organized religion was of high importance. He struggled with formal Christian dogmas, such as the truth of the Trinity, but kept his doubts private because a public disagreement could have threatened his academic appointment at Cambridge University, an institution of the Anglican Church. Most professors there were expected in time to become ordained ministers, but Newton carefully avoided this step. In spite of Newton's misgivings about particular religious elements of belief, his writings show that he was a profoundly religious man, and late in life he devoted years to historical analyses and calculations based on the Bible. Newton was brilliant, creative, a loner, and a supremely hard worker who was willing to pursue scientific investigations and calculations day and night without food or sleep. He was a fast learner who could adapt and perform well when faced with many varied problems or scientific questions. He was also temperamental and prone to argument. He recognized how complex the universe is, and how little we know of it. Of his own numerous magnificent scientific accomplishments, he once wrote late in life, "I know not what I may appear to the world, but to myself I appear to have been only like a boy playing on the seashore, and diverting myself in now and then finding a smoother pebble or a prettier shell than the ordinary, whilst the great ocean of truth lay all undiscovered before me."

In his *Opticks*, published in 1704, he criticized other contemporary scientists who were trying to banish God, the First Cause, from the proper understanding of the world. "Latter Philosophers banish the Consideration of such a Cause out of natural Philosophy," he wrote, "feigning Hypotheses for explaining all things mechanically and referring other Causes to Metaphysics." But Newton viewed this purely mechanical approach as flawed. Newton instead wanted to deduce "Causes from Effects till we come to the very first Cause." He was comfortable with gravity's mysterious action at a distance, for example, and was content to describe how gravity acted in mathematical detail while admitting that the precise mechanisms whereby gravity exerts its effects remained unexplained. Newton wanted not merely to "Unfold the Mechanism of the World," but he also wanted to learn "Whence is it that Nature doth nothing in vain; and whence arises all that Order and Beauty which we see in the World."

One of my favorite collections of essays, *The Immense Journey*, by naturalist and anthropologist Loren Eiseley, makes scientific points elegantly with marvelous prose while encouraging in the reader a sense of awe and appreciation of the mystery of our existence. Thought of by some as a modern Thoreau, all of Eiseley's books are superb. Eiseley echoes some of Newton's longings for ultimate understanding. "There is no logical reason for the existence of a snowflake any more than there is for evolution," he wrote, "It is an apparition from that mysterious shadow world beyond nature, that final world which contains – if anything contains – the explanation of men and catfish and green leaves." Eiseley was not enamored of organized religion, but his keen scientific mind also encompassed a profound mystical sense. "Man is not as other creatures..." he observed, "Without the sense of the holy, without compassion, his brain can become a gray stalking horror – the deviser of Belsen."

Appendix A

General and Career Advice

I have worked with medical students, interns, residents and endocrine fellows over many years, and I enjoyed brainstorming with them and advising them as they considered what to do with their lives and careers. So I thought I would add a section to this book that summarizes some of my advice. My observations served in many cases as a starting point for a thoughtful discussion with these young people. I also constantly updated my recommended reading list, and would ask you to consider reading some of my favorites.

General Advice About Choosing a Career

Know yourself (This takes time and effort.)
Give yourself time to wander in libraries – pick up and read whatever interests you.
Wander in museums (this takes time and planning).
Buy books that interest you and take them home.
Make an effort to read broadly.
Leave the TV and computer off for a while each day.
Read biographies of people you admire.
Write a short biography of someone you admire.
Seek out conversations with interesting people.
Travel when you can and keep expenses low.
Keep in close contact with your parents and siblings.
Call your parents on holidays and birthdays.
Get details of your family history from older relatives.
Participate in a religious community, even if you are an "atheist."
Retain a capacity for awe and admit the great mystery of existence.
Genuinely try to be a good person.
Recognize that you are a "scientific" person – this should shape your entire view of life.
Pay attention to how your mind and memory work – what quirks do you have?
Have a hobby (Learn to play chess well and join a club, but don't spend excessive time on this game).
Pay attention to and learn to optimize the rhythms of your body.

Have goals for your life, even if general, and think about them every day.
"I will have an interesting life, I will love and be loved, and I will do something of value for the world."

Seek a life-partner who shares many of your core values.

Guard your health – you are in this for the long-term.
Get adequate sleep.
Watch your diet.
Floss your teeth.
No smoking or illicit drugs.
Use alcohol sparingly.
Get adequate exercise, especially walking.
Avoid unnecessary risks (e.g., motorcycles).
Avoid excess sun exposure – wear a hat.
Take a daily calcium and vit D supplement.
Drink plenty of water.

Be open to chance events.

Work hard, and do the best you can at whatever you are doing at the moment.
Believe sincerely in the pursuit of excellence.
Be honest.
Be friendly.
Be a team player.
Be genuine.
Be willing to sacrifice.
Be courageous but sensible.
Lead by example.
Care about other people.
Don't preach, but communicate what you believe.

Money is VERY important, not as an END, but as a TOOL.
Forgo consumerism in order to save and invest every dollar you can – you will need those funds to achieve your goals.
Be frugal.
Avoid debt except for education and a sensible mortgage.
Donate small amounts regularly to good charities.
Be a regular blood donor.
When the right time comes, be prepared to use your savings as a powerful tool.

Avoid rash career changes, but after a time, be ready to make a change to better align your work with your goals. Be courageous, and use your resources to make a change that appears to be right.

For medical students or trainees who may be reading this book, I next offer a little personal advice about the pros and cons of taking a job in the biotech or pharmaceutical industry:

Advantages of a Career in the Pharmaceutical Industry

* Work on the cutting edge of science and clinical medicine with the newest potential medications.
* Plenty of resources to support the projects with no need to write grants.
* Able to attend any scientific or medical meeting worldwide if it is useful for the project.
* Make personal contacts with key academic researchers and top doctors and scientists globally.
* Exercise creativity in strategic planning, study design, data analysis, report writing, oral and written presentations.
* Can still interact with basic science colleagues as well as clinical colleagues.
* Work with high quality colleagues: smart, verbal and interesting people with a wide range of backgrounds.
* Good salary and benefits without wrangling with insurance companies or billing systems.
* Although there are important project deadlines and busy periods, there is usually no difficulty taking time off for holidays and vacations.
* Time available to read journals and texts, and stay up on the latest in science and medicine.
* Can still engage in teaching activities within one's project teams or in the company.
* Easy to move from one company to another – ample opportunity for a change of scene if desired.

Disadvantages of a Career in the Pharmaceutical Industry

* Little or no direct patient contact (unless one sets up a local clinical activity).
* Usually one no longer publishes as a first author or a key author, or gives major presentations at scientific meetings – the goal is not to enhance one's own prestige as a leader in medicine, but instead is the success of the project.
* Not directly part of a university – usually no academic appointment, with little opportunity for teaching medical students, residents or fellows.
* Must take care about confidential and proprietary information.
* Some people harbor negative views of the pharma industry, and may change the way they think about you.

Aczel, Amir, *Descartes' Secret Notebook: A True Tale of Mathematics, Mysticism, and the Quest to Understand the Universe*, Broadway books, New York 2005

—, *Entanglement: The Unlikely Story of How Scientists, Mathematicians, and Philosophers Proved Einstein's Spookiest Theory*, Plume Peguin, New York 2001

—, *The Jesuit & The Skull: Teilhard de Chardin, Evolution, and the Search for Peking Man*, Riverhead Books, New York 2007

—, *The Mystery of the Aleph*, Simon & Schuster, Pocket Books, New York, 2000

—, *Uranium Wars*, Palgrave Macmillan, New York, 2009

Adler, Mortimer, *The Angels and Us*, MacMillan, New York 1982

—, *The Difference of Man and the Difference It Makes*, Fordham University Press, New York 1993

—, *How to Think About God: A Guide for the 20th Century Pagan*, MacMillan, New York 1980

—, *Philosopher At Large: An Intellectual Autobiography 1902-1976*, MacMillan, New York 1977

—, *A Second Look in the Rearview Mirror*, MacMillan, New York 1992

—, *Six Great Ideas*, Macmillan, New York, 1981

—, *Truth in Religion: The Plurality of Religions and the Unity of Truth*, Self-published. Chicago 1990

Adler, Mortimer and Van Doren, Charles, *How To Read A Book*, Simon & Schuster, New York 1972 edition

Bartusiak, Marcia, *The Day we Found the Universe*, Vintage Books, Random House, New York 2009

Beyer, Rick, *The Greatest Science Stories Never Told*, Harper Collins, New York 2009

Bliss, Michael, *Banting: A Biography*, University of Toronto Press, Toronto 1992 edition

—, *The Discovery of Insulin*, University of Chicago Press, Chicago, 1982

Boorstin, Daniel, *Cleopatra's Nose: Essays on the Unexpected*, Vintage Books, Random House, New York 1994

—, *The Discoverers*, Random House, New York, 1983

Brady, Frank, *Endgame: Bobby Fischer's rise and Fall – From America's Brightest Prodigy to the Edge of Madness*, Broadway Paperbacks, New York 2011

Cadbury, Deborah, *The Dinosaur Hunters*, Fourth Estate, London, 2000

Cain, Susan, *Quiet: The Power of Introverts in a World That Can't Stop Talking*, Broadway Books, New York 2012

Cathcart, Brian, *The Fly in the Cathedral*, Farrar, Straus and Giroux, New York, 2005

Christianson, Gale, *Fox At The Wood's Edge: A Biography of Loren Eiseley*, Henry Holt & Company, New York 1990

Cochran Gregory and Harpending, Henry, *The 10,000 Year Explosion: How Civilization Accelerated Human Evolution,* Basic Books, New York, 2009

Collins, Francis, *The Language of God: A Scientist Presents Evidence for Belief*, Free Press, Simon & Schuster, New York 2006

Darwin, Charles, *The Autobiography of Charles Darwin*, Nora Barlow, ed. W. W. Norton, New York 1958

—, *On the Origin of Species*, Atheneum, New York, 1967

—, *The Voyage of the Beagle*, Bantam Books, New York 1958

Davidson, Keay, *Carl Sagan: A Life*, John Wiley & Sons, New York 1999

Davis, Joel, *Flyby: The Interplanetary Odyssey of Voyager 2*, Atheneum, New York, 1987

Dawkins, Richard, *The Devil's Chaplain: Reflections on Hope, Lies, Science and Love*, Mariner Books, Houghton Miflin Company, Boston 2004

—, *The Extended Phenotype: The Long Range of the Gene*, Oxford University Press, Oxford 1999

—, *The Selfish Gene*, Oxford University Press. Oxford, 1989 edition

de Kruif, Paul, *Microbe Hunters*, Harvest Book, Harcourt Brace, 1926

Drake, Stillman, *Discoveries and Opinions of Galileo*, Doubleday Anchor Books, Garden City, NY, 1957

Eiseley, Loren, *All the Strange Hours: The Excavation of a Life*, Charles Scribner's Sons, New York 1975

—, *Darwin and the Mysterious Mr. X: New Light on the Evolutionists*, E. P. Dutton, New York 1979

—, *Darwin's Century: Evolution and the Men Who Discovered It*, Anchor Doubleday, Garden City 1961

—, *The Firmament of Time*, Atheneum, New York 1970

—, *The Immense Journey*, Vintage Books, New York, 1959

—, *The Man Who Saw Through Time: Francis Bacon and the Modern Dilemma*, Charles Scribner's Sons, New York 1973

—, *The Night Country*, Charles Scribner's Sons, New York, 1971

—, *The Star Thrower*, Harcourt, Brace Jovanovich, San Diego 1978

—, *The Unexpected Universe*, Harcourt Brace Jovanovich, San Diego 1969

Feynman, Richard, *The Meaning of It All*, Penguin, London, 1999

—, *Perfectly Reasonable Deviations from the Beaten Track*, Basic Books, New York 2005

—, *Surely You're Joking, Mr. Feynman*, W. W. Norton & Co., New York, 1985

Franklin, Benjamin, *The Autobiography of Benjamin Franklin*, Introduction, Daniel Aaron, Vintage Books, Toronto, 1990

Galison, Peter, *Einstein's Clocks, Poincare's Maps*, W. W. Norton, New York 2003

Gamow, George, *One Two Three...Infinity: Facts and Speculation of Science*, Bantam Books, New York 1967 edition

Gardner, Martin, *Science: Good, Bad and Bogus*, Prometheus Books, Buffalo 1989

—, *The Whys Of A Philosophical Scrivener*, St. Martin's Griffin, New York 1999 edition

Gardner, Martin, ed., *Great Essays in Science*, Washington Square, New York, 1957

Geison, Gerald, *The Private Science of Louis Pasteur*, Princeton University Press, Princeton, 1995

Gilder, Joshua and Anne-Lee, *Heavenly Intrigue*, Anchor Books, New York, 2004

Gladwell, Malcolm, *David and Goliath: Underdogs, Misfits and the Art of Battling Giants*, Little, Brown & Company, New York 2013

—, *Outliers: The Story of Success*, Back Bay Books, Little Brown & Company, New York 2008

—, *The Tipping Point: How Little Things Can Make a Big Difference*, Little, Brown & Company, New York 2000

—, *What the Dog Saw*, Little, Brown & Company, New York 2009

Glenn, John and Taylor, Nick, *John Glenn: A Memoir*, Bantam Books, New York, 1982

Gottschall, Jonathan, *The Storytelling Animal: How Stories Make Us Human*, Houghton Mifflin Harcourt, New York 2012

Gould, Stephen Jay, *Bully for Brontosaurus*, W. W. Norton, New York 2001

—, *Dinosaur in a Haystack*, Crown Trade Paperbacks, New York 1995

—, *Eight Little Piggies: Reflections in Natural History*, W. W. Norton, New York 1993

—, *Ever Since Darwin*, W. W. Norton, New York 1977

—, *The Flamingo's Smile*, W. W. Norton, New York 1985

—, *Full House: The Spread of Excellence From Plato To Darwin*, Harmony Books, New York 1996

—, *Hen's Teeth and Horse's Toes*, W. W. Norton, New York 1983

—, *I Have Landed*, Three Rivers Press, New York 2003

—, *The Individual in Darwin's World*, Edinburgh University Press 1990

—, *Leonardo's Mountain of Clams and the Diet of Worms*, Vintage, London 1998

—, *Time's Arrow Time's Cycle: Myth and Metaphor in the Discovery of Geological Time*, Harvard University Press, Cambridge 1987

—, *An Urchin in the Storm*, W. W. Norton, New York 1987

—, *Wonderful Life: The Burgess Shale and the Nature of History*, W. W. Norton, New York 1989

Gorst, Martin, *Measuring Eternity*, Broadway Books, New York, 2001

Gratzer, Walter, *Eurekas and Euphorias*, Oxford University Press, Oxford, 2002

Guillen, Michael, *Five Equations That Changed The World: The Power and Poetry of Mathematics*, Hyperion, New York 1995

Harre, Rom, *Great Scientific Experiments*, Phaidon, Oxford, 1981

Hawking, Stephen, *A Brief History of Time: From the Big Bang to Black Holes*, Bantam Books, New York 1988

Hellman, Hal, *Great Feuds in Science*, John Wiley & Sons, New York, 1998

Horgan, John, *Rational Mysticism: Spirituality Meets Science in the Search for Enlightenment*, Mariner Books, Houghton Mifflin Company, Boston 2003

Isaacson, Walter, *Benjamin Franklin: An American Life*, Simon & Schuster, New York 2003

Jaffe, Bernard, *Crucibles: The Story of Chemistry*, Fawcett, Greenwich, 1957

Johanson, Donald and Wong, Kate, *Lucy's Legacy: The Quest for Human Origins*, Three Rivers Press, New York 2010

Kahneman, Daniel, *Thinking Fast and Slow*, Farrar, Straus & Giroux, New York 2011

Kushner, Harold, *When Bad Things Happen To Good People*, Avon, New York, 1981

Leakey, Richard, and Lewin, Roger, *Origins Reconsidered: In Search of What Makes Us Human*, Anchor Doubleday, New York 1992

Levenson, Thomas, *Newton and the Counterfeiter*, Mariner Books, Boston, 2009

Lightman, Alan, *The Discoveries*, Vintage Books, Random House, New York, 2005

—, *A Sense of the Mysterious*, Vintage Books, 2005

Livio, Mario, *Brilliant Blunders*, Simon & Schuster, New York 2013

Masfield, Stephen, *Lincoln's Battle with God*, Thomas Nelson, Nashville 2012

Mayer, Richard, *Thinking, Problem Solving, Cognition*, W. H. Freeman, New York 1992

Medawar, Jean, A Very Decided Preference: Life With Peter Medawar, W. W. Norton, New York 1990

Medawar, Peter, *The Threat and the Glory: Reflections on Science and Scientists*, Oxford University Press, Oxford 1991

Meyers, Morton, *Happy Accidents: Serendipity In Modern Medical Breakthroughs*, Arcade Publishing, New York 2007

—, *Prize Fight: The Race and the Rivalry to be the First in Science*, Palgrave MacMillan, New York 2012

Miller, Kenneth, *Finding Darwin's God: A Scientist's Search for Common Ground Between God and Evolution*, Cliff Street Books, New York 1999

Mullis, Kary, *Dancing Naked in the Mind Field*, Vintage Books, Random House, New York 1998

Nagel, Ernest and Newman, James, *Gödel's Proof*, New York University Press, New York 2001

Preston, Diana and Michael, *A Pirate of Exquisite Mind: Explorer, Naturalist, and Buccaneer – The Life of William Dampier*, Berkley Books, New York 2005

Salsburg, David, *The Lady Tasting Tea: How Statistics Revolutionized Science in the Twentieth Century*, Henry Holt Co., New York, 2001

Sandage, Tom and Lane, Allen, *The Neptune File*, Penguin Group, New York, 2000

Sebag-Montefiore, Hugh, *Enigma: The Battle for the Code*, John Wiley & Sons, Hoboken 2000

Shore, William, ed., *Mysteries of Life and the Universe: New Essays from America's Finest Writers on Science*, A Harvest Book, Harcourt Brace & Company, San Diego, 1992

Simpson, George Gaylord, *Concession to the Improbable: An Unconventional Autobiography*, Yale University Press, New Haven 1978

—, *The Meaning of Evolution*, Yale University Press, New Haven, 1967

—, *This View of Life: The World of an Evolutionist*, Harcourt, Brace & World, New York 1964 edition

Smith, John Maynard, *Did Darwin Get It Right?: Essays on Games, Sex and Evolution*, Chapman & Hall, New York 1992

Sobel, Dava, *Galileo's Daughter*, Penguin, New York, 2000

Squyres, Steve, *Roving Mars*, Hyperion, New York, 2005

Stone, Alex, *Fooling Houdini: Magicians, Mentalists, Math Geeks & the Hidden Powers of the Mind*, Harper Collins 2012

Swisher, Charles; Curtis, Garniss; Lewin, Roger, *Java Man: How Two Geologists' Dramatic Discoveries Changed Our Understanding of the Evolutionary Path to Modern Humans*, Scribner, New York 2000

Sykes, Bryan, *The Seven Daughters of Eve*, W. W. Norton & Co., New York, 2001

Taleb, Nassim, *The Black Swan: The Impact of the Highly Improbable*, Random House, New York 2007

Thomas, Lewis, *The Fragile Species*, MacMillan, New York 1992

—, *Late Night Thoughts on Listening to Mahler's Ninth Symphony*, Penguin Books, New York 1983

—, *The Lives of a Cell: Notes of a Biology Watcher*, Penguin Books, New York, 1974

—, *The Medusa and the Snail*, Penguin Books, New York 1979

—, *The Medusa and the Snail: More Notes of a Biology Watcher*, Penguin Books, London, 1995

—, *The Youngest Science*, Penguin Books, New York 1983

van Oosterzee, Penny, *Where World's Collide: The Wallace Line*, Cornell University Press, Ithaca 1997

Wade, Nicholas, *Before the Dawn: Recovering the Lost History of Our Ancestors*, Penguin Books, New York 2006

Waller, John, *Einstein's Luck*, Oxford University Press, Oxford, 2002

Watson, James, *The Double Helix,* Simon & Schuster, Touchstone, New York, 2001

Wells, Spencer, *Deep Ancestry*, National Geographic, Washington, DC 2007

—, *The Journey of Man: A Genetic Odyssey*, Random House, New York 2003

Wright, Robert, *Three Scientists and Their Gods: Looking for Meaning in an Age of Information*, Harper & Row, New York 1989

Yourgrau, Palle, *A World Without Time: The Forgotten Legacy of Gödel and Einstein*, Basic Books, New York 2005

Zimmerman, Robert, *The Universe in a Mirror: The Saga of the Hubble Space Telescope and the Visionaries Who Built It*, Princeton University Press, Princeton 2008

Appendix C

Magner Publications of Interest

The purpose of this book is to tell an interesting story – an American scientific case-study. The tale includes family crises and triumphs, struggles and achievements in school, pursuit of hobbies and outside interests, and challenges in scientific and medical arenas. The latter can be technical and may seem a bit obscure to some readers. The science is best documented in the original laboratory notebooks, records of meeting abstracts and conversations, and publications that were rejected and accepted. But all of that could never be captured in detail.

With limited time for this book project, and while trying to accommodate what would be of interest to general scientifically-educated readers, I wanted to reproduce publications that were important to my career and also might be of interest. My strategy was to provide an excerpt from my CV to show a complete list of publications, but then to selectively present full-length publications. Unfortunately, several of my most interesting publications cannot be included in this book because I could not nail down all the required permissions for reproduction. Several publishers were really not helpful at all, and for other publishers use of the Copyright Clearance Center with computerized approvals was helpful in some cases. For other permissions I worked with helpful individuals at publishers / journals, and I truly thank those people for making republication of an interesting paper possible.

Note that for all the republished articles, the copyright remains with the publishers, and no reproduction in whole or part may be made without written permission.

I want to call out the following publishers and individuals who were particularly helpful when working with me to secure the necessary permissions for reproduction:

Karger; European Thyroid Journal: Silvia Meier
Biological Bulletin: Carol Schachinger and Victoria Gibson
Wolters Kluwer; The Endocrinologist: Ronesha Battle
Journal of Biological Chemistry
Association for the Study of Internal Secretions; Endocrinology
Endocrine Society; J Clin Endocrinol Metab
Mary Ann Liebert Inc.; Thyroid: Karen Ballen
Springer; Journal of Endocrinological Investigation
The Scientist: Mary Beth Aberlin

Publications Listed in C.V.

1. Magner JA. Radiation biology: An explosive topic. Resident and Staff Physician 1981 Feb;104-111. Reprinted with permission in Medical Times: 1981 Aug 40s-45s, 1981 Aug.

2. Magner JA, Weintraub BD. Thyroid-stimulating hormone (TSH) subunit processing and combination in microsomal subfractions of mouse pituitary tumor. J Biol Chem 1982;257:6709-6715.

3. Magner JA. Information in the signal peptide? J Theor Biol 1982;99:831-833.

4. Kohl EA, Magner JA, Persellin ST, Vaughan GM, Kudzma DJ, Friedberg SJ. Improved control of non-insulin-dependent diabetes mellitus by combined halofenate and chlorpropamide therapy. Diabetes Care 1984;7:19-24.

5. Magner JA, Rogol AD, Gorden P. Reversible growth hormone deficiency and delayed puberty triggered by a stressful experience in a young adult. Am J Med 1984;76:737-742.

6. Ronin C, Stannard BS, Rosenbloom IL, Magner JA, Weintraub BD. Glycosylation and processing of high mannose oligosaccharides of thyroid-stimulating hormone subunits: Comparison to non-secretory cell glycoproteins. Biochemistry 1984;23:4503-4510.

7. Magner JA, Ronin C, Weintraub BD. Carbohydrate processing of thyrotropin differs from that of free alpha subunit and total glycoproteins in microsomal subfractions of mouse pituitary tumor. Endocrinology 1984;115:1019-1030.

8. Mazzone T, Papagiannes E, Magner J. Early kinetics of human macrophage apolipoprotein E synthesis and incorporation of carbohydrate precursors. Biochem Biophys Acta 1986;875:393-396.

9. Murata Y, Magner JA, Refetoff S. The role of glycosylation on the molecular conformation and secretion of thyroxine binding globulin. Endocrinology 1986;118:1614-1621.

10. Magner JA, Novak W, Papagiannes E. Subcellular localization of fucose incorporation into mouse thyrotropin and free alpha-subunits: Studies employing subcellular fractionation, and inhibitors of the intracellular translocation of proteins. Endocrinology 1986;119:1315-1328.

11. Magner J, Papagiannes E. Studies of double-labeled mouse thyrotropin and free alpha-subunits to estimate relative fucose content. Proceedings of the Society for Experimental Biology and Medicine 1986;183:237-240.

12. Gesundheit N, Magner JA, Chen T, Weintraub BD. Differential sulfation and sialylation of secreted mouse thyrotropin subunits: Regulation by thyrotropin-releasing hormone. Endocrinology 1986;119:455-463.

13. Vogel DL, Magner JA, Sherins RJ, Weintraub BD. Biosynthesis, glycosylation and secretion of rat luteinizing hormone alpha and beta subunits: Differential effects of orchiectomy and gonadotropin-releasing hormone. Endocrinology 1986;119:202-213.

14. Magner JA, Petrick P, Menezes-Ferreira M, Stelling M, Weintraub BD. Familial generalized resistance to thyroid hormones: Report of three kindreds and correlation of patterns of affected tissues with the binding of [125I]triiodothyronine to fibroblast nuclei. Journal of Endocrinological Investigation 1986;9:459-470.

15. Magner JA, Papagiannes E. Structures of high-mannose oligosaccharides of mouse thyrotropin: Differential processing of alpha versus beta subunits of the heterodimer. Endocrinology 1987;120:10-17.

16. Magner JA, Papagiannes E. The subcellular sites of sulfation of mouse thyrotropin and free alpha subunits: Studies employing subcellular fractionation and inhibitors of the intracellular translocation of proteins. Endocrine Research 1987;13(4):337-361.

17. Magner JA, Clark W, Allenby P. Congestive heart failure and sudden death in a young woman with thyrotoxicosis. Western Journal of Medicine 1988;149:86-91.

18. Magner JA, Papagiannes E. Blockade by brefeldin A of intracellular transport of secretory proteins in mouse pituitary cells: Effects on the biosynthesis of thyrotropin and free alpha-subunits. Endocrinology 1988;122:912-920.

19. Schneider AB, McCurdy A, Chang T, Dudlak D, Magner JA. Metabolic labeling of human thyroglobulin with [35S]sulfate: Incorporation into chondroitin 6-sulfate and endoglycosidase F-susceptible carbohydrate units. Endocrinology 1988;122:2428-2435.

20. Perkel VS, Liu AY, Miura Y, Magner JA. The effects of brefeldin A on the high-mannose oligosaccharides of mouse thyrotropin, free alpha-subunits, and total glycoproteins. Endocrinology 1988;123:310-318.

21. Miura Y, Perkel VS, Magner JA. Rates of processing of the high-mannose oligosaccharide units at the three glycosylation sites of mouse thyrotropin and the two sites of free alpha subunits. Endocrinology 1988;123:1296-1302.

22. Miura Y, Perkel VS, Magner JA. Differential susceptibility to N-glycanase at the individual glycosylation sites of mouse thyrotropin and free alpha-subunits. Endocrinology 1988;123:2207-2213.

23. Perkel VS, Miura Y, Magner JA. Brefeldin A inhibits oligosaccharide processing of glycoproteins in mouse hypothyroid pituitary tissue at several subcellular sites. Proceedings of the Society for Experimental Biology and Medicine 1989;190:286-293.

24. Magner JA. Assay of sulfotransferase in subcellular fractions of hypothyroid mouse pituitary and liver tissue. Biochemical Medicine and Metabolic Biology 1989;41:81-83.

25. Miura Y, Perkel VS, Papenberg KA, Magner JA. Concanavalin A, lentil and ricin lectin affinity binding characteristics of human thyrotropin: Differences in the sialylation of TSH in sera of euthyroid, primary and central hypothyroid patients. J Clin Endocrinol Metab 1989;69:985-995.

26. Miura Y, Perkel V, Magner JA. Susceptibility to endoglycosidase F and H at the individual glycosylation sites of mouse thyrotropin and free alpha-subunits. Hormone and Metabolic Research 1990;22:369-373.

27. Magner JA. Thyroid-Stimulating Hormone: Biosynthesis, Cell Biology, and Bioactivity. Endocrine Reviews 1990;11:354-385.

28. Johnson MJ, Miura Y, Rubin D, Magner JA. Processing to endoglycosidase H-resistant thyrotropin subunits occurs in the presence of brefeldin-A: Evidence favoring the recycling of Golgi membranes to the rough endoplasmic reticulum in mouse thyrotrophs. Thyroid 1991;1:185-194.

29. Magner J, Klibanski A, Fein H, Smallridge R, Blackard W, Young Jr., W., Ferriss, J.B., Murphy, D., Kane, J. and Rubin, D.: Ricin and lentil lectin-affinity chromatography reveals oligosaccharide heterogeneity of thyrotropin secreted by twelve human pituitary tumors. Metabolism 1992;41:1009-1015.

30. Magner JA, Kane J, Chou ET. Intravenous TRH releases human TSH that is biochemically different from basal TSH. J Clin Endocrinol Metab 1992;74:1306-1311.

31. Magner JA, Miura Y, Rubin D, Kane J. Structures of high-mannose and complex oligosaccharides of mouse TSH and free alpha-subunits after in vitro incubation of thyrotropic tissue with TRH. Endocrine Research 1992;18:175-199.

32. Magner JA, Kane J. Binding of thyrotropin to lentil lectin is unchanged by thyrotropin-releasing hormone administration in three patients with thyrotropin-producing pituitary adenomas. Endocrine Research 1992;18:163-173.

33. Magner J, Schluep J, Miura Y, Wezeman F. Fucosylation of glycoproteins begins in the rough endoplasmic reticulum of mouse active thyrotrophs. Thyroid 1993;2:337-344.

34. Francis TB, Smallridge RC, Kane J, Magner JA. Octreotide changes serum TSH glycoisomer distribution as assessed by lectin chromatography in a TSH macroadenoma patient. J Clin Endocrinol Metab 1993;77:183-187.

35. Harel G, Kane JP, Shamoun DS, Magner JA, Szabo M. Effect of thyroid hormone deficiency on glycosylation of rat TSH secreted in vitro. Hormone and Metabolic Research 1993;25:278-280.

36. Magner JA. TSH-mediated hyperthyroidism. Endocrinologist 1993;3:289-296.

37. Magner JA, West RL. Lymphocytic hypophysitis. West J Med 1994;160:462-464.

38. Helton TE, Magner JA. Sialyltransferase mRNA increases in thyrotrophs of hypothyroid mice: an in situ hybridization study. Endocrinology 1994;134:2347-2353.

39. Magner J, Daughtry S, Lengerich E, Stoodt G. How primary care physicians in North Carolina assess and counsel their diabetic patients. North Carolina Med J 1994;55:275-278.

40. Daughtry SB, Magner J. Physician standards of diabetes care: results from the North Carolina Diabetes Control Pilot Project. North Carolina Med J 1994;55:281-283.

41. Magner JA. Biosynthesis, cell biology, and bioactivity of thyroid-stimulating hormone: update 1994. Endoc Rev Monographs 1994;3:55-60.

42. Magner J, Gerber P. Urticaria due to blue dye in Synthroid tablets. (letter). Thyroid 1994;4:341.

43. Magner JA, Snyder DK. Methimazole-induced agranulocytosis treated with recombinant human granulocyte colony-stimulating factor (G-CSF). Thyroid 1994;4:295-296.

44. Helton TE, Magner JA. β 1, 4-galactosyltransferase and α-mannosidase II messenger ribonucleic acid levels increase with different kinetics in thyrotrophs of hypothyroid mice. Endocrinology 1994;135:1980-1985.

45. Harel G, Shamoun DS, Kane JP, Magner JA, Szabo M. Prolonged effects of tumor necrosis factor -α on anterior pituitary hormone release. Peptides 1995; 16:641-645.

46. Trojan J, Schaaf L, Weis G, Bergmann A, Helton TE, Magner JA, Usadel KH. Isolation and characterization of different subfractions of human serum thyrotropin (hTSH). Exp Clin Endocrinol 1994;102:33-37.

47. Helton TE, Magner JA. β-Galactoside α-2,3-sialyltransferase messenger RNA increases in thyrotrophs of hypothyroid mice. Thyroid 1995;5:315-317.

48. Schaff L, Trojan J, Helton TE, Usadel KH, Magner JA. Serum thyrotropin (TSH) heterogeneity in euthyroid subjects and patients with subclinical hypothyroidism: the core fucose content of TSH-releasing hormone-released TSH is altered, but not the net charge of TSH. J Endocrinol 1995;144:561-567.

49. Cansler CL, Latham JA, Brown PM, Chapman III WHH, Magner JA. Duodenal obstruction in thyroid storm. Southern Medical Journal 1997; 90:1143-1146.

50. Magner J, Roy P, Fainter L, Barnard V, Fletcher Jr P. Transiently decreased sialylation of thyrotropin (TSH) in a patient with the euthyroid sick syndrome. Thyroid 1997; 7:55-61.

51. Rosenstock J, Brown A, Fischer J, Jain A, Littlejohn T, Nadeau D, Sussman A, Taylor T, Krol A, Magner J. Efficacy and safety of acarbose in metformin-treated patients with type 2 diabetes. Diabetes Care 1998;21:2050-2055.

52. Kelley DE, Bidot P, Freedman Z, Haag B, Podlecki D, Rendell M, Schimel D, Weiss S, Taylor T, Krol A, Magner J. Efficacy and safety of acarbose in insulin-treated patients with type 2 diabetes. Diabetes Care1998;21:2056-2061.

53. Magner JA. Thyroid-stimulating hormone-mediated hyperthyroidism. Endocrinologist 2004;14(4): 201 – 211.

54. Magner JA. Emil Fischer (1852-1919): The stereochemical nature of sugars. Endocrinologist 2004;14(5): 239 – 244.

55. Robbins R, Driedger A, Magner J and the Thyrogen Compassionate Use Investigator Group. Recombinant human TSH-assisted radioiodine therapy for patients with metastatic thyroid cancer who could not elevate endogenous TSH or be withdrawn from thyroxine. Thyroid 2006; 16 (11): 1121-1130.

56. Jonklaas J, Sarlis N, Litofsky D, Ain K, Bigos T, Brierley J, Cooper D, Haugen B, Ladenson P, Magner J, Robbins J, Ross D, Skarulis M, Maxon H, Sherman S. Outcomes of patients with differentiated thyroid carcinoma following initial therapy. Thyroid 2006; 16 (12): 1229-1242.

57. Magner JA. Seymour D. Van Meter, MD (1865-1934): The Texan who wielded a scalpel in Denver and left a lasting legacy. The Endocrinologist 2007; 17 (2): 71-77. Reprinted in slightly revised form in Thyroid 2007; 17 (8): 779 - 785.

58. Braverman L, Kloos RT, Law Jr B, Kipnes M, Dionne M, Magner J. Evaluation of various doses of recombinant human thyrotropin in patients with multinodular goiters. Endocrine Practice 2008; 14 (7): 832-839.

59. Magner J. Problems associated with the use of Thyrogen in patients with a thyroid gland. (letter) N Engl J Med 2008; 359: 1738-1739.

60. Ross DS, Litofsky D, Ain KB, Bigos T, Brierly JD, Cooper DS, Haugen BR, Jonklaas J, Ladenson PW, Magner J, Robbins J, Skarulis M, Maxon HR, Sherman SI. Recurrence after treatment of micropapillary thyroid cancer. Thyroid 2009; 19: 1043-1048.

61. Elisei R, Schlumberger M, Driedger A, Reiners C, Kloos RT, Sherman SI, Haugen B, Corone C, molinaro E, Grasso L, Leboulleux S, Rachinsky I, Luster M, Lassman M, Busaidy NL, Wahl RL, Pacini F, Cho SY, Magner J, Pinchera A, Ladenson PW. Follow-up of low-risk differentiated thyroid cancer patients who underwent radioiodine ablation of postsurgical thyroid remnants after either recombinant human thyrotropin or thyroid hormone withdrawal. J Clin Endocrinol Metab 2009; 94: 4171-4179.

62. Jonklaas J, Cooper D, Ain K, Bigos T, Brierley J, Haugen B, Ladenson P, Magner J, Ross D, Skarulis M, Steward D, Maxon H, Sherman S. Radioiodine therapy in patients with stage I differentiated thyroid cancer (letter). Thyroid 2010; 20:1423-1424.

63. Graf H, Fast S, Pacini F, Pinchera A, Leung A, Vaisman M, Reiners C, Wemeau J, Huysmans D, Harper W, Driedger A, Noemberg de Souza H, Castagna M, Antonangeli L, Braverman L, Corbo R, Duren C, Proust-Lemoine E, Edelbroek M, Marriott C, Rachinsky I, Grupe P, Watt T, Magner J, Hegedus L. Modified-release recombinant human TSH (MRrhTSH) augments the effect of 131-I therapy in benign multinodular goiter: Results from a multicenter international, randomized, placebo-controlled study. J Clin Endocrinol Metab 2011; 96(5): 1368-1376.

64. Jonklaas J, Nogueras-Gonzalez G, Munsell M, Litofsky D, Ain K, Bigos S, Brierley J, Cooper D, Haugen B, Ladenson P, Magner J, Robbins J, Ross D, Skarulis M, Steward D, Maxon H, Sherman S. The impact of age and gender on papillary thyroid cancer survival. J Clin Endocrinol Metab 2012; 97(6): E878-887. doi: 10.1210/jc.2011-2864. Epub 2012 Apr 10.

65. Drozd V, Leonova T, Mitjukova T, Lushchik M, Kortiko S, Magner JA, BikoJ, Reiners C. Recombinant human thyrotropin to help confirm lack of evidence of radiation-induced differentiated thyroid cancer in young women seeking pregnancy. Nucl Med Rev Cent East Eur 2012; 15: 108-112.

66. Braverman L, Magner J. Introduction to the recombinant human TSH (rhTSH) symposium articles. Endocr Practice 2013; 19 (1): 137-138.

67. McLeod D, Cooper D, Ladenson P, Ain K, Brierley J, Fein H, Haugen B, Jonklaas J, Magner J, Ross D, Skarulis M, Steward D, Maxon H, Sherman S. Thyroid 2014; 24 (1): 35-42.

68. Bartenstein Peter, Calabuig Elisa Caballero, Maini Carlo Ludovico, Mazzarotto Renzo, Muros de Fuentes M Angustias, Petrich Thorsten, Rodrigues Fernando José Cravo, Vallejo Casas Juan Antonio, Vianello Federica, Basso Michela, Balaguer Marcelino Gómez, Haug Alexander, Monari Fabio, Sánchez Vaňó Raquel, Sciuto Rosa, Magner James. High-risk patients with differentiated thyroid cancer T4 primary tumors achieve remnant ablation equally well using rhTSH or thyroid hormone withdrawal. Thyroid 2014; 24 (1):480-487.

69. Fast S, Hegedus L, Pacini F, Pinchera A, Leung AM, Vaisman M, Reiners C, Wemeau JL, Huysmans D, Harper W, Rachinsky I, Noemberg de Souza H, Castagna MG, Antonangeli L, Braverman LE, Corbo R, Duren C, Proust-Lemoine E, Marriott C, Driedger A, Grupe P, Watt T, Magner J, Purvis A, Graf H. Long-term efficacy of modified-release recombinant human TSH (MRrhTSH) augmented radioiodine (131-I) therapy for benign multinodular goiter. Results from a multicenter international, randomized, placebo-controlled dose-selection study. Thyroid 2014; 24 (4):727-735.

70. Magner J. Historical Note: Many steps led to the 'discovery' of thyroid-stimulating hormone. Eur Thyroid J 2014; 3 (2):95-100.

Abstracts

1. Magner J, Eberhard A, Nealson K. Characterization of bioluminescent bacteria by studies of their inducers of luciferase synthesis. Biol Bull October 1972;143:469.

2. Magner JA, Weintraub BD. Thyrotropin (TSH) subunit processing and combination in subcellular microsomal fractions. Program of the American Thyroid Association 1981;T-32.

3. Magner JA, Stannard BS, Weintraub BD. Processing of thyrotropin (TSH) carbohydrate units: Relation to subcellular site, subunit combination, transport and secretion. Program of the Endocrine Society 1982;No. 883.

4. Magner J, Ronin C, Weintraub B. Structures of oligosaccharide units of thyrotropin subunits in microsomal fractions. Program of the Endocrine Society 1983;No. 22.

5. Vogel DL, Magner JA, Sherins RJ. Biosynthesis of LH-alpha and -beta subunits in intact and orchiectomized rats. Program of the Endocrine Society 1983;No. 144.

6. Magner JA, Ronin C, Weintraub BD. Carbohydrate processing of thyrotropin subunits differs from that of non-TSH glycoproteins in microsomal fractions. Program of the American Thyroid Association 1983;No. 79.

7. Magner JA, Papagiannes E, Weintraub BD. Sialic acid is present in mouse pituitary tumor thyrotropin alpha and beta subunits. Program of the American Thyroid Association 1984;T48.

8. Magner J, Murata Y, Refetoff S. Structures of oligosaccharides (CHO) in precursors of human thyroxine-binding globulin (TBG). Program of the American Thyroid Association 1984;T45.

9. Mazzone, T. and Magner, J.: Biosynthesis of Apolipoprotein E by human macrophages: Studies with monensin and endoglycosidase H. (abstract). Arteriosclerosis 1984;4:522a.

10. Magner J, Papagiannes E. Subcellular localization of TSH and free α-subunit processing in mouse pituitaries. Program of the Endocrine Society 1985;No. 1254.

11. Papagiannes E, Magner J. Accumulation of fucosylated TSH alpha-subunit precursors in monensin-treated mouse tumor cells. Program of the Endocrine Society 1985;No. 702.

12. Chen T, Papagiannes E, Magner J. Sialic acid is present in mouse pituitary thyrotropin alpha and beta subunits. Program of the Western Section 1986;AFCR, 21A.

13. Magner JA, Papagiannes E. Effects of CCCP and monensin on mouse thyrotropin biosynthesis: Direct analyses of subcellular fractions. Program of the Endocrine Society 1986;No. 791.

14. Magner JA, Papagiannes E. Structures of high-mannose oligosaccharides of mouse thyrotropin: Differential processing of alpha versus beta subunits. Program of the American Thyroid Association 1986.

15. Magner JA, Gorman M, Salvo B, Papagiannes E. The subcellular sites of sulfation of mouse thyrotropin and free alpha subunits. Program of the Endocrine Society 1987.

16. Magner JA, Papagiannes E. Blockade by brefeldin A of intracellular transport of thyrotropin and free alpha subunits in mouse pituitary cells. Program of the American Thyroid Association 1987.

17. Papagiannes E, Magner J. Assay of sulfotransferase in subcellular fractions of hypothyroid mouse pituitaries. Program of the American Thyroid Association 1987.

18. Perkel VS, Liu AY, Miura Y, Magner JA, The effects of brefeldin A on the high-mannose oligosaccharides of mouse thyrotropin, free alpha-subunits and total glycoproteins. Program of the Endocrine Society 1988.

19. Miura Y, Perkel VS, Magner JA. Differential processing at asparagine glycosylation sites of mouse thyrotropin and free alpha-subunits. Program of the Eighth International Congress of Endocrinology, Kyoto 1988;No. 04-19-016.

20. Perkel VS, Miura Y, Magner JA. Effects of the inhibitors brefeldin A, carboxyl cyanide m-chlorophenylhydrazone and monensin on the processing of oligosaccharides of TSH, free alpha-subunits and cellular glycoproteins. Program of the American Thyroid Association 1988;No. 89.

21. Miura Y, Perkel VS, Zeunert P, Magner JA. Rates of processing of the high-mannose oligosaccharide units, and differential susceptibility to N-glycanase, at the individual glycosylation sites of mouse thyrotropin and free alpha-subunits. Program of the American Thyroid Association 1988;No. 90.

22. Perkel VS, Papenberg KA, Miura Y, Magner JA. Concanavalin A and lentil lectin binding characteristics of human thyrotropin from sera of hypothyroid and euthyroid subjects. Program of the Endocrine Society 1989;No. 1828.

23. Miura Y, Johnson MJ, Perkel V, Magner JA. Qualitatively different forms of human TSH in sera of euthyroid, primary and central hypothyroid patients: Analyses by ricin and McKenzie bioassay. Program of the Endocrine Society 1989;No. 632.

24. Miura Y, Johnson MJ, Magner JA. Sialylation and sulfation of mouse thyrotropin subunits secreted by thyrotropic tumor and hypothyroid pituitaries. Program of the American Thyroid Association, San Francisco 1989;No. 154.

25. Johnson MJ, Miura Y, Magner JA. Evidence of Golgi-RER membrane recycling in mouse thyrotropic tissue: Endo H-resistant free α-subunits appear in the presence of brefeldin A (BFA). Program of the American Thyroid Association San Francisco 1989;No. 94.

26. Johnson MJ, Miura Y, Rubin D, Magner JA. Endo H-resistant TSH subunits appear in the presence of brefeldin-A (BFA): Evidence of Golgi to RER membrane recycling in mouse thyrotrophs. Program of the Endocrine Society Atlanta 1990;No. 1232.

27. Magner JA, Kane J. TSH secreted in vitro by a human pituitary tumor is highly sialylated in spite of unresponsiveness to TRH. Program of the Endocrine Society Atlanta 1990;No. 1235.

28. Magner J, Klibanski A, Fein H, Smallridge R, Blackard W, Kane J. Ricin lectin-affinity chromatography reveals oligosaccharide heterogeneity of thyrotropin secreted by eight human pituitary tumors. Program of the 10th International Thyroid Congress, The Hague 1991;No. 257.

29. Magner JA, Wezeman F, Schluep J. Autoradiographic demonstration that a Golgi-posttranslational processing step (fucosylation) partially shifts to the rough endoplasmic reticulum in active mouse thyrotrophs: Implications for the physiologic modulation of TSH oligosaccharide structure. Program of the Endocrine Society, Washington, D.C. 1991;No. 822.

30. Kane J, Magner JP. Human TSH released by intravenous TRH is biochemically different than basal TSH. Program of the American Thyroid Association, Boston, 1991;No. 104.

31. Harel G, Shamoun DS, Kane JP, Magner JA, Szabo M. Effects of chronic exposure to TNF-alpha on rat anterior pituitary hormone secretion in vitro. Program of the Endocrine Society, San Antonio, 1992;No. 666.

32. Harel G, Kane JP, Shamoun DS, Magner JA, Szabo M. Effects of thyroid hormone deficiency on glycosylation of rat TSH secreted in vitro. Program of the American Thyroid Association, Rochester, 1992;No. 166.

33. Manasco PK, Blithe DL, Rose SR, Gelato MC, Magner JA, Nisula BC. Thyrotropin abnormalities in central hypothyroidism. Program of the Serono Symposium on Glycoprotein Hormones, 1993.

34. Helton TE, Magner JA. Sialyltransferase mRNA increases in thyrotrophs of hypothyroid mice: an in situ hybridization study. Program of the American Thyroid Association, 1993;Tampa.

35. Schaaf L, Trojan J, Weis G, Helton TE, Magner JA, Usadel KH. Thyrotropin (TSH) isoform distribution in patients with primary hypothyroidism compared to intrapituitary TSH. Program of the 38th Symposium, German Society of Endocrinology (DGE), Würzburg 1994 March.

36. Magner JA, Kane J, Scherberg N. Circadian variation in circulating TSH oligosaccharides: Observations from frequent blood sampling in four human subjects. Program of the American Thyroid Association 1994, Chicago.

37. Helton TE, Magner JA. Galactosyltransferase and mannosidase II mRNA levels increase with different kinetics in thyrotrophs of hypothyroid mice. Program of the American Thyroid Association 1994, Chicago.

38. Helton, TE, Magner JA. β-Galactoside α-2, 3 sialyltransferase mRNA increases in thyrotrophs of hypothyroid mice. Program of the Endocrine Society, 1995.

39. Magner JA, Menke JB. Potential thyroid hormone response elements (TREs) within the DNA sequences of glycosyltransferases: Implications for the hormonal modulation of TSH glycosylation. Program of the 11th International Thyroid Congress, Toronto, 1995.

40. Cansler C, Lathan J, Magner J. Duodenal obstruction in thyroid storm. Program of the North Carolina American College of Physicians, Raleigh, 1996.

41. Magner J, Roy P, Fainter L, Barnard V, Fletcher P. Changes in TSH bioactivity/immunoactivity ratio and sialylation in patients with euthyroid sick syndrome. Program of the American Thyroid Association, San Diego, 1996.

42. Magner J, Roy P, Fainter L, Barnard V, Fletcher P. Altered thyrotropin (TSH) biochemistry in poorly nourished hospitalized patients. Program of the North Carolina Institute of Nutrition, Chapel Hill, 1996.

43. Magner J, Roy P. Altered thyrotropin (TSH) biochemistry in poorly nourished hospitalized patients. Program of the North Carolina Institute of Nutrition, Chapel Hill, 1997.

44. Kelley DE, Magner J, Krol A, Taylor T. Efficacy and safety of acarbose in patients with type 2 diabetes inadequately controlled with insulin therapy. Program of the American Diabetes Association, Abstract # 0348, Chicago, 1998.

45. Rosenstock J, Magner J, Krol A, Taylor T. Efficacy and safety of acarbose in patients with type 2 diabetes inadequately controlled with metformin. Program of the American Diabetes Association, Abstract # 1357, Chicago, 1998.

46. Magner JA. Use of rhTSH to ablate thyroid remnants and to follow patients for residual thyroid cancer. 48th Annual Meeting of the Japan Thyroid Assn., Tokyo, November, 2005

47. Compston A, Margolin D, Haas J, Magner J, Gonzales G, Valente W, Coles A. Two year interim analysis of thyroid abnormalities in a trial of alemtuzumab vs high-dose interferom-beta-1a, for treatment of relapsing-remitting multiple sclerosis. 22nd Congress of the European Committee for Treatment and Research in Multiple Sclerosis, Madrid, September, 2006

48. Magner JA, Kipnes MS, Kloos RT, Law BM, Braverman LE. Cardiac effects of Thyrogen (rhTSH) in multinodular goiter (MNG) patients: A cautionary note. 77th Annual Meeting of the American Thyroid Assn., Phoenix, 2006 and Thyroid 16 (10): 1072, 2006.

49. Elisei R, Corone C, Driedger A, Haugen B, Kloos R, Magner J, Pacini F, Luster M, Schlumberger M, Sherman S, Pinchera A, Ladenson P. Follow-up of differentiated thyroid cancer patients who underwent radioiodine ablation of postsurgical thyroid remnants after recombinant human thyrotropin or thyroid hormone withdrawal. Annual Meeting of the European Thyroid Assn., Leipzig, 2007.

50. Saurabh S, Litofsky D, Ain K, Brierly J, Cooper D, Haugen B, Jonklaas J, Ladenson P, Magner J, Maxon H, Robbins J, Skarulis M, Steward D, Sherman S. Hurthle cell carcinoma of the thyroid: prognostic factors in the National Thyroid Cancer Treatment Cooperative Study (NTCTCS). 79th Annual Meeting of the American Thyroid Assn., Chicago, 2008.

51. Ross D, Litofsky D, Ain K, Bigos T, Brierley J, Cooper D, Haugen B, Jonklaas J, Ladenson P, Magner J, Robbins J, Skarulis M, Maxon H, Steward D, Sherman S. Recurrence after treatment of micropapillary thyroid cancer. 79th Annual Meeting of the American Thyroid Assn., Chicago, 2008.

52. Jonklaas J, Litofsky D, Munsell M, Ain K, Bigos T, Brierley J, Cooper D, Haugen B, Ladenson P, Magner J, Robbins J, Ross D, Skarulis M, Steward D, Maxon H, Sherman S. Effect of gender on differentiated thyroid cancer survival in the National Thyroid Cancer Treatment Cooperative Study Group Registry. 79th Annual Meeting of the American Thyroid Assn., Chicago, 2008.

53. Graf H, Fast S, Pacini F, et al. Modified-release recombinant human TSH (MRrhTSH) augments the effect of 131-I in moderately-sized benign multinodular goiters. Results from a global, randomized, placebo-controlled study. Annual Meeting of the American Thyroid Assn., Palm Beach, Florida, 2009.

54. McLeod DS, Cooper DS, Ladenson PW, Ain KB, Bigos ST, Brierly JD, Fein HG, Haugen BR, Jonklaas J, Magner J, Ross DS, Skarulis DL, Steward DL, Maxon HR, Sherman S. Prognosis of differentiated thyroid cancer in relation to at-diagnosis TSH and thyroglobulin status. Annual Meeting of the American Thyroid Assn., Quebec City, Quebec, 2012.

55. Bartenstein Peter, Calabuig Elisa Caballero, Maini Carlo Ludovico, Mazzarotto Renzo, Muros de Fuentes M Angustias, Petrich Thorsten, Rodrigues Fernando José Cravo, Vallejo Casas Juan Antonio, Vianello Federica, Basso Michela, Balaguer Marcelino Gómez, Haug Alexander, Monari Fabio, Sánchez Vaňó Raquel, Sciuto Rosa, Magner James. High-risk patients with differentiated thyroid cancer T4 primary tumors achieve remnant ablation equally well using rhTSH or thyroid hormone withdrawal. Annual Meeting of the European Thyroid Assn., Leiden, The Netherlands, 2013.

56. Carhill Aubrey, Litofsky Danielle, Ain Kenneth, Brierly James, Cooper David, Fein Henry, Haugen Bryan, Jonklaas Jacqueline, Ladenson Paul, Magner James, Ross Douglas, Skarulis Monica, Steward David, Xing Mingxhao, Maxon Harry, Sherman Steven. Long-term moderate thyroid hormone suppression therapy is associated with improved outcomes in differentiated thyroid carcinoma: National Thyroid Cancer Treatment Cooperative Study Group Registry Analysis 1987-2012. Annual meeting of the American Thyroid Assn., Coronado, CA, 2014.

Editorials

1. Magner JA. The nuclear arms race and the physician. (letter). N. Engl. J. Med. 1981;305:222.

2. Magner JA. Nuclear war and the 1985 Nobel Peace Prize (letter). N. Engl. J. Med. 1986;315:831.

3. Magner JA. The inherent uncertainty of nature is a basis for religion. The Scientist 2 (24):9, December 26, 1988.

4. Magner JA. Book Review. Molecular Endocrinology. Basic concepts and clinical correlations, by B.D. Weintraub. The Endocrinologist , 1996;6:69-70.

5. Magner JA. Smallpox (letter). N.Engl. J. Med. 1996;335:900.

6. Magner JA. Transiently decreased sialylation of thyrotropin in a patient with the euthyroid sick syndrome (letter). Thyroid 1997;7:807-808.

7. Magner J. Thyrotropin in San Diego: Echoes after nearly a century (letter). Thyroid 2014; 24:1551.

Contributions to Textbooks

1. Weintraub BD, Stannard BS, Magner JA, Ronin C, Taylor T, Joshi L, Constant RB, Menezes-Ferreira M, Petrick PA, Gesundheit N. Glycosylation and post-translational processing of thyroid-stimulating hormone: Clinical implications. Rec Prog. Hormone Res. 1985;41:577-606.

2. Magner JA. Weintraub BD. Thyroid-stimulating hormone biosynthesis In Braverman L.E., and Ingbar S.H., (Eds): The Thyroid, Fifth Edition, J.B. Lippincott, 1986, pp. 271-287.

3. Magner JA. Thyroid-Stimulating Hormone: Structure and Function. In Ekholm R., Kohn L.D.,Wollman S. (Eds.): Control of the Thyroid Gland, Plenum Press, 1989, pp. 27-103.

4. Magner JA, Kilbanski A, Fein H, Smallridge R, Blackard W, Young W, Kane J, Rubin D. Ricin and lenti lectin-affinity chromatography reveals oligosaccharide heterogeneity of thyrotropin secreted by human pituitary tumors. In Gordon A, Gross J, Hennemann G. (Eds.): Progress in Thyroid Research, A.A. Balkema, Rotterdam, 1991, pp. 155-158.

5. Wondisford FE, Magner JA, Weintraub BD. Chemistry and Biosynthesis of Thyrotropin. In Braverman, L.E. and Utiger, R.D. (Eds.): The Thyroid, Sixth Edition, J.B. Lippincott, Philadelphia, 1991, pp 257-276.

6. Magner JA. Thyrotropin. In Haeberli, A. (Ed.). Human Protein Data, VCH Publishers, Weinheim, 1992.

7. Magner JA. Hypothyroidism. In Rakel, R.E. (Ed.): Conn's Current Therapy. W.B. Saunders, 1993, pp. 613-619.

8. Trojan J, Schaaf L, Weis G, Bergmann A, Helton T, Magner J, Usadel K. Isolation and characterization of different subfractions of human serum thyrotropin (hTSH). International Workshop on Recent Advances in Thyroid Diagnostics, Henning Symposium Schilddruse, Heidelberg, 1993.

9. Manasco PK, Blithe DL, Rose SR, Gelato MC, Magner JA, Nisula BC. Thyrotropin abnormalities in central hypothyroidism. In Lustbader, J.W., Puett, J.D. and Ruddon, R. (eds): Glycoprotein Hormones: Structure, Function and Clinical Implications, Springer-Verlag, New York, 1994, pp. 343-348.

10. Wondisford FE, Magner JA, Weintraub BD. Chemistry and biosynthesis of thyrotropin. In Braverman LE and Utiger RD (eds): The Thyroid, Seventh Edition, JB Lippincott, Philadelphia, 1996, pp. 190-207.

11. Magner JA. Pituitary-thyroid relationships, In Bittar, EE and Bittar, N (eds): Principles of Medical Biology, Volume 10A, JAI Press, Greenwich, 1997, pp. 165-189.

12. Magner J, Amatruda J. Alpha-glucosidase inhibitors in the treatment of diabetes. In Olefsky, Taylor and LeRoith (eds): Diabetes Mellitus, Second Edition, Lippincott Williams & Wilkins, New York, 1994, pp. 797-803.

Authored Books

Magner J. Chess Juggler: Balancing Career, Family and Chess in the Modern World. Russell Enterprises, Milford, CT, 2011.

Appendix D

Selected Articles

Woods Hole Abstract

My academic advisor at University of Illinois, Judy Willis, informed me that there would be a Marine Ecology course given during the summer of 1972 at Woods Hole, Massachusetts that might be of interest to me. Dr. Ralph Wolfe at University of Illinois often taught in that course and supervised research projects there in view of his microbiology interests. I was accepted into the program to stay at Woods Hole that summer to attend the lectures and work on a research project for a few weeks with Anatol Eberhard and Ken Nealson, two experts in bacterial bioluminescence. As an Illinois-bred, landlocked, budding biologist, it would be a pleasure to spend time at the ocean – the likely cradle of life where a great diversity of life forms had appeared over billions of years.

The several instructors gave fascinating lectures, often completed later with a walk along a beach or tidal pool to provide real life illustrations. Note that the nineteenth century naturalist, Louis Agassiz, who spent time doing research at Woods Hole, famously directed his students to "Study nature, not books." Dr. Wolfe, for example, took our small class on an evening walk into a swampy area. Wearing high boots, he stepped out into the muck and by probing the muddy bottom with a stick, demonstrated how bubbles of gas could be released from the mud. Although the smell was bad, the biology was fascinating, as the gas was largely coming from methane-producing bacteria in the mud. Dr. Wolfe had published on the biochemistry and physiology of the methanoarchaea, and had developed means for cultivating these microorganisms in the lab.

In addition to lectures, each student tried to complete some aspect of a small research project during the summer. Nealson and Eberhard were interested in the biochemistry of bioluminescent bacteria, which could live freely under some circumstances, although often the bacteria were symbionts in partnership, so to speak, with larger animals. The bacteria were carried in nurturing small organs within the skin of fish or other marine animals that made use of their light-producing ability. When the number of bacteria growing in an organ reached an adequate level, the low-light production increased substantially by induction of the luciferase system, which made use of oxygen and biochemistry to produce light. Induction was due to the action of a chemical substance that accumulated in the liquid outside the growing bacteria, and the bacteria also in some cases needed to degrade any inhibitors in the surrounding liquid. Over millions of years natural selection operated on the marine animals such that light in these animal organs became a vital feature of signaling for mating, attracting prey, confusing predators or other purposes – recall that as one descends below the surface the majority of the vast volume of the ocean is in perpetual darkness.

Everything about working with bioluminescent bacteria was entirely new to me, but I easily reproduced the well-known phenomenon that ordinary seawater plated on agar – an appropriate growth medium with a marine level of salt grew up small colonies of bacteria that appeared as match-head-sized white fuzzy spots of the surface of the agar. The key point was that if one took the petri dish into a dark closet, one or two of the fifty or so bacterial colonies glowed eerily in the dark, producing their own light! These were "free-living strains" of bioluminescent bacteria, although it was possible that they were escaped symbionts. A caveat is that over the years there have been reports that fresh water sometimes contained bioluminescent bacteria, but that was controversial. Those observations have been attributed by some researchers to marine bacteria that over geologic time may have escaped and adapted to some extent to lower amounts of salt. The main thrust of my summer project was to grow freshwater isolates as well as marine bioluminescent bacteria each in a liquid medium, then collect the "conditioned media." Each conditioned medium should contain the molecular inducer secreted by that specific type of bacterium. I then started new liquid cultures of each type of bacterium at low density (no light production), and added back an amount of medium that had been conditioned by that type or a different type of bacterium to see if the inducer molecules would cross-react biologically to cause earlier than expected production of light (at relatively low bacterial density) by one or more types of bacteria. The many steps in a given experiment could not easily be stopped at a convenient point, so I found that I sometimes had to start an experiment at a very early hour, and then perform laboratory steps during many hours in order to get useful results – but it was fun, and the abstract describes the basic results. This was my first scientific abstract.

Since my summer experience in 1972 the field of bioluminescence has grown. Biochemically-produced light is now a useful tool in a number of biological models and assays, with light being used to report the occurrence and amount of a desired biochemical event.

Characterization of bioluminescent bacteria by studies of their inducers of luciferase synthesis. JAMES MAGNER, ANATOL EBERHARD AND KENNETH NEALSON.

In 1970, Mitchell and Hastings proposed on the basis of the decay kinetics of luciferases isolated from different strains of bacteria, that the luminous bacteria consist of two distinct groups, the free living and the symbiotic types. Eberhard, working with one strain of each group has shown that the luminous bacteria produce a small molecule which accumulates in the medium and results in induction of the synthesis of the luminescent system, and that the inducers produced by the two different strains did not cross react with respect to enzyme induction. We chose to examine this property of inducer cross reaction in order to determine whether it might be used as a tool for which to examine the relatedness of luminous bacteria. To do this, we chose two strains, one a local Woods Hole free living isolate, and one a purported freshwater luminous strain (*Vibrio albensis*) obtained from Scotland. The latter was of particular interest, as luminosity is thought to be a property which is confined to marine bacteria. With regard to this problem, it was found that *V. albensis* would grow on a medium with no sodium chloride, but that it's optimum of growth occurred at 3% salt, characteristic of other marine forms. With regard to the inducers of the strains, it was found that both the freshwater isolate from Woods Hole, and *V. albensis* produced an inducer which cross reacted unambiguously with the free living type (MAV). Since the inducers from the two types of bacteria differ in many other respects, it may be quite reasonable that they have evolved to be useful in separate niches, and that characterization of the bacteria by the type of inducer would be a good systematic approach to understanding their ecology.

Abstract from Magner, J. et al. 1972 Biol. Bull. 143: 469. Reprinted with permission from the Marine Biological Laboratory, Woods Hole, MA.

My First Important Scientific Publication

In the summer of 1980 I was budding with enthusiasm as I started work in Dr. Bruce Weintraub's laboratory at NIH as a major part of my endocrinology fellowship. Years earlier I had loved my undergraduate student laboratory experiences in Urbana, IL. During the summer between my junior and senior years of college I had gained a bit more experience by working in a research laboratory briefly in Woods Hole, Massachusetts; that summer project resulted in my first quite brief scientific abstract. I was hoping that with this experience under my belt that my work with thyroid-stimulating hormone (TSH) in Dr. Weintraub's lab would result in my first important scientific publication. And it did, but not without some challenges.

As requested by Dr. Weintraub, I undertook a project to attempt to isolate very early precursors of the α- and β-subunits of mouse TSH. From July through October, 1980 I made use of techniques new to me: a mouse transplantable tumor model that made TSH, pulse-chase radioactive labeling of tissues using ^{35}S-methionine, subcellular fractionation to isolate ribosomes hopefully still with attached TSH subunit precursor molecules, immunoprecipitation of the subunits, SDS-gel electrophoresis, and then analyses of the gels. Disconcertingly, through October all of my gels turned out blank. I tried adding a drug, puromycin, that might keep the nascent protein chains from running off the ribosomes. We also tried using specific antisera to denatured TSH α- and β-subunits because the very early proteins might not yet have folded properly, but to no avail. There were dozens of potential reasons why my experiments were not working, and I could not solve the issues.

So I raised the idea of shifting my project to the study of subunit precursors somewhat later during biosynthesis – the glycoproteins would then be properly folded, and might be in higher prevalence in the cells. Weintraub agreed, so I adjusted my subcellular fractionation technique to try to separate later subcellular compartments, such as rough endoplasmic reticulum (RER) from Golgi. But in November and December, 1980 these new efforts also resulted in blank gels! I reflected on potential technical issues and planned some experimental design adjustments for January, 1981. By good luck the tumor source that I used in January for my new type of experiment was rich enough in TSH production that the gels showed great data – prior failures apparently were because of tumors that made too small of a quantity of TSH.

Important background information is that as α-subunits are synthesized the protein portion first has one sugar chain added that raises the apparent molecular weight of α-subunits on a gel from 11K to 18K. Then during the next few minutes α-subunits have a second sugar chain added that further increases their weight from 18K to 21K. In contrast, the 11K β-subunits have only one sugar chain added making their final weight 18K. Note that a radioactive gel band at the 18K location theoretically could contain a mix of partially assembled α-subunits (one sugar chain) plus β-subunits (also one sugar chain), whereas a 21K gel band can only represent α-subunits.

But there is another important detail about this publication other than having used fortuitously a richer source of TSH subunits. As I had pondered the design of the January experiment, I realized that if I tried a novel sequence of use of the antisera for immunoprecipitation of the subunits I might be able to get some very unique cell biology data. I decided to reverse the routine order of the antisera – the routine order Weintraub always had used for years, and that he had prescribed for me. I postulated that my reversal might detect quantitatively the gradual combination of the TSH subunits over time during the pule-chase tissue incubation. Let me explain why.

The α-subunit was known to come from a different gene than did the β-subunit, the RNAs of the two subunits were transcribed separately, and the two subunits presumably combined later somewhere in the cell. It was also known that the tumor cells commonly synthesized limiting amounts of β-subunits with an excess of α-subunits. One can represent the still free as well as the combined TSH subunits present in a given cell compartment sample (such as a sample of RER at an early time of labeling) diagrammatically like this: (α α α α α α αβ β β β). In this depiction at an early time of synthesis, there are 7 uncombined α-subunits, there is one intact TSH molecule having both an α- and a β-subunit, and there are also 3 uncombined β-subunits. If the anti-α antiserum is used first in the routine manner, followed later by the anti-β antiserum, the radioactively labeled molecules captured sequentially by the two antisera will have been sorted into two groupings for later analysis, as follows:

(1) Anti-α yields this: (α   α   α   α   α   α   α   αβ)

(2) Then use of the supernatant later with anti-β gives a sample containing the following: (β   β   β)

Note that in illustration (1) a single β-subunit is depicted being co-precipitated with all the other α-subunits, since in an intact TSH molecule one β-subunit is hydrogen bonded to one α-subunit. The highly specific anti-α serum is not making a mistake; the serum is bringing along a β-subunit as the serum correctly binds to an α-subunit in an intact TSH molecule. Subsequent use of the anti-β serum on that supernatant then isolates any left-over subunits as shown in (2). These are simply all the remaining β-subunits, and there are no α-subunits remaining in the specimen to be brought along with any of those β-subunits. Recall that a mature α-subunit (weight 21K) is heavier than a β-subunit (weight 18K), meaning that mature α-subunits can be distinguished from β-subunits on SDS gels, whereas immature α-subunits (weight 18K) cannot be distinguished from β-subunits on these gels. So in the gel analysis of (1), the single β-subunit will be lost in the same gel band at 18K as any remaining immature α-subunits (18K). And some mature free α-subunits (weight 21K) that have never combined with a β-subunit will be mixed with the less common α-subunit (weight 21K) that had previously combined with a β-subunit. Thus, the problem with using the anti-α serum first on the specimen is that during the gel analyses of the final specimens with all subunits denatured to allow standard gel migrations (all subunits are freed, with no subunits sticking together any longer), the amount of in vivo combination of TSH subunits originally present in the cell compartment will be obscured.

Reversing the order of antisera use in the original cell sample (α   α   α   α   α   α   α   αβ   β   β   β) will sort the molecules differently, however, and in a much more valuable manner, as follows:

(1) Anti-β yields this: (αβ   β   β   β)

(2) Then use of the supernatant later with anti-α gives a sample containing only α-subunits that had originally been in the cell compartment as free α-subunits, as follows: (α   α   α   α   α   α   α)

Note that by changing the order of the antisera and sorting the radioactive molecules differently, every α-subunit (weight 21K) present in (1) is known to have been bound to a β-subunit (weight 18K) in an intact TSH molecule. The SDS gel analysis of (1) will have a peak of easily visible heavy α-subunits and of lighter β-subunits, and it is certain that every α-subunit had once been bound to a β-subunit. Of crucial importance, the 21K peak can only represent α-subunits that had been previously combined with a β-subunit! That 21K peak cannot be contaminated with mature but free α-subunits that had never previously combined with β-subunits. During a pulse-chase experiment, the 21K gel peak of α-subunits that had been immunoprecipitated by "grabbing their β-subunit handles" will be seen to gradually increase in a quantitative manner with time reflecting ongoing combination in the cells of α- with β-subunits. Specimen (2), on the other hand, will allow an analysis of just pure free α-subunits as a footnote to the experiment, merely for completeness.

This reversal of order of the antisera was a crucial idea, and proved to be the icing on the cake once I had obtained in January labeled tissue that actually contained a sufficient quantity of subunits to analyze. The experiment provided novel insights about the timing and subcellular location of the combination of the α- and β-subunits into intact TSH during biosynthesis.

There is a final personal story about this experiment. I had struggled from July through mid-January with no useful experimental results to show for my efforts. In mid-January I performed the pulse-chase radioactive labeling of the new batch of tumor tissue, ran the ultracentrifugation steps to get the subcellular cell compartments, completed the serial immunoprecipitation steps on the subcellular fractions, loaded the priceless final specimens onto the SDS gel (on January 22), turned on the electric current and went home with great anticipation to acquire the completed SDS gel in the morning. And very early on January 23 my wife went into labor with our first child! In spite of her labor, letting my specimens be lost by failing to retrieve the gel in time off the machine was not an option. Fortunately for me, Glenda understood the situation, and she allowed me to run to the lab to retrieve my specimens, then we went to the hospital to have the baby. All of the key data in this paper (Figs 1, 2, and 3) would have been lost if I had not retrieved that gel.

Free to Decide

THE JOURNAL OF BIOLOGICAL CHEMISTRY
Vol. 257, No. 12, Issue of June 25, pp. 6709–6715, 1982
Printed in U.S.A.

Thyroid-stimulating Hormone Subunit Processing and Combination in Microsomal Subfractions of Mouse Pituitary Tumor*

(Received for publication, December 17, 1981)

James A. Magner and Bruce D. Weintraub

From the Clinical Endocrinology Branch, National Institute of Arthritis, Diabetes, and Digestive and Kidney Diseases, National Institutes of Health, Bethesda, Maryland 20205

Mouse pituitary thyrotropic tumor minces were labeled with [^{35}S]methionine and fractionated into rough microsomes, intermediate, and low density smooth microsomes. Thyroid-stimulating hormone subunits were mainly in rough microsomes after a 10-min pulse, but with increasing chase times the proportion in smooth microsomes increased. In rough microsomes, small amounts of an α subunit precursor of M_r = 11,000 and larger amounts of an α form of M_r = 18,000 were rapidly processed to a form of M_r = 21,000, while small amounts of a β subunit precursor of M_r = 11,000 were processed to a form of M_r = 18,000. Most of the M_r = 18,000 and M_r = 21,000 subunit forms were converted by endoglycosidase H to forms of M_r = 11,000 to 12,000. Small amounts of endoglycosidase H-resistant forms appeared in low density smooth microsomes after a 30-min chase. Subunit combination was not detected at 10 min; combination was first detected at 20 min and increased progressively to a maximum of 61% of β in the low density smooth microsomes at 60 min of chase. Although α of M_r = 11,000 and 18,000, and β of M_r = 11,000, were not detected in thyroid-stimulating hormone, both endoglycosidase H-sensitive and -resistant α subunit of M_r = 21,000 and β subunit of M_r = 18,000 were found combined. Thus, the rough endoplasmic reticulum (ER) contains only small amounts of nonglycosylated subunits (M_r = 11,000). The major subunit precursors contain one high mannose oligosaccharide (M_r = 18,000), with a second unit being added only to α in the rough ER. Combination of α (M_r = 21,000) with β (M_r = 18,000) begins in the rough ER but occurs predominantly in the smooth ER/Golgi. Oligosaccharides of both combined and uncombined subunits are processed from high mannose to complex forms predominantly in the smooth ER/Golgi.

Recent studies of thyroid-stimulating hormone biosynthesis in cell-free systems (1–5) have indicated that nonglycosylated and uncombined α and β pre-subunits are synthesized from separate messenger RNAs. In intact cells, glycosylation precedes, and appears necessary for α-β subunit combination (6), but the intracellular sites of carbohydrate processing, subunit combination, and the relationship of these events were previously unknown for TSH[1] or any glycoprotein hormone. In the present study, we have applied subcellular fractionation techniques to define these sites in cells synthesizing TSH, and have employed the enzyme endoglycosidase H to characterize the nature of the carbohydrate moieties of both combined and uncombined subunits immunoprecipitated from various fractions. We propose a model that may be generally applicable to TSH and gonadotropin biosynthesis.

MATERIALS AND METHODS

Mouse pituitary thyrotropic tumors were induced and transplanted as previously described (7). One to four tumors (average tumor = 3 g) were minced to 1- to 2-mm pieces with steel scalpel blades, and preincubated for 30 min at 37 °C in moist 5% CO_2, 95% air in sterile tubes containing methionine-free and serum-free Dulbecco's Modified Eagles Medium, supplemented with 10 mM 4-(2-hydroxyethyl)-1-piperazineethanesulfonic acid, 2 mM glutamine. In continuous labeling experiments, tumor minces were incubated for either 10 min or 60 min after addition of 500 μCi/ml of L-[^{35}S]methionine (Amersham/Searle, 800 to 1,200 Ci/mmol). Incubations were terminated by chilling on ice. Alternatively, tumor minces were incubated for 20 min after addition of 200 μCi/ml of [^{35}S]methionine, followed by incubations of 0 min, 10 min, 30 min, or 60 min after addition of excess unlabeled methionine to a final concentration of 0.01% (w/v). Incubations were terminated by adding additional chase media chilled to 0 °C. Tumor minces were centrifuged at 500 × g for 3 min at 4 °C, washed once, and then resuspended in small volumes of ice-cold 0.6 M sucrose in water. After 10 strokes of a Dounce glass homogenizer, the homogenates were centrifuged at 1,000 × g for 10 min at 4 °C. The supernatants were centrifuged at 10,000 × g for 15 min at 4 °C, and the 10,000 × g supernatants were applied to top-loaded sucrose step gradients consisting of 5 ml of 2.0 M sucrose, 10 ml of 1.35 M sucrose, 10 ml of 0.86 M sucrose, and then 10 ml of specimen in 0.6 M sucrose. Similar gradients have been used by others for subfractionation of liver and other tissues (8–13). After centrifugation in an SW27 rotor at 75,000 × g for 9 h at 4 °C, three visible bands formed near interfaces 2.0 M/1.35 M, 1.35 M/0.86 M, and 0.86 M/0.6 M sucrose which we have termed the heavy, intermediate, and light fractions, respectively. Visible bands were transferred to fresh cellulose nitrate SW27 rotor tubes, and diluted dropwise with ice-cold 0.15 M Tris-HCl buffer, pH 8.0, to remove proteins nonspecifically adherent to the microsomal vesicles (14). Vesicles were pelleted at 75,000 × g for 90 min at 4 °C and aliquots were either fixed for electron microscopy or lysed for further study.

EM was performed by Dr. Bernhard Kramarsky (Electronucleonics, Inc., Columbia, MD). Specimens were fixed in 2.5% glutaraldehyde in a 0.2 M sodium cacodylate buffer at pH 7.4 for 1 h at 4 °C, and then rinsed with excess cacodylate buffer. After pelleting at 100,000 × g for 1 h, specimens were incubated for 30 min at 4 °C in 1% tannic acid in cacodylate buffer, and then post-fixed with Dalton's chrome-osmium for 1 h, followed by incubation in 1% aqueous uranyl acetate for 1 h. Low viscosity epoxy resin (NC 1010, Polaron Co., Lexington, PA) was used for embedding. Sections were made with an Ultratome III (LKB), placed on 300-mesh copper grids, stained with uranyl acetate and lead citrate, and viewed with a Siemens Elmiskop 1 A. EM of vesicles in sucrose gradient fractions revealed ratios of rough to smooth ER/Golgi[2] vesicles of > 90:10 for the heavy, < 20:80 for the

---

* The costs of publication of this article were defrayed in part by the payment of page charges. This article must therefore be hereby marked "*advertisement*" in accordance with 18 U.S.C. Section 1734 solely to indicate this fact.

[1] The abbreviations used are: TSH, thyroid-stimulating hormone; CG, choriogonadotropin; LH, luteinizing hormone; ER, endoplasmic reticulum; SDS, sodium dodecyl sulfate; EM, electron microscopy.

[2] No effort was made to distinguish smooth ER from Golgi vesicles. Enzyme markers may not be specific in this distinction in thyrotropic cells (see "Discussion").

intermediate, and < 10:90 for the light density fraction, in agreement with results for other tissues (9–13).

Portions of pellets not destined for EM were resuspended in a few milliliters of buffer containing 0.15 M sodium chloride, 0.02 M Tris-HCl, 0.01 M EDTA, 1% (w/v) Triton X-100, and 100 units/ml of aprotinin, pH 7.6. Solubilized radioactivity was precipitated with rabbit anti-bovine LH-α, anti-bovine TSH-β, and nonimmune serum as previously described (6), and then analyzed by SDS-polyacrylamide gel electrophoresis.

Subunits immunoprecipitated from certain fractions were pooled in order to ensure adequate substrate, and then each specimen was divided into equal 0.018-ml portions for incubation either with or without endoglycosidase H (provided by Dr. Frank Maley, New York State Dept. of Health, Albany). Subunits were initially present in an elution buffer containing 0.1 M Tris, 0.02 M EDTA, 0.01% (w/v) Bromphenol blue, 0.7 M sucrose, 1% (w/v) SDS, 5% (w/v) 2-mercaptoethanol, pH 9.5. To each 0.018-ml specimen was added 0.036 ml of 0.3 M citrate, pH 5.5. Then 0.0225 ml of 0.1 M citrate buffer containing 2 mM phenylmethylsulfonyl fluoride, 100 units/ml of aprotinin, pH 5.5, with or without 10 mIU of endoglycosidase H, was added to the specimens, followed by an incubation at 37 °C for 16 h.

Subunits were analyzed by electrophoresis in SDS-polyacrylamide slab gels using a 5% polyacrylamide stacking gel (1 cm) and a 12 to 20% linear gradient resolving gel (9 cm) as previously described (4). The following protein standards (2 to 5 μg each obtained from Calbiochem or Sigma) were mixed with each sample immediately prior to gel electrophoresis to serve as internal molecular weight markers: carbonic anhydrase (29,000), soybean trypsin inhibitor

(20,000), myoglobin (17,000), and cytochrome c (12,000). Coomassie brilliant blue (Eastman)-stained gels were sliced into 1- or 2-mm sections, solubilized, and counted in 10 ml of a toluene-based, detergent-containing solution (Ultrafluor, National Diagnostics) as previously described (6). All data have been corrected for radioactive decay.

RESULTS

Data from a continuous labeling experiment are shown in Fig. 1. Microsomal vesicles from the light fraction contained proportionately more radioactivity after 60 min compared to 10 min. Small amounts of an α species of $M_r = 11,000$ and larger amounts of α forms of $M_r = 18,000$ and 21,000 were well defined at 10 min; by 60 min the α species of $M_r = 21,000$ predominated, and the $M_r = 11,000$ species was not detected. At 10 min a β species of $M_r = 18,000$, as well as a trace of a species of $M_r = 11,000$, were seen. At 60 min a species of $M_r = 21,000$ was also apparent in the anti-β precipitations; we have previously demonstrated by acid-dissociation techniques and confirmed in the present study that this radioactivity actually represents α subunit of $M_r = 21,000$ from intact TSH precipitated through its β subunit and then dissociated by heat and reduction prior to electrophoresis (6). The percentage of limiting β combined into intact TSH in each fraction

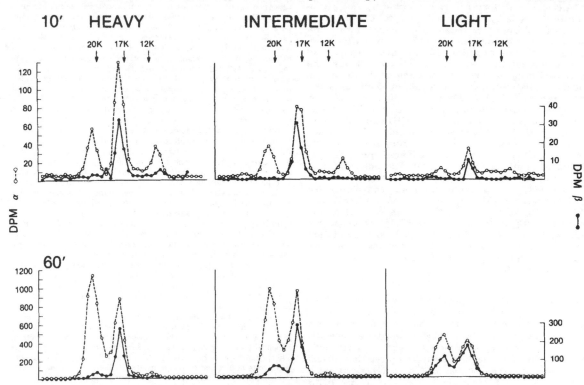

Fig. 1. **Immunoprecipitation of [35S]methionine-labeled TSH-α and TSH-β from sucrose step gradient fractions of continuously labeled thyrotropic tumor minces.** Tumor minces were continuously labeled for either 10 min or 60 min and homogenates were subfractionated as described under "Materials and Methods." Radioactivity immunoprecipitated by anti-bovine LH-α (*open circles*) and anti-bovine TSH-β (*closed circles*) from sucrose gradient fractions was analyzed by SDS-polyacrylamide gel electrophoresis. Gradient fractions from near interfaces 2.0 M/1.35 M, 1.35 M/0.86 M, and 0.86 M/0.6 M sucrose are designated heavy, intermediate, and light density fractions, respectively, and were enriched for rough ER (>90%), smooth ER/Golgi (>80%), and smooth ER/Golgi (>90%) vesicles, respectively. Internal molecular weight markers ($M_r = 12,000$–20,000) identified by Coomassie brilliant blue stain were included in each lane of slab gels and used to align figures. Radioactivity precipitated by nonimmune sera (not shown) was invariably at background levels as previously shown (6).

was calculated using a previously determined (6) α to β methionine ratio of 3 to 2. No β was combined with α in any fraction at 10 min, but at 60 min 10% of β subunits were combined with α in the heavy, 26% in the intermediate, and 41% in the light fraction. At 60 min the molar ratio of α:β was 7:1, 6:1, and 3:1 in these fractions, respectively.

In order to validate further the directional flow of radioactivity through these compartments, a pulse-chase labeling scheme was employed. Shown in Fig. 2 is the absolute radioactivity observed on gel lanes after immunoprecipitation of heavy, intermediate, and light sucrose fractions at each pulsechase time. As evidenced by the species of $M_r = 21,000$ precipitated by anti-β, some subunit combination (19%, see Table I) had already occurred at 20-min pulse, 0-min chase in the heavy fraction. After 60 min of chase the light fraction was a subcellular compartment highly enriched in combined subunits (61% of β subunits combined). The precursor-product relationship between α forms of $M_r = 18,000$ and $M_r = 21,000$ noted previously in unfractionated cells (6, 15) was evident.

Fig. 3 shows the percentage of distribution of various molecular weight varieties of α and β. With increasing chase time the percentage of subunits in the heavy fraction, the rough ER, declined, whereas the percentage of subunits in the light fraction, the smooth ER/Golgi, increased. Processing of α and

TABLE I
Calculated percentages of β subunit combined with α in gradient fractions

The species of $M_r = 21,000$ in an anti-β precipitation was used as an indicator of subunit combination (see text). The ratio of the methionine content of α:β is 3:2. The percentage of β combined with α was calculated for each fraction as follows:

$$\% \,\beta \text{ combined} = \frac{\text{dpm of } M_r = 21,000 \text{ species}}{3/2 \times \text{dpm of } M_r = 18,000 \text{ species}} \times 100\%$$

	β subunit in intact TSH				
	10 min, 0 min	20 min, 0 min	20 min, 10 min	20 min, 30 min	20 min, 60 min
			%		
Heavy	0	19	21	42	43
Intermediate	0	12	13	19	24
Light	0	18	24	41	61

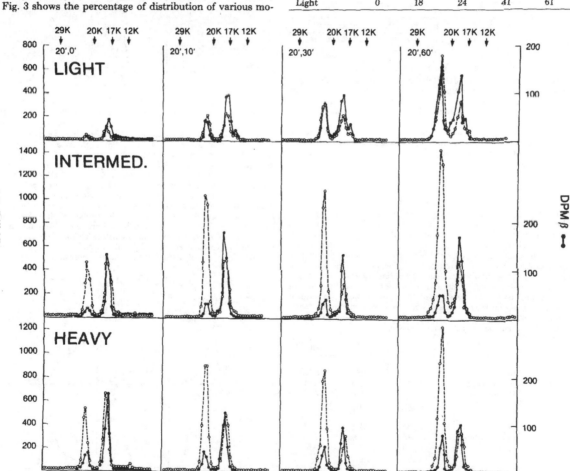

FIG. 2. **Immunoprecipitation of [³⁵S]methionine-labeled TSH-α and TSH-β from sucrose step gradient fractions of thyrotropic tumor minces labeled in pulse-chase fashion.** Tumor minces were pulse-labeled for 20 min followed by a chase of 30,000-fold excess unlabeled methionine for 0 min, 10 min, 30 min, or 60 min, and homogenates were subfractionated as described under "Materials and Methods." Radioactivity immunoprecipitated by antibovine LH-α (*open circles*) and anti-bovine TSH-β (*closed circles*) from sucrose gradient frations enriched in rough ER (*HEAVY*), smooth ER/Golgi (*INTERMED.*), and smooth ER/Golgi (*LIGHT*), was analyzed by SDS-polyacrylamide gel electrophoresis.

Subcellular Sites of TSH Subunit Processing and Combination

β precursors to higher molecular weight forms was noted in the heavy fraction. It was of interest that β subunits appeared to be chased toward the light fraction more rapidly than α. The calculated α/β molar ratios at various chase times in heavy, intermediate, and light density fractions are listed in Table II.

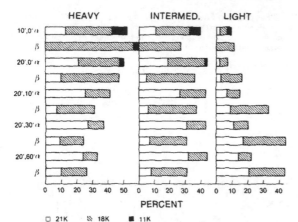

FIG. 3. **Percentage of distribution in microsomal fractions of various molecular weight varieties of TSH-α and TSH-β.** The sum of radioactivity of TSH-α or TSH-β subunits in the three microsomal fractions at a given labeling time was normalized to 100%. The first time designation (10 min or 20 min) indicates the minutes that tumor minces were pulse-labeled. The second time designation indicates the chase incubation time with excess unlabeled methionine. The species of M_r = 21,000 precipitated by anti-β is TSH-α originally in intact TSH.

TABLE II

Molar ratio of α/β in each subfraction

Total α (M_r = 21,000 + 18,000 + 11,000) and β (M_r = 18,000 + 11,000) radioactivity on gel lanes derived from Fig. 2 was used to calculate the molar ratio of subunits in each microsomal subfraction at various chase times after a 20-min pulse. This calculation (2/3 α dpm + β dpm) was based on the relative methionine content of subunits (α/β = 3/2) as determined in previous studies (6). Total radioactivity of both subunits increased during the chase as noted in previous studies (6, 25); this may reflect delayed equilibration of intracellular methionine specific activity and completion of nascent chains initiated during the pulse. There was no evidence for degradation of either subunit during the chase, which would have been reflected in a decrease in total radioactivity.

Chase	Subfraction	α	β	α/β molar ratio
min		*dpm*		
0	Light	565.	165.	2.28
0	Intermediate	3,707.	391.	6.31
0	Heavy	4,265.	464.	6.12
		8,537.	1,020.	
10	Light	1,790.	378.	3.15
10	Intermediate	5,346.	496.	7.18
10	Heavy	5,085.	383.	8.84
		12,221.	1,257.	
30	Light	2,164.	416.	3.46
30	Intermediate	4,576.	374.	8.15
30	Heavy	3,986.	228.	11.64
		10,726.	1,018.	
60	Light	3,896.	553.	4.69
60	Intermediate	7,521.	546.	9.17
60	Heavy	5,717.	378.	10.07
		17,134.	1,477.	

Subunits immunoprecipitated from certain fractions were incubated either with or without endoglycosidase H, an enzyme which cleaves the bond between the two proximal *N*-acetylglucosamines of precursor high mannose oligosaccha-

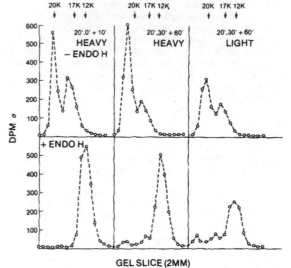

FIG. 4. **Endoglycosidase H sensitivity of TSH-α subunits.** [³⁵S]Methionine-labeled TSH-α subunits were immunoprecipitated from sucrose gradient fractions and several specimens were pooled to ensure adequate substrate; the designation *Light 20',30'+60'* indicates that subunits immunoprecipitated by anti-bovine LH-α from the gradient fraction near the 0.86 M/0.6 M sucrose interface (enriched in smooth ER/Golgi) after tumor slices had been pulse-labeled for 20 min followed by a chase incubation of 30 min, were pooled with subunits from that gradient fraction after a 20-min pulse and 60-min chase. Thus, sensitivity to the enzyme was compared for subunits from rough ER at early times, rough ER at relatively late times, and smooth ER/Golgi at relatively late times. Each of the three specimens was equally divided, and incubated either with (*bottom*) or without (*top*) endoglycosidase H (*ENDO H*). Incubation products were then analyzed by SDS-polyacrylamide gel electrophoresis.

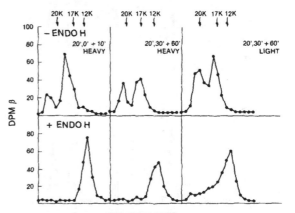

FIG. 5. **Endoglycosidase H sensitivity of TSH subunits immunoprecipitated from microsomal fractions by anti-bovine TSH-β.** [³⁵S]Methionine-labeled subunits of TSH were immunoprecipitated from sucrose gradient fractions by anti-bovine TSH-β. Specimens were pooled in the same manner as described for Fig. 4, equally divided, and incubated with (*bottom*) or without (*top*) endoglycosidase H (*ENDO H*). Incubation products were then analyzed by SDS-polyacrylamide gel electrophoresis.

The Journal of Biological Chemistry

rides but not of mature complex oligosaccharides (16). α subunit sensitivity to endoglycosidase H is illustrated in Fig. 4. All α subunits in the heavy fractions at early times were endoglycosidase H-sensitive; both α species of $M_r = 18,000$ and 21,000 were shifted to a species of $M_r = 11,000$, consistent with the weight of protein core subunit plus one or two N-acetylglucosamines. By 30 to 60 min of chase, 13% of α subunits were endoglycosidase H-resistant in the heavy fractions, and 28% were endoglycosidase H-resistant in the light fractions. In the analogous experiment using pooled radioactivity from anti-β precipitations (Fig. 5), species of $M_r = 21,000$ in the control incubations represented α subunit from intact TSH. All combined α, as well as combined and uncombined β subunits, in the heavy fractions were sensitive to endoglycosidase H. In the pooled light fractions from 30- and 60-min chases, a definite shoulder representing resistant forms was apparent. Of α subunits from intact TSH in this fraction, 78% were not yet processed to resistant mature oligosaccharides.

DISCUSSION

The mouse pituitary thyrotropic tumor is a useful model system for studying the biosynthesis of the glycoprotein hormone TSH. As has been described elsewhere (7), radiothyroidectomized LAF female mice develop neoplasms of pituitary thyrotrophs which can be transplanted subcutaneously into other hypothyroid recipients. In the resulting benign tumors as much as one-third of the protein synthesized is TSH subunits (4); in the present studies TSH subunits comprised about 15% of the protein synthesized (data not shown). The tumors have been shown to have morphologic and biochemical features as well as endocrine responsiveness similar to non-neoplastic, stimulated thyrotrophs (17).

The α subunit of bovine (18) and mouse (19) TSH contains 96 amino acids and has two complex-type oligosaccharides linked to asparagines 56 and 82; the 113-amino acid bovine TSH β subunit has one complex-type oligosaccharide linked to asparagine 23 (18). In the intact cell (6), nonglycosylated presubunits, which are seen in cell-free synthesis (1–5), are not detected due to rapid co-translational cleavage of the signal peptide, but glycosylated forms are detected including α of $M_r = 18,000$ and 21,000 (for which a precursor-product relationship has been demonstrated), and a β form of $M_r = 18,000$. Because the relative incorporation of labeled sugars into the two α subunit forms differed, these species were believed to reflect post-translational modifications of carbohydrate moieties (6). However, the intracellular sites of subunit precursor processing and combination were unknown.

In the current studies, tissue minces rather than enzyme-dispersed cells were employed in order to avoid possible enzyme-induced changes in membrane densities that might have affected the subcellular fractionation. Since central necrosis of clumps of cells was theoretically possible during prolonged incubations, these studies focused on early processing events in microsomal subfractions. One drawback of using the relatively short chase times was that labeled subunits were not completely chased out of any compartment. As shown in Fig. 3, at 20-min pulse, 60-min chase, 33% of α subunit precursors and 26% of β subunit precursors remained in the rough ER. Weintraub and Stannard[3] have demonstrated that about 50% of labeled subunits remain within thyrotropic tumor-dispersed cells even after an 18-h chase period, and that most subunits in whole cell lysates, as well as virtually all in the media, at that late time have endoglycosidase H-resistant carbohydrate.

It was not possible to reliably distinguish vesicles of smooth ER from Golgi vesicles by morphology, and the notation "smooth ER/Golgi" was adopted to designate components enriched in the light and intermediate density sucrose fractions. However, since EM of intact tumor cells disclosed very little identifiable smooth ER, most smooth vesicles in our fractions probably were derived from Golgi. The adequacy of a subfractionation method may, in general, be assessed by morphological and/or enzyme markers. EM of vesicles from microsomal fractions at gradient interfaces 1.35 M/2.0 M, 0.86 M/1.35 M, and 0.6 M/0.86 M revealed ratios of rough:smooth/Golgi vesicles of > 90:10, < 20:80, and < 10:90, respectively. Thus, our method was deemed adequate on morphologic grounds in that there was only about 10% cross-contamination between the extreme sucrose fractions; the intermediate fraction was enriched in smooth ER/Golgi, but was more contaminated with rough ER than the light fraction. We chose not to employ enzyme markers as a measure of adequacy of separation in these initial studies because of serious questions regarding the specificity of such markers in thyrotropic (20) as well as other (21–24) cells. Moreover, the sequential flow of radioactivity (Fig. 3) from the heavy, through the intermediate, and to the light fraction during pulse-chase experiments was consistent with the assigned identities.

The yield of subunits for analysis was about 10%, as determined by immunoprecipitation of various preparative fractions by Dr. Suzanne Rowgacz in our laboratory.[4] Because gentle homogenization was necessary to preserve microsomal vesicles, 50% (range 40–65%) of immunoprecipitable subunits (data not shown) were lost in preparation of the 10,000 × g supernatant. Another 30% of subunits were lost by the washing effect of the step gradient, and 10% were lost in the Tris buffer wash which was necessary to ensure removal of nonspecifically adsorbed proteins. However, there was no evidence of differential recovery of subunits at different chase times.

Our data suggest that separate forms of α and β subunit precursors are rapidly and probably co-translationally glycosylated with one high mannose unit in the rough ER. This initial glycosylation produces α and β subunit precursors of $M_r = 18,000$. Co-translational glycosylation, *i.e.* covalent addition of carbohydrate to nascent proteins still attached to ribosomes, is not proven by the current studies, but is likely for TSH subunit precursors since prior studies (6, 25) of unfractionated thyrotrophs have demonstrated that the precursors of $M_r = 18,000$ predominate after pulse times as short as 1 min. Co-translational glycosylation has been well demonstrated in other biosynthetic systems (26–29). The small amounts of precursors of $M_r = 11,000$ are likely to represent unglycosylated core protein because in prior studies (6) forms of $M_r = 11,000$ predominated in whole cell lysates and media when thyrotrophs were incubated with tunicamycin, a substance which prevents the *en bloc* glycosylation of proteins at asparagine sites. Moreover, the conversion of precursors of $M_r = 18,000$ to forms of $M_r = 11,000$–12,000 (Figs. 4 and 5) by endoglycosidase H is consistent with this scheme. TSH subunit precursors of $M_r = 11,000$ were better detected in the present experiments than in past studies because we had enriched for very early forms in the heavy density sucrose fractions; these forms were detected predominantly in the rough ER at early chase times, and may represent nascent chains that had not yet been glycosylated.

Furthermore, our data suggest that the rough ER is also the site of the post-translational addition of a second high mannose unit to the α subunit precursor of $M_r = 18,000$; this glycosylation, probably at the asparagine at position 82 near the carboxyl terminus, results in an endoglycosidase H-sensi-

---

[3] B. Weintraub and B. Stannard, unpublished results.

[4] S. Rowgacz, J. Magner, and B. Weintraub, unpublished results.

tive α form of M_r = 21,000. The quantal precursor-product relationship between α forms of M_r = 18,000 and 21,000 was again demonstrated in the present studies. The post-translational nature of this conversion is suggested by the gradual predominance of the heavy form during 5- to 10-min chase periods in prior studies of unfractionated cells (6, 25), and the quantal nature of the shift in molecular weight is consistent with the proposed *en bloc* glycosylation. This tentative identification of α subunit precursors of M_r = 18,000 as being glycosylated at one site, and α precursors of M_r = 21,000 as being glycosylated at two sites is also consistent with the finding that both forms reverted to apparently the same form of M_r = 11,000–12,000 after incubation with endoglycosidase H, a weight consistent with the protein core subunit plus one or two N-acetylglucosamines.

Our fractionation techniques revealed an increase in subunits with complex-type, endoglycosidase H-resistant carbohydrate in the smooth ER/Golgi (Figs. 4 and 5). At the longest chase time employed, only 22% of α subunits in the light fraction had become endoglycosidase H-resistant. Experiments in our laboratory[3] have demonstrated that virtually all secreted TSH, as well as secreted free α subunit, is endoglycosidase H-resistant. Use of dispersed cells, longer chase times, and analysis of secretory granule as well as plasma membrane fractions may clarify whether processing of carbohydrate is completed prior to secretion within the Golgi, as opposed to post-Golgi compartments. We find that subunit precursors processed from endoglycosidase H-sensitive to resistant forms exhibit little change in their apparent molecular weights on SDS-polyacrylamide gels; thus, there appear to be two different forms of α of M_r = 21,000, one endoglycosidase H-sensitive and one resistant. Similarly, there are two varieties of β of M_r = 18,000, one endoglycosidase H-sensitive and one resistant. We also recognize that microheterogeneity of carbohydrate due to trimming or addition of residues is likely within each class.

The prevalence of subunit combination in each microsomal fraction at each chase time was determined by use of a specific anti-TSH β, which has been shown to have less than 1% cross-reactivity with the α subunit (6). Since there is no form of β of M_r = 21,000, that peak of radioactivity in gels of anti-β precipitates represented α subunit of M_r = 21,000 from intact TSH that had been precipitated through the β subunit; the α and β subunits were dissociated by heat and reduction prior to electrophoresis. Using whole cell lysates, acid-dissociation experiments as well as cross-precipitation experiments which employed first anti-β sera and then anti-α sera (6) have shown this species of M_r = 21,000 to be α. It was again proven in microsomal fractions (data not shown) that prior acid-dissociation of TSH into separate α and β subunits specifically abolished the appearance of the species of M_r = 21,000 in anti-β precipitations.

α forms of M_r = 21,000 of both endoglycosidase H-sensitive and -resistant varieties, as well as β forms of M_r = 18,000 of both sensitive and resistant varieties, were observed in intact TSH (Figs. 4 and 5). However, α precursors of M_r = 11,000 and 18,000 were not observed combined in TSH. Combination of high mannose forms of α of M_r = 21,000 with β of M_r = 18,000 begins in the rough ER and continues in the smooth ER, Golgi, and post-Golgi compartments, where carbohydrate processing of combined and uncombined subunits is completed; attainment of endoglycosidase H resistance (*i.e.* processed complex-type carbohydrate) is not a prerequisite for subunit combination. However, it is not possible to infer from the available data whether only certain variants of endoglycosidase H-sensitive forms may be capable of combining. Much carbohydrate processing, mainly trimming of glucose

and mannose residues may occur, yet such variants may remain endoglycosidase H-sensitive, as judged by studies in other glycoprotein systems (30). One might speculate that if the three oligosaccharides of TSH are processed from high mannose to complex forms in random order, several major subclasses of intracellular TSH might exist (α-complex, complex, β-high mannose, etc.), each with identical amino acid composition but differing in carbohydrate composition. In fact, heterogeneity of TSH has been observed (31–34), and in human (35) and whale (36) preparations these forms have been demonstrated to differ primarily in mannose content.

The present studies also provide insight into the intracellular transport of newly synthesized subunits. The α subunit precursor was produced in excess of the β subunit precursor. There was no evidence for significant amounts of degradation of either subunit. As seems clear from the relative shifts of radioactivity from heavy to light density sucrose fractions during the pulse-chase study (Fig. 3), free and combined β subunit precursors may move to the Golgi faster than free α subunit precursors. We speculate that the post-translational interaction of membrane-bound glycosylating enzymes with free α subunit precursors at the time of their second glycosylation retards the exit of α precursors from the rough ER compared to β precursors, which do not have a second high mannose unit added. Moreover, subunits which have combined in the rough ER seemed to move to the Golgi more rapidly than uncombined subunits.

Our model of TSH biosynthesis, depicted in Fig. 6, may be contrasted with that of Chin *et al.* (25), whose data derived from unfractionated cellular homogenates. Both laboratories have identified the same species of α and β subunits except for the small amounts of presumably nonglycosylated subunits of M_r = 11,000 which we noted primarily in the rough ER. However, the models differ in several major respects. First,

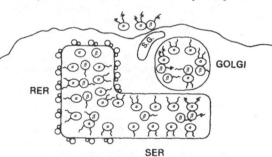

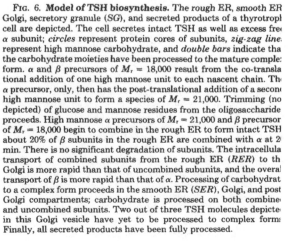

FIG. 6. **Model of TSH biosynthesis.** The rough ER, smooth ER, Golgi, secretory granule (*SG*), and secreted products of a thyrotroph cell are depicted. The cell secretes intact TSH as well as excess free α subunit; *circles* represent protein cores of subunits, *zig-zag lines* represent high mannose carbohydrate, and *double bars* indicate that the carbohydrate moieties have been processed to the mature complex form. α and β precursors of M_r = 18,000 result from the co-translational addition of one high mannose unit to each nascent chain. The α precursor, only, then has the post-translational addition of a second high mannose unit to form a species of M_r = 21,000. Trimming (not depicted) of glucose and mannose residues from the oligosaccharide proceeds. High mannose α precursors of M_r = 21,000 and β precursor of M_r = 18,000 begin to combine in the rough ER to form intact TSH; about 20% of β subunits in the rough ER are combined with α at 2 min. There is no significant degradation of subunits. The intracellular transport of combined subunits from the rough ER (*RER*) to the Golgi is more rapid than that of uncombined subunits, and the overall transport of β is more rapid than that of α. Processing of carbohydrate to a complex form proceeds in the smooth ER (*SER*), Golgi, and post-Golgi compartments; carbohydrate is processed on both combined and uncombined subunits. Two out of three TSH molecules depicted in this Golgi vesicle have yet to be processed to complex forms. Finally, all secreted products have been fully processed.

unlike Chin *et al.* we find no selective degradation of β subunits; we find α/β molar ratios > 1 in all fractions at all time points, resulting from increased α synthesis rather than β degradation (see Table II). Another difference between the models is that we find that endoglycosidase H-sensitive, high mannose forms of α and β begin to combine in the rough ER, whereas Chin *et al.* speculated that subunit combination did not occur until carbohydrate moieties were processed to a "mature" form in the Golgi. These workers first noted the sensitivity of TSH subunits to endoglycosidase H in unfractionated cell lysates at late times (37). Sensitivity to endoglycosidase H at late times has also been noted by Ruddon *et al.* for intracellular forms of human CG subunits (38, 39). These and other workers (40) observed no degradation of either human CG subunit. However, the sites of intracellular processing and combination were not addressed in any of these studies.

With respect to co-translational glycosylation and subsequent processing of carbohydrate moieties, our model is consistent with the general scheme proposed by others (41, 42). However, the apparent delayed addition of the second high mannose group to the α subunit is, to our knowledge, unusual for glycoproteins thus far studied. Also, the rate of processing of carbohydrate to complex forms is relatively slow as compared to systems such as vesicular stomatitis virus in which 70% of the coat glycoprotein is endoglycosidase H-resistant in about 60 min (43).

With respect to subunit combination, our model may be contrasted with those nonhormone glycoproteins which contain multiple subunits covalently linked by disulfide bonds. Studies employing tunicamycin have suggested that the co-translational assembly of subunits to form immunoglobulins (44–47), fibrinogen (48), haptoglobin (49), and procollagen (50, 51) is not impaired by the lack of asparagine-linked carbohydrate, although eventual secretion of nonglycosylated molecules is variably affected. On the contrary, at least the inner or "core" carbohydrate residues appear necessary for combination of TSH α and β (6). This may be related to the fact that the TSH subunits are not covalently linked and may require a specific conformation for subunit interaction that depends on glycosylation.

By applying subcellular fractionation techniques, we have been able to assign specific steps in mouse tumor TSH biosynthesis to specific microsomal locations. Although these studies should be extended to non-neoplastic cells, our current model may be generally applicable to TSH and gonadotropin biosynthesis, as well as to the biosynthesis of certain other glycoproteins containing noncovalently bound subunits.

REFERENCES

1. Chin, W. W., Habener, J. F., Kieffer, J. D., and Maloof, F. (1978) *J. Biol. Chem.* **253**, 7985–7988
2. Kourides, I. A., and Weintraub, B. D. (1979) *Proc. Natl. Acad. Sci. U. S. A.* **76**, 298–302
3. Vamvakopoulos, N. C., and Kourides, I. A. (1979) *Proc. Natl. Acad. Sci. U. S. A.* **76**, 3809–3813
4. Giudice, L. C., Waxdal, M. J., and Weintraub, B. D. (1979) *Proc. Natl. Acad. Sci. U. S. A.* **76**, 4798–4802
5. Giudice, L. C., and Weintraub, B. D. (1979) *J. Biol. Chem.* **254**, 12679–12683
6. Weintraub, B. D., Stannard, B. S., Linnekin, D., and Marshall, M. (1980) *J. Biol. Chem.* **255**, 5715–5723
7. Blackman, M. R., Gershengorn, M. C., and Weintraub, B. D. (1978) *Endocrinology* **102**, 499–508
8. Uhr, J. W., and Schenkein, I. (1970) *Proc. Natl. Acad. Sci. U. S. A.* **66**, 952–958
9. Eriksson, L. C., DePierre, J. W., and Dallner, G. (1978) *Pharmacol. Ther. Part A Chemother. Toxicol. Metab. Inhibitors* **2**, 281–317
10. Dallner, G. (1978) *Methods Enzymol.* **52**, 71–83
11. Ehrenreich, J. H., Bergeron, J. J. M., Siekevitz, P., and Palade, G. E. (1973) *J. Cell Biol.* **59**, 45–72
12. Bergeron, J. J. M., Borts, D., and Cruz, J. (1978) *J. Cell Biol.* **76**, 87–97
13. Tartakoff, A., and Vassalli, P. (1977) *J. Cell Biol.* **83**, 284–299
14. Autuori, F., Svensson, H., and Dallner, G. (1975) *J. Cell Biol.* **67**, 687–699
15. Weintraub, B. D., and Stannard, B. S. (1978) *FEBS Lett.* **92**, 303–307
16. Kobata, A. (1979) *Anal. Biochem.* **100**, 1–14
17. Marshall, M. C., Williams, D., and Weintraub, B. D. (1981) *Endocrinology* **108**, 908–915
18. Pierce, J. G., and Parsons, T. F. (1981) *Annu. Rev. Biochem.* **50**, 465–495
19. Chin, W. W., Kronenberg, H. M., Dee, P. C., Maloof, F., and Habener, J. F. (1981) *Proc. Natl. Acad. Sci. U. S. A.* **78**, 5329–5333
20. Pelletier, G., and Puviani, R. (1973) *J. Cell Biol.* **56**, 600–605
21. Andersson, G. N., and Eriksson, L. C. (1981) *J. Biol. Chem.* **256**, 9633–9639
22. Jarasch, E. D., Kartenbeck, J., Bruder, G., Fink, A., Marré, D. J., and Franke, W. W. (1979) *J. Cell Biol.* **80**, 37–52
23. Howell, K. E., Ito, A., and Palade, G. E. (1978) *J. Cell Biol.* **79**, 581–589
24. Ito, A., and Palade, G. E. (1978) *J. Cell Biol.* **79**, 590–597
25. Chin, W. W., Maloof, F., and Habener, J. F. (1981) *J. Biol. Chem.* **256**, 3059–3066
26. Kiely, M. L., McKnight, G. S., and Schimke, R. T. (1976) *J. Biol. Chem.* **251**, 5490–5495
27. Bergman, L. W., and Kuehl, W. M. (1977) *Biochemistry* **16**, 4490–4497
28. Bergman, L. W., and Kuehl, W. M. (1978) *Biochemistry* **17**, 5174–5180
29. Bergman, L. W., Harris, E., and Kuehl, W. M. (1981) *J. Biol. Chem.* **256**, 701–706
30. Ruddon, R. W., Bryan, A. H., Hanson, C. A., Perini, F., Ceccorulli, L. M., and Peters, B. P. (1981) *J. Biol. Chem.* **256**, 5189–5196
31. Shome, B. D., Brown, D. M., Howard, S. M., and Pierce, J. G. (1968) *Arch. Biochem. Biophys.* **126**, 456–466
32. Giudice, L. C., and Pierce, J. G. (1977) *Endocrinology* **101**, 776–781
33. Davy, K. M. M., Fawcett, J. S., and Morris, C. J. O. R. (1977) *Biochem. J.* **167**, 279–280
34. Yora, T., Matsuzaki, S., Kondo, Y., and Ui, N. (1979) *Endocrinology* **104**, 1682–1685
35. Jacobson, G., Roos, P., and Wide, L. (1977) *Biochim. Biophys. Acta* **490**, 403–410
36. Tamura-Takahasi, H., and Ui, N. (1976) *Endocrinol. Jpn.* **23**, 511–516
37. Chin, W. W., and Habener, J. F. (1981) *Endocrinology* **108**, 1628–1633
38. Ruddon, R. W., Hanson, C. A., and Addison, N. J. (1979) *Proc. Natl. Acad. Sci. U. S. A.* **76**, 5143–5147
39. Ruddon, R. W., Hanson, C. A., Bryan, A. H., Putterman, G. J., White, E. L., Perini, F., Meade, K. S., and Aldenderfer, P. H. (1980) *J. Biol. Chem.* **255**, 1000–1007
40. Dean, D. J., Weintraub, B. D., and Rosen, S. W. (1980) *Endocrinology* **106**, 849–858
41. Waechter, C. J., and Lennarz, W. J. (1976) *Annu. Rev. Biochem.* **45**, 95–112
42. Kornfeld, R., and Kornfeld, S. (1980) in *Glycoproteins and Proteoglycans* (Lennarz, W. J., ed) pp. 1–34, Plenum Press, New York
43. Tabas, I., Schlesinger, S., and Kornfeld, S. (1978) *J. Biol. Chem.* **253**, 716–722
44. Weitzman, S., and Scharff, M. D. (1976) *J. Mol. Biol.* **102**, 237–252
45. Hickman, S., and Kornfeld, S. (1978) *J. Immunol.* **121**, 990–996
46. Hickman, S., Kulczycki, A., Jr., Lynch, R. G., and Kornfeld, S. (1977) *J. Biol. Chem.* **252**, 4402–4408
47. Sidman, C. (1981) *J. Biol. Chem.* **256**, 9374–9376
48. Nickerson, J. M., and Fuller, G. M. (1981) *Proc. Natl. Acad. Sci. U. S. A.* **78**, 303–307
49. Haugen, T. H., Hanley, J. M., and Heath, E. C. (1981) *J. Biol. Chem.* **256**, 1055–1057
50. Duksin, D., and Bornstein, P. (1977) *J. Biol. Chem.* **252**, 955–962
51. Bornstein, P. (1980) in *Biology of Collagen* (Vüdik, A., and Vuust, J., eds) pp. 61–75, Academic Press, New York

Familial Generalized Resistance to Thyroid Hormone

During my endocrinology fellowship at the National Institutes of Health (1980-1983), my priorities were (1) develop basic science laboratory expertise and develop a resume that would support successful basic science grant applications in the thyroid field, (2) learn clinical endocrinology by seeing routine types of endocrinology patients, and (3) participate in clinical research as the opportunity might arise. Young physicians who are currently interested in endocrinology fellowship training need to realize that in the USA nearly all endocrine training programs are quite good for learning routine clinical endocrinology, but a fewer number can also offer an excellent basic science experience as well as clinical research experience, so one must carefully consider the details of what is offered by each program.

Priority (1) was achieved, but regarding (2), it is true that during those three years the variety and number of routine clinical patients that I saw were somewhat limited. There were exotic and rare cases, such as acromegaly, as these were drawn to the tertiary center. But the usual bread-and-butter cases that would commonly be seen by an endocrinologist in a medium-sized Midwest city, for example, were fewer than in many training programs. I supplemented my clinical learning by reading case reports and clinical textbooks of endocrinology, including several books like a wonderful short case book by Dr. Ernie Mazzaferri that I had seen during residency training. (Many years later when I took the job with Genzyme I met several times with Dr. Mazzaferri for Genzyme business. He was pleased to hear how my exposure to his practical case book, which he had written during his endocrinology fellowship, influenced my decision to go into endocrinology. He signed my yellowed and dog-eared copy.)

Regarding priority (3) clinical research, I naturally had an opportunity to see some unusual thyroid patients referred to the NIH, and I participated with Dr. Weintraub in his protocol for the clinical evaluation of three extended families with the genetic syndrome of resistance to thyroid hormone. Such patients generally presented to their local physicians with a few mild symptoms, a slightly enlarged thyroid gland, and some unusual thyroid blood tests that seemed not to make much sense at first. Dr. Weintraub's clinical protocol allowed affected patients and certain family members to be tested, and affected patients had a variety of thyroid-related clinical measurements made, including some old metabolic tests popular decades before but rarely used anymore in the 1980s, such as measurement of basal metabolic rate. In affected patients, some body tissues seemed to be in a mildly hyperthyroid state, whereas other tissues seemed to be in a mildly hypothyroid state. As I departed the NIH in 1983 for Chicago, Dr. Weintraub possessed several years of rather unique clinical data gathered by several people, but no one had the time or inclination to organize, carefully assess, and publish these disparate data. When Dr. Weintraub asked if I would do it, and offered me first-author status if I pulled it all together, I had to agree, even though I would be very busy in the next year setting up my own research laboratory and trying to start a career in Chicago. One simply must say yes to certain opportunities, and make the time to do the job.

My efforts resulted in a paper published in a European journal in 1986, which by then was my third year working in Chicago. Because of that publication, I was asked through the years to write short book chapters or give small talks about this topic, especially as the thyroid field became more interested with the discovery of mutations in the nuclear receptors for thyroid hormone that caused the several syndromes of resistance to thyroid hormone.

J. Endocrinol. Invest. 9: 459, 1986

Familial generalized resistance to thyroid hormones: report of three kindreds and correlation of patterns of affected tissues with the binding of [^{125}I] triiodothyronine to fibroblast nuclei

J.A. Magner, P. Petrick, M.M. Menezes-Ferreira, M. Stelling, and B.D. Weintraub

The Molecular, Cellular, and Nutritional Endocrinology Branch, National Institute of Arthritis, Diabetes, Digestive and Kidney Diseases, Bethesda, MD 20205 and Michael Reese Hospital, University of Chicago, Chicago, IL 60616, USA

ABSTRACT. We here report three kindreds with a total of 19 persons affected with central and peripheral resistance to thyroid hormones: one kindred with 10 affected persons is the largest reported to date. Male to male transmission of the syndrome was evident in two kindreds, consistent with an autosomal dominant mode of inheritance. During several years of follow up, the degree of resistance to thyroid hormones did not ameliorate. Within a given kindred, a given tissue or tissues was consistently more resistant to thyroid hormone than other tissues. The pattern of tissues most affected in one kindred differed from that of another kindred, perhaps reflecting the inherited underlying molecular defects. Members of kindred A frequently had bone involvement, and several had learning disabilities and recurring infections, while most members of kindreds B and C had little bone involvement, but marked hepatic and cardiac resistance to thyroid hormones. Kinetic studies of the binding of [^{125}I] triiodo-L-thyronine to nuclei from skin fibroblasts from affected patients from each of the kindreds demonstrated decreased maximum binding as compared to normal fibroblasts, but there was no correlation between this parameter and other features of the disease. Four of the 19 patients had previously been treated inappropriately with antithyroid therapies, demonstrating how the syndrome may be readily confused with Graves' disease by some clinicians. Behavior or school performance improved in all children treated with thyroid hormones, and a growth spurt was documented in six children, but objective improvement in IQ scores was not demonstrated, suggesting that initiation of hormone therapy at an early age may be important for maximum benefit.

INTRODUCTION

The syndrome of generalized thyroid hormone resistance, characterized by refractoriness to the action of endogenous and exogenous T_3 and T_4, was initially reported by Refetoff et al. (1) in two siblings in whom the peripheral thyroid hormone action suggested hypo- or euthyroidism despite elevated blood levels of free thyroid hormones. Subsequently, these patients were noted to have inappropriately normal or elevated TSH levels, consistent with pituitary resistance to thyroid hormones. These patients also had hearing impairment and stippled epiphyses, and an autosomal recessive mode of inheritance was postulated. Since then, other patients with generalized tissue resistance have been reported, some sporadic but most familial, with an autosomal dominant mode of inheritance with variable expression within a single family (2). These patients lack hearing impairment or stippled epiphyses. One variant of thyroid hormone resistance, initially described by Gershengorn and Weintraub (3) and confirmed in several subsequent reports (4), was selective pituitary resistance in which the patients had elevated thyroid hormone and TSH levels but with a peripheral hyperthyroid state. A single case of selective peripheral but not pituitary resistance was described by Kaplan et al. (5).

The molecular basis for these disorders is unknown, but is believed to involve one or more cellular defects in thyroid hormone action. Within a given patient, certain tissues appear to be more affected than others as judged by parameters of the peripheral action of thyroid hormones. Patients from a given kindred presumably have the same putative molecular defect. The study of large kindreds rather than families with only two or three affected members is vital, because it is only by evaluating many patients from a single kindred that one can assess whether the varying degree of resistance of

Key-words: Resistance to thyroid hormones, hormone resistance, triiodothyronine.

Correspondence: Dr. James Magner, Division of Endocrinology, Michael Reese Hospital, 31st Street and Lake Shore Drive, Chicago, IL 60616, USA.

Received February 25, 1986; accepted August 5, 1986.

459

J.A. Magner, P. Petrick, M.M. Menezes-Ferreira, et al.

several tissues represents a significant consistent pattern. Moreover, by comparing the clinical and biochemical features of patients from several large kindreds, one can ascertain whether the patterns of tissue resistance are the same or different, and also determine by *in vitro* studies whether the kindreds manifest the same or different molecular defect(s).

Because the interaction of thyroid hormone with its nuclear receptor is a major step in the mediation of thyroid hormone action, several authors have attempted to identify alterations of T_3 nuclear receptor binding in affected patients using either lymphocytes (6-13, 19) or cultured fibroblasts (7, 14-19).

The results of these equilibrium binding studies have been highly variable, but in general no consistent differences between cells from patients and cells from normal subjects were found. Recently, we demonstrated (20) that kinetic analysis for $[^{125}I]T_3$ nuclear uptake was a more powerful technique than equilibrium analysis for studies of fibroblasts from patients with generalized thyroid hormone resistance.

We now report our clinical and biochemical evaluations of members of three large kindreds with this syndrome, including one family with the largest number of affected members reported to date. We compare and contrast the patterns of tissue resistance observed for members of a given kindred, and also note that the kindreds differ as to which tissues are consistently most affected. Moreover, we correlate these clinical features with *in vitro* T_3 nuclear receptor binding studies of fibroblasts from these patients.

MATERIALS AND METHODS

Clinical Evaluation of Patients

Routine clinical, radiologic, nuclear medicine and laboratory studies were performed at the Clinical Center of the National Institutes of Health. Basal metabolic rate determinations were sometimes obtained at the Naval Medical Center, Bethesda, MD. Serum T_3, T_4, and TSH

concentrations were measured by previously described methods (3). Free T_4 (FT_4) and FT_3 concentrations in the serum were determined by equilibrium dialysis (Nichols Institute, San Pedro, CA). Sex hormone binding globulin (TEBG) was measured as previously described (21). Details of the tests used to measure thyroid hormone action in these subjects have been reported (16).

Binding Studies

Fibroblasts obtained from skin punch biopsy were cultured, and prepared for the binding assay as previously described (16). The kinetics of $[^{125}I]T_3$ nuclear uptake, and the nuclear binding of $[^{125}I]T_3$ at equilibrium were measured as previously reported (20). Fibroblasts from seventeen normal subjects, each of whom had normal serum T_3, T_4, FT_4, TSH and TRH test results, served as controls. Various binding parameters were derived or calculated as described (20); the kinetic binding studies yielded the maximum binding (B_{max}), the slope at the origin (λ), and the apparent association rate constant (k_{+1}), while the total number of receptors (Ro), and the equilibrium dissociation constant (K_d) were measured in the equilibrium binding studies.

RESULTS

Clinical Evaluations

Patient A IV 9, the propositus of kindred A (Fig. 1), is the product of a consanguineous marriage of first cousins, and has been previously reported in part (16). This white male had several episodes of pneumonia as a child, and at age 6 10/12 an elevated T_4 of 24.3 μg/dl, but absence of goiter, were noted. He was described as "hyperactive", with pulse 80-100/min. The thyroid enlarged to three times normal size during several months of therapy with propylthiouracil. The drug was discontinued, and resting pulses of 80 to 93/min were noted with T_4 level 17.9 μg/dl, FT_4 4.3 ng/dl, 24 h thyroidal radioiodine uptake 87%, basal TSH 7.0 μU/ml, TSH 30

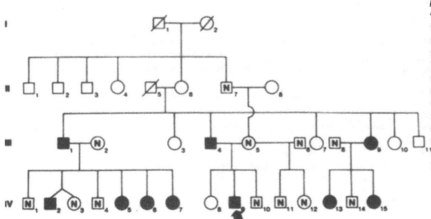

Fig. 1 - Kindred A. *Solid figures represent patients affected clinically and biochemically with peripheral and central resistance to thyroid hormones. In most instances elevated total and free thyroxine levels in serum, and inappropriate responses of TSH after administration of TRH were documented. Figures labeled with N represent persons evaluated clinically and biochemically, and found not to be affected with the syndrome. Open figures represent persons alive but not evaluated. Slashed figures represent deceased persons. With ten af-*[...]*transmission of the syndrome are evident,*[...]*only two other published kindreds (19, 22).*

min after 250 μg TRH 42.6 μU/ml, and thyroxine binding globulin (TBG) 26 μg/ml. The impression of peripheral and pituitary resistance to thyroid hormone was confirmed by other studies (Tables 1 and 2).

Family studies disclosed that nine additional kindred members were affected with the syndrome, and two instances of male to male transmission were detected, a pattern consistent with an autosomal dominant mode of inheritance.

The thyroid function studies and parameters of the peripheral action of thyroid hormone are given in Table 3. In all cases, TSH responded briskly to the intravenous administration of TRH in the face of elevated levels of free thyroid hormones, and free α-subunit levels (not shown) were not elevated out of proportion to TSH. Six cousins of the propositus were found to be affected. Patient AIV2, born April 7, 1969, weighed 1.9 kg at birth, while his twin sister weighed 2.6 kg. He gained weight poorly in the neonatal period, and was hospitalized for pneumonia as a small child. His sister, patient AIV5, weighed 3.1 kg at birth on February 12, 1977, and gained weight poorly for several weeks. She was hospitalized several times for pneumonia and tonsillitis, and although a goiter was noted at age 3, there

were no symptoms of hyper- or hypothyroidism. There was no history of hepatitis or jaundice. On physical exam at age 5 10/12 years she was in the tenth and seventh percentile for height and weight, respectively. The thyroid was diffusely enlarged to twice normal size, the liver was enlarged with edge palpable 4 cm below the right costal margin, and the spleen was palpable. Serum levels of total bilirubin were normal, the transaminases were mildly elevated, alkaline phosphatase was 441 U/l, and LDH was 465 U/l. A liver/spleen scan showed homogeneous uptake of isotope in an enlarged liver and spleen. Patient AIV6, born September 16, 1978, weighed 3.2 kg at birth and had transient hyperbilirubinemia. She was believed to have excessive "clumsiness" as judged by her parents. Patient AIV7, born June 12, 1980, grew poorly at less than the fifth percentiles in height and weight, and suffered episodes of pneumonia and diarrhea. Patient AIV13 weighed 2.6 kg at birth on April 20, 1976, and was born six weeks premature. Mild liver enlargement was noted as an infant, and she had frequent episodes of tonsillitis and otitis media. A small goiter was noted at age 4 years, and she was described as "hyperactive". Physical exam at age 7 years 4 months disclosed scarred

Table 1 - *Patient AIV9: thyroid function studies.*

Date mo/yr	Therapy	Duration of therapy	T_3 (ng/dl) 62-200[3]	T_4 (μg/dl) 5.7-11.3	FT_4 (ng/dl) 1.0-2.3	Basal TSH (μU/ml) 0.8-6.0	Max TSH[2] (μU/ml) 10-30	131I 4 h 6-18	Uptake (%) 24 h 8-32
4/79	None	—		24.3					
4/80	PTU and Propranolol	1 yr	456	7.9					
1/81	Same	1 9/12 yr	486	9.4		37	319		
2/81	None	1 mo	332	17.9	4.3	7.0	43	82	87
6/81	None	1 mo	416	23.2		2.8			
7/81	T_3 25 μg BID	1 mo	650	16.1		2.6			
9/81	T_3 50 μg BID	2 mo	790	10.3		2.0			
11/81	T_3 75 μg BID	2 mo	1110	15.9		1.3	1.4		
1/82	T_3 50 μg BID	2 mo	550	13.6	3.7	1.1	1.2	12	9
4/82	None	1 mo	295	18.2		2.0			
5/82	T_4 0.2 mg/d	1 mo	345	18.6	7.1	1.7	18		
10/82	Same	6 mo	326	25.3	6.6	2.7	14	21	42
4/83	Same	1 yr	232	28.3		2.2			
12/83	Same	1 8/12 yr	300	25.0	5.6	1.2	6.0	11	15
4/84	Same	2 yr	344	25.1		0.7			
10/84	Same	2 1/2 yr	416	25.7		1.9			

[1]Propylthiouracil (PTU) 200 mg/d, and propranolol 80 mg/d.
[2]Maximum serum TSH level after TRH administration.
[3]Normal range for euthyroid controls.

461

J.A. Magner, P. Petrick, M.M. Menezes-Ferreira, et al.

Table 2 - *Patient AIV9: Parameters of peripheral action of thyroid hormones. See Table 1 for concomitant blood levels of thyroid hormones.*

Date mo/yr	Resting pulse (beats/min)	QKD[1] (msec)	BMR[2] (%)	Chrono-logical age (yr)	Bone age (yr)	TEBG[9] (μg/dl)	Choles-terol[10] (mg/dl)	IQ[3]	Height [cm (%ile)]	Weight [kg (%ile)]	Goiter size (xnl)
4/79	100							4			1xnl
4/80	80			7 10/12	4 6/12						2xnl
2/81	80- 93	184	+ 24	8 8/12	5 6/12	1.08	161	68[5]	126 (20)	22.5 (<5)	3xnl
1/82	96-100			9 7/12	7 0/12	1.72	134	71[6]	129 (12)	24.0 (5)	2xnl
4/82	101-112								132 (25)	26.4 (10)	2xnl
10/82	82-107	196	- 8	10 4/12	8 0/12	1.72	175	7	135 (25)	26.8 (10)	1xnl
12/83	80- 83	173	- 46	11 6/12	10 0/12	1.38	172	72[8]	143 (30)	30.5 (10)	1xnl
4/84	76								147 (40)	32.8 (16)	1xnl
10/84	84							11	149 (40)	34.3 (20)	1xnl

[1]Pulse arrival time. Normal ranges for boys of height 130 cm, 130-190 msec; 140 cm, 140-200 msec; 150 cm, 145-205 msec (27).
[2]Basal metabolic rate, normal range - 20 to + 20%.
[3]Full scale IQ as determined by the Wechsler Intelligence Scale for Children - Revised.
[4]The patient was "hyperactive", with poor school performance.
[5]Verbal IQ 70, performance IQ 69, poor school performance.
[6]Verbal IQ 74, performance IQ 72, poor school performance.
[7]School performance began to improve in May, 1982, about four weeks after therapy with T_4 0.2 mg/d was begun. By October, "hyperactivity", in the classroom was less, and school performance continued to improve.
[8]Verbal IQ 68, performance IQ 81, poor school performance improved.
[9]Normal range for males, ages 2-11 yr, 1.0-3.3 μg/dl (11).
[10]Normal range for boys, 120-200 mg/dl (28).
[11]School performance improved.

tympanic membranes, inflamed tonsils, a small goiter and a slightly enlarged liver. Patient AIV15 weighed 2.8 kg at birth on March 29, 1981. She had normal growth and development.

Three adults in the kindred were affected. Patient AIII1 is a 35-year-old white male with an unremarkable history and physical examination. Patient AIII4 was unavailable for examination, but reportedly had no symptoms of hyperthyroidism in spite of an elevated serum thyroxine level. Patient AIII9 is a 29-year-old white female who had frequent bouts of tonsillitis as a child, grew slowly, and performed poorly in elementary school. Menarche was at age 11, her periods were normal, and she had three pregnancies. The physical examination was unremarkable.

Patient BIV5, the propositus of kindred B; (Fig. 2) was delivered by Caesarean section on April 7, 1969. Her mother had diabetes mellitus. The birth weight was 2.8 kg, and she grew and developed normally, but was described as "hyperactive". Therapy with methylphenidate hydrochloride was instituted at age 5 yr, but eleven months later the serum PBI was found to be elevated at 10.8 μg/dl, although no goiter was present. Propylthiouracil and pemoline were prescribed during a three-year period, but the child remained "hyperactive", the thyroid grew to several times normal size, and serum T_4 levels ranged from 9.0-13.2 μg/dl, while random TSH levels were 4.5 and 10.5 μU/ml. At age 9 yr 2 mo a subtotal thyroidectomy was performed, and one

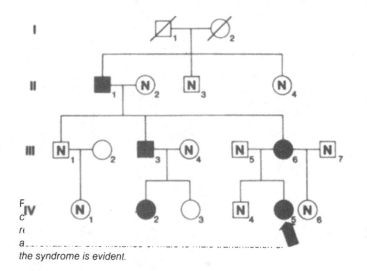

the syndrome is evident.

month later on no medicines the T_4 was 10 μg/dl with T_3RU 38.8%. By age 10 yr 11 mo regrowth of the goiter was evident, with T_4 level 11.5 μg/dl and TSH 35 μU/ml. Four months later the goiter had increased substantially in size, the "hyperactivity" had worsened, yet the pulse was 84/min. Blood-work disclosed T_4 14.6 μg/dl and T_3RU 36.9%, and methimazole was prescribed. At age 11 yr 7 mo, while taking 10 mg

462

Table 3 - *Summary of kindred A studies.*

Patient	Therapy	T3 (ng/dl) 62-200	T4 (μg/dl) 5.7-11.3	FT4 (ng/dl) 1.0-2.3	Basal TSH (μU/ml) 0.8-6.0	Max TSH[1] (μU/ml) 10-30	131I Uptake 4h (6-18)	131I Uptake 24h (8-32)	Pulse (beats/min)	QKd[2] (msec)	BMR[3] (%)	C.A.[4] (yr)	Bone Age (yr)	TEBG (μg/dl)	Cholesterol (mg/dl)	IQ[5]	Height cm (%ile)	Weight kg (%ile)	Infections	Goiter
III1	None	262	22.6	4.5	2.7		26	36	64		+17	35			283	85[6]	169	62	-	-
	None	213	23.7		2.5	15.8						36								
	T3 50 μg/d, 1 mo																			
III4	None	348	19.5		1.5	11.4						36								
	None	294	22.7									32								
III9	None	232	15.2	4.0	3.7	37.2	22	38	92		+57	29		0.38	147	7	150(<5)	50(20)	-	-
IV2	None	268	20.6	4.8	3.8	32.4	15	35	70-90		-3	13 6/12	13 6/12	1.46	103	8	140(<5)	32.5(<5)	+	-
	None	279	22.5		2.9	23.4						14 0/12								
	T3 50 μg/d, 1 mo	416	15.3		1.9	17.9						14 1/12								
IV5	None	181	30.4	6.4	43.3	352.	27	13	86-94		-20	5 8/12	3 3/12	1.39	141	9	106(10)	15.2(7)	+	+
	T3 50 μg/d, 1 mo	641	8.8		57.1	709.						6 3/12								
	T3 75 μg/d, 3 mo	1051	15.2		2.0	16.0						6 6/12								
	T3 50 μg/d, 5 mo	414	11.7	1.8	23.5	>92.	38	36	100-116	155	-28	6 1/12	4 2/12		56	82[10]				
	T3 50 μg/d, 6 mo		9.4		24.0							7 0/12		3.04						
IV6	None	278	13.1	2.8	2.5	35.4	11	10	90-104		-27	4 1/12	2 6/12	2.51	120		97(12)	15.1(30)	+	+
	T3 50 μg/d, 1 mo	465	2.6		1.1	1.5														
	T3 75 μg/d, 3 mo	867	5.7		0.7	0.7														
	T3 50 μg/d, 5 mo	331	1.5		2.3	1.1	2	4	110-130	132	-15	5 4/12	3 1/12	12.6	71	98[11]	108(35)	16.9(15)		
	T3 75 μg/d, 1 mo		2.1		0.8															
IV7	None	286	23.9	4.5	5.4	43.7	35	46	100-130			2 4/12	1 9/12	1.29	186		81(<5)	9.6(<5)	+	-
	T3 25 μg/d, 1 mo	793	13.8		2.6	17.2														
	T3 50 μg/d, 3 mo	413	13.3		<1.1	11.9														
	T3 25 μg/d, 5 mo	400	21.8	4.5	6.3									3.95						
	T3 25 μg/d, 6 mo		19.1		4.2	27.5														
IV9	(See Tables 1 and 2)						47	41	104-114	118	-22	3 7/12	2 6/12		124	12	90(<5)	11.4(<5)	+	+
IV13	None	364	20.0		3.3	26.0	21	37	94		+14	7 4/12	5 9/12	2.44	168	105[13]	117(15)	15.8(<5)	+	+
	T3 25 μg/d, 4 mo	407	16.1	4.5	3.6	20.8	13	31	100			8 3/12	6 3/12	1.69	191		121(18)	20.1(5)		
IV15	None	198	19.6	4.2	3.8	30.7	14	39	102-128			2 5/12	1 6/12		140	14	83(<5)	10.3(<5)	-	-
	T3 12.5 μg/d, 4 mo	448	19.4	4.6	3.5	19.8	20	31	113	200		3 4/12	3 3/12	3.96	137		91(7)	12.3(8)		

[1] Maximum serum TSH level after TRH administration; [2] Pulse arrival time. Normal ranges for children of height 80 cm, 90-150 msec; 90 cm, 100-160 msec; 100 cm, 105-165 msec; 110 cm, 115-175 msec; 120 cm, 120-180 msec; 130 cm, 130-190 msec; 140 cm, 140-200 msec; 150 cm, 145-205 msec (27); [3] Basal metabolic rate normal range -20% to +20%; [4] Chronologic age; [5] Full scale IQ as determined by the Wechsler Intelligence Scale for Children - Revised; [6] Full scale IQ as determined by the Wechsler Adult Intelligence Scale; [7] Poor elementary school performance; [8] Poor elementary school performance, word reversals while reading; [9] Good kindergarten student; [10] Verbal IQ 72, Performance IQ 72, Performance IQ 105, poor language skills; [11] Verbal IQ 96, good first grade student; [11] Verbal IQ 91, Performance IQ 96, [12] McCarthy Scales for Children's Abilities: General cognitive index 72 (4%ile); [13] Verbal IQ 96, above average student; [14] Bailey Scales of Infant Development 15-20%ile.

463

J.A. Magner, P. Petrick, M.M. Menezes-Ferreira, et al.

methimazole twice daily, the T_4 was 8.5 μg/dl, T_3RU 33%, and TSH > 100 μU/ml; the methimazole was discontinued. At age 12 yr 3 mo, the T_4 was 13.7 μg/dl, basal TSH 19.5 μU/ml and TSH 30 min after TRH was > 40 μU/ml. Subsequently the FT_4 was found to be elevated at 3.0 ng/dl, and the patient was referred to the National Institutes of Health for further evaluation. On physical examination at age 12 yr 11 mo, the patient was well developed, with pulse 66/min, weight 43.3 kg (40%ile), and height 159 cm (65%ile). The right lobe of the thyroid was slightly enlarged, and contained an irregular mass 2 cm in diameter. Thyroid function studies, and measurements of the peripheral action of thyroid hormone are summarized in Table 4.

Family screening disclosed that four additional members of the kindred were affected, and one instance of male to male transmission was discovered. A cousin, patient BIV2, weighed 2.8 kg at birth on March 19, 1973 after a 37-week gestation. She suffered an episode of periorbital cellulitis at age 2, and had frequent bouts of otitis media, but her growth and development were normal, and she ranked in the top 2% of her third grade class academically. The physical examination was unremarkable. Patient BII1 is a 63-year-old white male who had no history of goiter or thyroid symptoms, although the history was positive for peripheral vascular disease, adult onset diabetes mellitus, hypertriglyceridemia, hyperuricemia, and peptic ulcer disease. He had a B.S. degree in engineering, and had been employed as a petroleum engineer for many years. On physical exam he was a well-developed cooperative man, height 180 cm, weight 62.2 kg, and the thyroid was normal in size.

Patient BIII3 is a 38-year-old male with a history of a cryptorchid testicle, "spastic colon", and frequent urinary tract infections. In 1974 he complained of anxiety, and a small goiter and elevated serum thyroxine were treated with one dose of radioactive iodine, followed six months later by therapy with L-thyroxine. In 1978 he complained of intermittent, sharp, tearing chest pains, but the blood pressure and a treadmill exercise test were normal. In 1980 abdominal surgery was performed for a ruptured appendix; surgical intervention was delayed several days because the white blood cell count had not been elevated. In 1981, while taking 0.3 mg L-thyroxine daily, he had no symptoms of thyroid disease, but screening blood tests disclosed T_4 17.2 μg/dl, FT_4 3.9 ng/dl, and basal TSH 30 μU/ml, which increased to 240 μU/ml 30 min after TRH. On physical examination he was well-developed and muscular, with BP 128/78, P 80/min. No thyroid tissue was palpable. A murmur of aortic insufficiency was present. Routine blood and urine studies were normal, and syphilis serology was negative. Echocardiography revealed that the aortic root was dilated to 43 mm in diameter, and propranolol was prescribed. Repeat echocardiography performed fourteen months later showed that the dilatation of the aortic root had increased slightly to 48 mm, and propranolol was continued.

Patient BIII6 is a 33-year-old woman who had normal growth and development, but who was treated as a child for "hyperactivity". At age 12 a goiter was noted, and radioiodine therapy was administered. At age 13 she noted polyuria, and insulin dependent diabetes mellitus was diagnosed. Her goiter gradually recurred, and at age 22 L-thyroxine 0.1 mg daily was prescribed. At age 30 she noted vague joint pains, and bilateral carpal tunnel syndrome.

Patients CI2, CII2, and CIII1 have been previously described by Wortsman et al. (18). Patient CII2 was evaluated in our clinic at age 56. She had no symptoms of thyroid disease, and had always been in good health. She was 155 cm tall and weighed 68 kg. The thyroid gland was diffusely enlarged to twice normal size. Her son, patient CIII1, was 26-year-old, had no symptoms of thyroid disease, and had been in good health. He had performed poorly in elementary school, and had required special education classes. He was 170 cm tall, and weighed 93 kg. The thyroid gland was slightly enlarged. Patient CIII2 was a 23-year-old man who had required surgery at age 10 because of an undescended right testicle. Peptic ulcer disease had been treated with cimetidine. He was an average student in high school, but had particular difficulty with mathematics. He had no symptoms of thyroid disease, and no goiter was present. The laboratory data are summarized in Table 5.

In most cases, the resistance to thyroid hormone of individual tissues of affected patients in the three kindreds was estimated (Table 6) while no thyroid hormones were administered, but while blood levels of thyroid hormones were frankly elevated. For patients who were taking synthroid for several years after thyroid ablation, resistance was gauged while they were

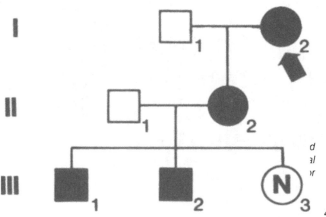

Table 4 - *Summary of kindred B studies.*

Patient	Therapy	T3 (ng/dl)	T4 (µg/dl)	FT4 (ng/dl)	Basal TSH (µU/ml)	Max TSH[1] (µU/ml)	131I Uptake (%) 4 h	131I Uptake (%) 24 h	Pulse (beats/min)	QKd[2] (msec)	BMR[3] (%)	C.A.[4] (yr)	Bone Age (yr)	TEBG[12] (µg/dl)	Cholesterol[13] (mg/dl)	IQ[5]	Height cm (%ile)	Weight <g (%ile)	Goiter
II1	None		21.8	5.1	1.5	6.3	16	39	61-66	191		63		0.52	185	6	180	66.2	+
	T3 25 µg/d, 7 mo	183	14.7		2.3	17.3													
	T3 25 µg/d, 17 mo	171	11.9	4.3	2.4	9.7			64	194	+12	64		0.71	192				+
III3	T4 0.3 mg/d, 1 yr	163	17.2	3.9	30.0	240.		6	64-80	180	−2	38		0.44	103		182	66.1	—[11]
	T4 0.3 mg/d, 2 yr	178	19.6		61.4														
	T3 50 µg/d, 3 mo	294	3.3		211.														
	T3 50 µg/d, 4 mo	261	3.1.		44.														
III6	T3 25 µg/d, 14 mo	172	2.3	0.7	121.	1020.	5	5	62		−1			0.81	93				—[11]
	T4 0.1 mg/d, 11 yr		12.9	2.8	3.7	67.	10	22	96	214		33		2.29	126	7	165	66.0	+[11]
	T4 0.1 mg/d+ T3 50 µg/d, 7 mo	152	10.9	2.4	5.0	65.	5	7	110	183	+33	34		0.68	118				+[11]
	Same, 17 mo	147	11.3		2.8	27.													
IV2	None	310	23.8	4.6	2.4	24.	15	38	60-94	162	−3	9 3/12	9	1.13	95	8	129(25)	25.6(25)	+
	T3 50 µg/d, 1 mo	548	15.9	2.8	2.6	16.8								1.63					+
	None, 6 mo	389	23.6	6.0	4.2	25.9			88		−1	11 2/12	10	0.76	96	121[9]	140(25)	32.5(25)	+
IV5	None	253	14.6	3.5	25.	>144.	21	26	66	202		12 11/12		1.69			159(65)	43.3(40)	+[11]
	T3 50 µg/d, 7 mo	222	11.9		8.5	210.										10			
	T3 50 µg/d, 17 mo	249	7.6	1.8	22.	136.	11	19	66	196	+9	14 4/12			165		166(75)	51.6(50)	+[11]

1 Maximum serum TSH level after TRH administration.
2 Pulse arrival time (27). Normal adult range 180-220 msec. See other tables for children's ranges.
3 Basal metabolic rate, normal -20% to +20%.
4 Chronologic age.
5 Full scale IQ as determined by the Wechsler Intelligence Scale for Children - Revised.
6 Engineer, IQ "above average", mild spatial dysfunction.
7 Luria IQ 102, rotations of spatial tasks.
8 Academically in top 2% of 3rd grade class.
9 Verbal IQ 119, Performance IQ 118, excellent spatial visualization.
10 Luria IQ 101, abnormal Bender Visual - Motor Gestalt, poor arithmetic ability, school behavior improved.
11 After thyroid ablative therapy.
12 Normal range for children, 1.0-3.3 µg/dl; adult males, 0.18-0.70 µg/dl; adult females 0.18-1.41 µg/dl (11).
13 Normal ranges: infant, 70-175 mg/dl; child, 120-200 mg/dl; adolescent, 120-210 mg/dl; adult, 140-310 mg/dl (28).

J.A. Magner, P. Petrick, M.M. Menezes-Ferreira, et al.

Table 5 - *Summary of kindred C studies.*

Patient	Age/ Sex	Therapy	T_3 (ng/dl) 62-200[6]	T_4 (μg/dl) 5.7-11.3	FT_4 (ng/dl) 1.0-2.3	Basal TSH (μU/ml) 0.8-6.0	Max[1] TSH (μU/ml) 10-30	131I Uptake (%) 4 h 6-18	24 h 8-32	Pulse (beats/ min)	TEBG[5] (μg/dl)	Choles- terol[5] (mg/dl)	IQ	Infec- tions	Goiter
I2[2]	74/F	None	251	22.4	6.6	6.6	26		42	80		317			+
II2	56/F	None	235	16.2	2.6	9.0	>40	15	30	76	0.63	230	3	—	+
III1	26/M	None	350	16.9	4.8	1.6	18.6	13	28	68	0.23	189	4	—	+
III2	23/M	None	268	14.3	4.1	2.6	16.0	20	39	68	0.33	154	3	—	+

[1]Maximum serum TSH level after TRH administration.
[2]From Wortsman et al. (18).
[3]Normal intelligence.
[4]Special education in elementary school.
[5]See legend to Table 4 for normal ranges.
[6]Normal range for euthyroid patients.

Table 6 - *Manifestations of resistance to thyroid hormones in various tissues. See text for criteria of tissue resistance.*

Patient	Bone	Liver	Brain	Heart	Body Metabolism	Pituitary
AIII1	—	+	+	⊕	+	+
AIII4						
AIII9	+	⊕	⊕	—	+	+
AIV2	+	+	⊕	⊕	+	+
AIV5	+	+	⊕	+	+	⊕
AIV6	+	+	—	—	+	+
AIV7	+	+	⊕	—	+	+
AIV9	+		⊕	+	+	+
AIV13	+	+	—	—	+	+
AIV15	+	+	—	—		+
BII1	—	⊕	—	⊕	+	+
BIII3	—	⊕	—	⊕	+	+
BIII6	—	—	+	—	+	+
BIV2	—	+	—	⊕	+	+
BIV5	—	+	+	⊕	+	+
CI2	—	⊕		⊕	+	+
CII2	—	⊕	—	⊕		+
CIII1	—	⊕	+	⊕		+
CIII2	—	⊕	—	⊕		+

— Minimal or no resistance or abnormality.
+ Moderate resistance or abnormality.
⊕ Severe resistance or abnormality.

taking their usual replacement dose, with blood levels of thyroid hormone in the normal or supranormal range. In many instances, the responses of peripheral tissues were evaluated while graded doses of T_3 and/or T_4 were administered to patients. The criteria used to gauge the thyroid hormone resistance of various peripheral tissues were as follows:

Bone:
+ Child: bone age retarded > 2 standard deviations (Gruelich and Pyle), or height < 5%ile.
+ Adult: adult height < 5%ile.

Brain:
(+) (severe): verbal or full scale IQ < 80, or general cognitive index of McCarthy Scales for Children's Activities < 5%ile, or exceptionally poor school performance but IQ testing not performed.
+ (moderate): history of inadequate school performance that necessitated formal special education, or

466

Table 7 - *Equilibrium and kinetic analysis of [^{125}I] T_3 nuclear binding in patients with familial generalized resistance to thyroid hormones: comparison with normal subjects and apparently normal siblings of affected families.*

Patient	Equilibrium analysis[1]			Kinetic analysis[2]		
	n°	Kd (x 10^{-10} M)	Ro (fmol/10^6 cells)	n°	λ (h^{-1})	B max (fmol/10^6 cells)
AIV9[3]	1	1.08-6.99	0.36-1.05	1	12.2	0.49
BIII6	2	2.00-6.00	1.50-5.40	0	—	—
BIV2	4	1.20-5.30	2.20-7,00	4	10.3 ±2.83	0.76±0.16
BIV3[4]	4	0.50-4.97	1.27-4.98	4	7.94±1.19	1.00±0.24
BIV5	1	1.00	2.50	0	—	—
CII2	5	1.20-3.80	0.80-7.90	4	3.75±1.22	0.80±0.08
CIII1	2	1.81-1.88	0.34-3.96	1	2.56	0.20
CIII2	2	0.87-2.13	0.38-1.28	1	3.32	0.12
CIII3[4]	1	0.83	2.54	1	8.04	1.00
Normal[5]	36	0.40-7.72	0.81-42.7	8	6.12±1.18	1.56±0.12

[1]Equilibrium analysis of data is expressed as minimal and maximal values of a non-parametric distribution.
[2]Kinetic analysis of data is expressed as mean ± SEM of a normal distribution.
[3]Two values given because plots of equilibrium binding were curvilinear.
[4]Normal siblings of affected families.
[5]Equilibrium analysis was performed in 17 cell lines from normal controls in 36 determinations and kinetic analysis included 6 cell lines in 8 determinations.

verbal or full scale IQ < 86 but > 80, or presence of subtle abnormalities of cognitive function (spatial relationships).

Heart:
(+) (severe): Mean resting pulse < 80.
+ (moderate): Mean resting pulse > 80 but < 90. (In many instances, the impression of cardiac thyroid hormone resistance was reinforced by measurements of QK_D).

Body metabolism:
+ (moderate): BMR < 120% of normal (+ 20%).

Pituitary:
(+) (severe): basal TSH > 40 μU/ml with marked TSH responses to TRH, but no prior history of thyroid surgery or radioactive iodine, and anti-thyroglobulin and anti-microsomal antibodies negative.
+ (moderate): maximal TSH > 15 μU/ml after TRH.

Liver:
(+) adult (severe): TEBG within the lower third of the normal range (male < 0.35 μg/dl, female < 0.70 μg/dl), or cholesterol > 300 mg/dl.
+ adult (moderate): TEBG within upper 2/3 of the normal range, or cholesterol > 240 mg/dl but < 300 mg/dl.
(+) child (severe): *Both* TEBG within the lower third of the normal range (< 1.7 μg/dl) *and* cholesterol > 200 mg/dl.
+ child (moderate): TEBG within upper 2/3 of the normal range (< 3.3 μg/dl but > 1.7 μg/dl), or TEBG within the lower third of the normal range but cholesterol < 200 mg/dl.

Parameters of the fibroblast nuclear uptake of [^{125}I]T_3 are summarized in Table 7.

The HLA type and dermatoglyphic pattern were determined for selected members of kindreds A and B, but no consistent associations were detected.

Karyotypes of several affected patients were normal. The diurnal variation of TSH secretion was assessed in several affected patients by determination of the serum TSH level at hourly intervals during a 24-h period; in all cases studied the pattern of the diurnal variation was normal, with peak TSH levels occurring between 23:00 and 01:00 h.

DISCUSSION

We here report three large kindreds with a total of 19 persons affected with central and peripheral resistance to thyroid hormones; kindred A, with 10 cases, is the largest to be reported to date. Both kindred A and B exhibit male to male transmission of the syndrome, a pattern reported previously in only two other kindreds (19, 22), a finding consistent with an autosomal dominant mode of inheritance. We believe that the consanguinity found in kindred A, and that reported in the family histories of other similar patients by others, may be coincidental. A tumor of pituitary thyrotrophs was not detected in any of our patients, even in elderly persons who had presumably been affected with the syndrome for decades; serum levels of free α-subunit were not elevated out of proportion to serum TSH levels, and the secretion of TSH could be suppressed by administration of thyroxine or triiodothyronine and

467

J.A. Magner, P. Petrick, M.M. Menezes-Ferreira, et al.

stimulated by TRH. During several years of follow-up evaluation, the degree of resistance to thyroid hormones was relatively constant in a given tissue in a given patient, whereas Refetoff et al. (23) reported progressive amelioration of the syndrome in some of their patients.

The clinical and biochemical manifestations of the resistance to thyroid hormone varied from patient to patient, and several tissues within a given patient also seemed to have differing degrees of resistance, a phenomenon that has been described previously by ourselves and others (2, 3, 23, 24). In this study, we report that this heterogeneity of tissue and patient resistance to thyroid hormones is not random. By evaluating relatively large numbers of patients within a given kindred, we found that a given tissue or tissues may be consistently more resistant to thyroid hormone than other tissues.

We also found that different kindreds had different patterns of affected tissues which "ran true" within a family, perhaps reflecting the underlying molecular mechanisms of the syndrome; presumably members of a given kindred have inherited the same molecular defect, which may differ from that in another kindred. Specifically, kindred A patients tended to have marked bone involvement, but only moderate hepatic and cardiac resistance. Moreover, an apparent deficit in immunity was present in at least six kindred A members, although environmental factors could not be ruled out as contributing to the infections. In contrast, members of kindreds B and C demonstrated more hepatic and cardiac resistance to thyroid hormones, and less bone resistance than did members of kindred A. Moreover, recurrent serious infections were not present in members of kindreds B and C. Of interest, but of uncertain significance, is that two of the four affected males in kindreds B and C (patients BIII3 and CIII2) had history of maldescent of a testis, a condition generally found in only 0.5 percent of males after one year of age (25).

The criteria by which we estimated the resistance of tissues to thyroid hormones are admittedly arbitrary, but were useful to categorize the tissue responses. Assessment of hepatic resistance to thyroid hormones in children was complicated by the broad normal range of TEBG and the generally lower levels of cholesterol in children than in adults; for these reasons, the criteria for hepatic resistance are rather complex. Another problematic area was the assessment of bone resistance to thyroid hormones in adults when no prior radiographs had been obtained to allow bone age to be estimated during development. The adults marked "negative" in Table 6 were greater than 5%ile in adult height, and had no history of being shorter than their peers during childhood. We acknowledge that delayed bone age may have been present in some of these patients, with subsequent "catch-up" growth.

Two parameters of thyroid hormone action, the basal metabolic rate and the serum level of TSH, seemed to be equally useful in screening affected patients from all three kindreds, and did not seem to be more abnormal in patients from a given kindred. Of note, screening using a commercial TSH assay may miss affected patients, since basal TSH levels in our patients were generally only slightly elevated. Four patients, AIV5, BIII3, BIV5, and CII2, had particularly high basal and stimulated TSH serum levels for the concomitant level of thyroid hormones, but the latter three patients had prior thyroid surgery or ^{131}I therapy. It remains unclear why prior antithyroid therapy should be associated with high levels of TSH when serum thyroid hormone levels were elevated to a degree similar to that of other patients, but this may be related to thyrotroph hyperplasia during past periods of iatrogenic hypothyroidism.

Patient AIV5 had no history of anti-thyroid therapy, and anti-thyroid antibodies were not detected; basal TSH levels > 25 $\mu U/ml$ have rarely been detected in patients with thyroid hormone resistance who had not undergone prior ablative therapy (24). This patient demonstrated no rise in serum T_3 at 120 min after TRH administration, but additional studies will be required to fully assess the bioactivity of her TSH.

Patient BIII3 developed a dilated aortic root in the absence of hypertension. It is uncertain at this time whether this might be related to the requirement of aortic smooth muscle cells for thyroid hormone. The occurrence of an aortic aneurysm in a patient exhibiting thyroid hormone resistance has not been previously reported.

It was difficult to ascertain whether the impaired cognitive function documented in six of the ten affected members of kindred A was wholly due to resistance to thyroid hormone, or in part due to cultural factors. More subtle cognitive dysfunction involving arithmetic ability and appreciation of spatial relationships was present in several affected members from all three kindreds.

Refetoff et al. (24) noted a reversible improvement in IQ of one child with thyroid hormone resistance while being treated with T_3. School performance improved in two of our patients after therapy with thyroid hormones, but IQ failed to improve; this raises the possibility that a delay in providing supplemental thyroid hormone to children affected with thyroid hormone resistance potentially leads to irreversible learning disabilities. Yet several children with the syndrome had good intellectual function; two of the brightest children, BIV2 and AIV13, had relatively high serum T_3 levels while on no therapy, suggesting that the spontaneously high T_3 levels may have had a protective effect.

A unique feature of this study is our attempt to correlate the pattern of the most affected tissues in a kindred with $[^{125}I]T_3$ binding parameters in studies of skin fibroblasts from these patients. As summarized in Table 7, the equilibrium analyses demonstrated only subtle differ-

468

ences between the patients and the normal control population. However, the kinetic analyses demonstrated significantly lowered B_{max} in affected patients in all three kindreds, and this parameter was also somewhat low in two putatively normal siblings that were tested. These data confirm and extend recently published studies from our laboratory (20). However, these preliminary studies indicate that there is no strong correlation between fibroblast $[^{125}I]T_3$ binding parameters and the pattern of affected tissues in a given patient or kindred. B_{max} was decreased in all five patients tested who were affected with the syndrome, but there was no convincing correlation between this parameter and other features of the disease. For example, patients CIII1 and CIII2, with the lowest of B_{max}, had no more evidence of brain or bone involvement than other patients with higher B_{max} values. Clearly, more patients must be tested to confirm this preliminarily finding. Wortsman et al. (18) previously reported that members of kindred C had decreased transport of thyroid hormones through the plasma membrane, but our findings suggest that there may also be a nuclear abnormality. It is possible that members of certain families may have greater abnormalities in fibroblast nuclear binding than members of other families.

Although fibroblasts derived from members of three different kindreds had similar properties in our studies, Murata et al. (26) found heterogeneity among patients' fibroblasts in studies using glycosaminoglycan biosynthesis as an index of specific resistance to T_3. They tested fibroblasts from six patients from five kindreds (one was patient CI2), and failed to demonstrate specific resistance to T_3 in fibroblasts from two patients, while fibroblasts from the remaining four patients were resistant to T_3. The fibroblasts from two patients in the same kindred behaved similarly, demonstrating resistance to T_3. Future studies testing fibroblasts from many clinically affected patients from a given kindred will be needed to determine whether this index of resistance to T_3 may vary among members of a kindred, or, alternatively, is consistently abnormal within certain kindreds but consistently normal in other kindreds.

Four of our patients (AIV9, BIII3, BIII6, and BIV5) had previously been treated with antithyroid therapies; two had received radioactive iodine therapy, and one had undergone subtotal thyroidectomy. This illustrates the frequency with which the syndrome of generalized resistance to thyroid hormones can be confused with true hyperthyroidism, an error that has previously been reported by ourselves and others (24). We believe that antithyroid therapy is misdirected in these patients, since high levels of circulating thyroid hormones are presumably needed to adequately supply resistant tissues with hormone. Further elevation of serum thyroid hormone levels by administration of exogenous thyroxine or triiodothyronine appeared to benefit several of our patients clinically. On therapy, a growth spurt

was documented in several children (AIV5, AIV6, AIV7, AIV9, AIV13, and AIV15), and hepatic enlargement and mildly abnormal serum liver function tests resolved in three patients (AIV5, AIV7, and AIV13). Behavior or school performance probably improved in all treated children, but was better documented in the older children than the preschool children. Because different tissues in a given patient may have differing degrees of resistance to thyroid hormones, no one level of serum hormone will induce euthyroidism in all tissues; the heart, especially, seems commonly to be less resistant than the other tissues.

Thus, especially in pediatric patients, we recommend that exogenous thyroid hormone therapy be prescribed to optimize growth and mental development; tachycardia may be suppressed with propranolol.

ACKNOWLEDGMENTS

We are grateful to Dr. Beverly White for evaluating dermatoglyphic patterns and karyotypes, Dr. Charles Eil for assistance with the fibroblast studies, and Drs. Sheldon Rubenfeld and Patrick Brosnan for helpful clinical evaluations of the patients. We are grateful to Dr. Samuel Refetoff for helpful discussions. Jan Smith provided expert secretarial assistance.

REFERENCES

1. Refetoff S., DeWind L.T., DeGroot L.J.
   Familial syndrome combining deaf-mutism, stippled epiphyses, goiter and abnormally high PBI: possible target organ refractoriness to thyroid hormone.
   J. Clin. Endocrinol. Metab. 27: 279, 1967.

2. Refetoff S.
   Syndrome of thyroid hormone resistance.
   Am. J. Physiol. 243: E88, 1982.

3. Gershengorn M.C., Weintraub B.D.
   Thyrotropin-induced hyperthyroidism caused by selective pituitary resistance to thyroid hormone: A new syndrome of "inappropriate secretion of TSH".
   J. Clin. Invest. 56: 633, 1975.

4. Weintraub B.D., Gershengorn M.C., Kourides I.A., Fein H.
   Inappropriate secretion of thyroid-stimulating hormone.
   Ann. Intern. Med. 95: 339, 1981.

5. Kaplan M.M., Swartz S.L., Larsen P.R.
   Partial peripheral resistance to thyroid hormone.
   Am. J. Med. 70: 1115, 1981.

6. Liewendahl K.
   Triiodothyronine binding to lymphocytes from euthyroid subjects and a patient with peripheral resistance to thyroid hormone.
   Acta Endocrinol. (Kbh.) 83: 64, 1976.

7. Bernal J., Refetoff S., DeGroot L.J.
   Abnormalities of triiodothyronine binding to lymphocytes and fibroblast nuclei from a patient with peripheral tissue resistance to thyroid hormone action.
   J. Clin. Endocrinol. Metab. 47: 1266, 1978.

469

J.A. Magner, P. Petrick, M.M. Menezes-Ferreira, et al.

8. Daubresse J.-C., Dozin-VanRoye B., DeNayer P., De-Vischer M.
   Partial resistance to thyroid hormones: reduced affinity of lymphocyte nuclear receptors for T_3 in two siblings.
   In: Stockigt J.R., Nagataki S. (Eds.), Thyroid research VIII.
   Australian Academy of Science, Canberra, 1980, p. 295.

9. Maxon H.R., Burman K.D., Premachandra B.N.
   Euthyroid, familial hyperthyroxinemia.
   N. Engl. J. Med. *302*: 1263, 1980.

10. Elewaut A., DeBaets M., Vermeulen A.
    Triiodothyronine binding to lymphocyte nuclei and plasma cyclic AMP response to intravenous glucagon in patients with peripheral resistance to thyroid hormones.
    Acta Endocrinol. (Kbh.) *97*: 54, 1981.

11. Cooper D.S., Ladenson P.W., Nisula B.C., Dunn J.F., Chapman E.M., Ridgway E.C.
    Familial thyroid hormone resistance.
    Metabolism *31*: 504, 1982.

12. Liewendahl K., Rosengard S., Lamberg B.A.
    Nuclear binding of triiodothyronine and thyroxine in lymphocytes from subjects with hyperthyroidism, hypothyroidism and resistance to thyroid hormone.
    Clin. Chim. Acta *83*: 41, 1978.

13. Maenpaa J., Liewendahl K.
    Peripheral insensitivity to thyroid hormones in a euthyroid girl with goiter.
    Arch. Dis. Child. *55*: 207, 1980.

14. Chait A., Kanter R., Green W., Kenny M.
    Defective thyroid hormone action in fibroblasts cultured from subjects with the syndrome of resistance to thyroid hormone.
    J. Clin. Endocrinol. Metab. *54*: 767, 1982.

15. Kaplowitz P.B., D'Ercole A.J., Utiger R.D.
    Peripheral resistance to thyroid hormone in an infant.
    J. Clin. Endocrinol. Metab. *53*: 958, 1981.

16. Eil C., Fein H.G., Smith T.J., Furlanetto R.W., Bourgeois M., Stelling M.W., Weintraub B.D.
    Nuclear binding of [^{125}I] triiodothyronine in dispersed cultured skin fibroblasts from patients with resistance to thyroid hormone.
    J. Clin. Endocrinol. Metab. *55*: 502, 1982.

17. Bantle J.P., Seeling S., Mariash C.N., Ulstrom R.A., Oppenheimer J.H.
    Resistance to thyroid hormones: a disorder frequently confused with Graves' Disease.
    Arch. Intern. Med. *142*: 1867, 1982.

18. Wortsman J., Premachandra B.N., Williams K., Burman K., Hay I.D., Davis P.J.
    Familial resistance to thyroid hormone associated with decreased transport across the plasma membrane.
    Ann. Intern. Med. *98*: 904, 1983.

19. Gheri R.G., Bianchi R., Mariani G., Toccafondi R., Cappelli G., Brat A., Borghi A., Giusti G., Forti G.
    A new case of familial partial generalized resistance to thyroid hormones: Study of 3,5,3'-triiodothyronine (T_3) binding to lymphocyte and skin fibroblast nuclei and *in vivo* conversion of thyroxine to T_3.
    J. Clin. Endocrinol. Metab. *58*: 563, 1984.

20. Menezes-Ferreira M.M., Eil C., Wortsman J., Weintraub B.D.
    Decreased nuclear uptake of [^{125}I] triiodo-L-thyronine in fibroblasts from patients with peripheral thyroid hormone resistance.
    J. Clin. Endocrinol. Metab. *59*: 1081, 1984.

21. Nisula B.C., Dunn J.F.
    Measurement of the testosterone binding parameters for both testosterone-estradiol binding globulin and albumin in individual serum samples.
    Steroids *34*: 771, 1979.

22. Brooks M.H., Barbato A.L., Collins S., Garbincius J., Neidballa R.G., Hoffman D.
    Familial thyroid hormone resistance.
    Am. J. Med. *71*: 414, 1981.

23. Refetoff S., DeGroot L.J., Bernard B., DeWind L.T.
    Studies of a sibship with apparent hereditary resistance to the intracellular action of thyroid hormone.
    Metabolism *21*: 723, 1972.

24. Refetoff S., Salazar A., Smith T.J., Scherberg N.
    The consequences of inappropriate treatment because of failure to recognize the syndrome of and peripheral tissue resistance to thyroid hormone.
    Metabolism *32*: 822, 1983.

25. Mau G., Schnakenburg K.V.
    Maldescent of the testes--an epidemiological study.
    Eur. J. Pediatr. *126*: 77, 1977.

26. Murata Y., Refetoff S., Horvitz A.L., Smith T.J.
    Hormonal regulation of glycosaminoglycan accumulation in fibroblasts from patients with resistance to thyroid hormone.
    J. Clin. Endocrinol. Metab. *57*: 1233, 1983.

27. Bercu B.B., Haupt R., Johnsonbaugh R., Rodbard D.
    The pulse wave arrival time (QK_d interval) in normal children.
    J. Pediatr. *95*: 716, 1979.

28. Behrman R.E., Vaughan V.C.
    Nelson's textbook of pediatrics (Appendix, Table 29-2, Reference ranges).
    W.B. Saunders, Philadelphia, 1983, p. 1832.

470

Labeled Sugars to Study TSH Biosynthesis

During most of my three years with Bruce Weintraub at NIH (1980-1983) I used a radioactively labeled amino acid, ^{35}S-methione, to perform pulse-chase experiments to study TSH biosynthesis. Analyses of the labeled TSH molecules were done using SDS-gel technology such that the ^{35}S-TSH still had its (unlabeled) sugars attached. In late-1982 a young French biochemist, Catherine Ronin, arrived to work for a year or so in Bruce Weintraub's laboratory, and she brought with her small vials of ^{14}C-labeled oligosaccharide standards. The availability of these standards made a new type of experiment possible – one could do pulse-chase labeling experiments with ^{3}H-mannose, for example, and then after getting the ^{3}H-TSH molecules in more pure solution using immunoprecipitation, one could use enzymes to cleave the labeled oligosaccharides from the TSH and analyze those smaller parts (they would look like branching trees if one could see molecules) using tall, thin chromatography columns that sized molecules. Vital was to spike each sample of experimentally derived ^{3}H-oligosaccharides with a mix of known ^{14}C-standard oligosaccharides when loading a sample onto a column. Liquid fractions coming serially out the bottom of a column would contain over time more or fewer oligosaccharides sorted by size, and one could presume in this context that if a ^{14}C-standard came off the column (eluted) in the same fraction as a ^{3}H-oligosaccharide of unknown structure that the ^{3}H-oligosaccharide had the same number of sugar residues as the co-eluting standard. We also developed a method using paper chromatography.

Catherine was to perform labeling experiments and then analyze TSH oligosaccharides in homogenates from whole cells, whereas my project would be a bit more detailed in some respects. I planned to perform the labeling experiments, homogenize the tissues, but then go one step further – I would use ultracentrifugation to analyze the TSH oligosaccharides in subcellular fractions, such as rough endoplasmic reticulum and Golgi, rather than just in whole cell homogenates. I also planned to use my unique technique of reversing the usual order of antibodies during the immunoprecipitation steps when purifying the TSH subunits, since I believed that I was getting more information by sorting the molecules more intelligently.

Because I was in my final year with Dr. Weintraub, I worked long hours and some Saturdays to get my data in hand before I left the NIH in June, 1983 to move to my new job in Chicago. While I set up my research laboratory in Chicago I wrote up my manuscript describing my findings using ^{3}H-mannose-labeled TSH oligosaccharides. I made Catherine and Bruce co-authors as we had agreed. Catherine was to make me a co-author on her paper per agreement. A small political problem, however, was that I had outpaced Catherine, as her experiments were lagging a bit. We both obtained very interesting results, and we both published in 1984 although my publication appeared in Endocrinology somewhat earlier than hers in Biochemistry. This was not actually a race but things just worked out in that order of publication, although I suspect that no other person in the entire world had any concern about the publication dates of these two papers. I used my ^{35}S-methione paper from J Biol Chem and this ^{3}H-mannose paper from Endocrinology to be the core of my first NIH grant application, and I was relieved and very proud to have the grant funded.

0013-7227/84/1153-1019$02.00/0
Endocrinology
Copyright © 1984 by The Endocrine Society

Vol. 115, No. 3
Printed in U.S.A.

Carbohydrate Processing of Thyrotropin Differs from that of Free α-Subunit and Total Glycoproteins in Microsomal Subfractions of Mouse Pituitary Tumor

JAMES A. MAGNER, CATHERINE RONIN,* AND BRUCE D. WEINTRAUB

Clinical Endocrinology Branch, National Institute of Arthritis, Diabetes, and Digestive and Kidney Diseases, National Institutes of Health, Bethesda, Maryland 20205

ABSTRACT. We have determined the structures of high mannose (Man) oligosaccharide units of TSH, free α-subunit, and non-TSH-related total glycoproteins (TP) within microsomal subfractions of mouse thyrotropic tumor. Tumor minces were incubated with D-[2-^{3}H]Man, homogenized, and subfractionated into rough endoplasmic reticulum (RER) as well as proximal and distal smooth endoplasmic reticulum/Golgi apparatus. TSH subunits and TP were precipitated from these fractions, and high Man units released by endoglycosidase H were analyzed by paper chromatography. $Glc_3Man_9GlcNAc_2$ (Glc = glucose; GlcNAc = N-acetylglucosamine) was not detected in TSH subunit precursors in any fraction, but was detected in TP. $Glc_1Man_9GlcNAc_2$ accumulated in TSH with chase, but only small amounts were detected in free α-subunit and TP. Trimming of $Man_9GlcNAc_2$ to $Man_8GlcNAc_2$ began in RER before 1 h for all species, but the rate of Man trimming was rapid for free α-subunit, moderate for TSH, and slow for TP. $Man_8GlcNAc_2$ was a rate-limiting step in processing for all species in the RER. $Man_5GlcNAc_2$ was a second major rate-limiting step in processing of free α-subunits only and accumulated in distal smooth endoplasmic reticulum/Golgi apparatus. Other studies in progress suggest that a function of the thyrotroph is to modulate the structure of TSH oligosaccharide units during biosynthesis to achieve mature hormone with physiologically appropriate metabolic clearance and intrinsic biological activity. The present study supports this notion, since we found that the qualitative nature and kinetics of processing differ for oligosaccharide units of TSH, free α-subunit and TP within the microsomes. (*Endocrinology* **115**: 1019–1030, 1984)

T SH IS a glycoprotein hormone composed of noncovalently linked α- and β-subunits which are initially synthesized from separate mRNAs (1–6). The α-subunit has two asparagine-linked carbohydrate units, and the β-subunit has one (7). Under some conditions, thyrotropic cells may secrete excess α-subunits (8–13) which remain uncombined.

Recent studies from our and other laboratories have suggested that carbohydrate units of TSH and other glycoprotein hormones may play important roles in their biosynthesis and action. High Man[1] precursor forms protect subunits from intracellular proteolysis and aggregation (14) and enable proper nascent chain folding to be attained so that the α-β-subunit combination may proceed (13, 14). The complex final forms influence metabolic clearance as well as the intrinsic biological activity of the hormone (for recent reviews, see Refs. 15–17). Prior subcellular fractionation studies in our laboratory (18) have demonstrated directly that the TSH α-β-subunit combination begins in the RER with precursors having high Man carbohydrate chains, which are not processed to final complex forms for several hours. We have recently identified the specific high Man structures on TSH subunit precursors in thyrotropic tumor homogenates and identified differences in the posttranslational processing of units on TSH subunits compared with total glycoproteins (19). These differences in processing appeared to be modulated by the endocrine and physiological milieu of the thyrotropic cells, suggesting that the biosynthetic machinery might be geared to process high Man units to a proper final complex form with an appropriate metabolic clearance or biological activity. In the present studies we directly examined subfractions of microsomes to learn the locations of oligosaccharide-processing steps and to determine the rate-limiting steps and kinetics of processing in various subfractions. We now report that within the microsomes of thyrotropic cells, the qualitative nature and kinetics of the processing of high Man units of TSH

Received February 7, 1984.
Address requests for reprints to: Dr. James A. Magner, Division of Endocrinology, Michael Reese Hospital and Medical Center, Lake Shore Drive at 31st Street, Chicago, Illinois 60616.
* Present address: Faculte' De Medecine, Secteur Nord, Boulevard Pierre Dramard 13326, Marseille, Cedex 3 France.
[1] The following abbreviations are used: Man, mannose; RER, rough endoplasmic reticulum; TP, non-TSH-related total glycoproteins; pSER/G, proximal smooth endoplasmic reticulum and Golgi apparatus; dSER/G, distal smooth endoplasmic reticulum and Golgi apparatus; Glc, glucose; GlcNAc, N-acetylglucosamine.

1019

and free β-subunits differ from those of free α-subunits, which also differ from those of TP.

Materials and Methods

Mouse pituitary thyrotropic tumors were induced and transplanted, as previously described (10). Four tumors (total tissue, 8.7 g) were minced to 1-mm^3 pieces with steel scalpel blades and preincubated for 30 min at 37 C in moist 5% CO_2-95% air in sterile tubes containing glucose-free Dulbecco's Modified Eagle's Medium, supplemented with 10 mM HEPES, 2 mM glutamine, and 5% hypothyroid calf serum (Rockland Farms, Gilbertsville, PA), so that the final glucose concentration was approximately 50 μg/ml. Tumor minces were incubated for 1 or 3 h at 37 C after addition of 625 μCi/ml D-[2-^{3}H]Man (New England Nuclear, Boston, MA; 13.4 Ci/mmol). Minces were centrifuged at 500 × g for 3 min at room temperature, washed once with excess medium, and either homogenized immediately or incubated for 2 h at 37 C in complete Dulbecco's Modified Eagle's Medium, supplemented as described above and containing 1 mM nonradioactive Man. Minces were homogenized and subfractionated by differential and sucrose gradient centrifugation, as described previously (18). After centrifugation in an SW27 rotor at 75,000 × g for 6 h at 4 C, three visible bands formed near interfaces 2.0 M/1.35 M, 1.35 M/0.86 M, and 0.86 M/0.6 M sucrose. Visible bands were transferred to fresh cellulose nitrate SW27 rotor tubes and diluted dropwise with ice-cold 0.25 M sucrose-0.15 M Tris-HCl buffer, pH 8.0, to remove proteins nonspecifically adherent to the microsomal vesicles. Vesicles were pelleted at 75,000 × g for 2 h at 4 C, and aliquots were either fixed for electron microscopy or lysed for further study.

Electron microscopy was performed by Dr. Bernhard Kramarsky (Electronucleonics, Inc., Columbia, MD), as previously described (18). Vesicles from the three interfaces noted above were greater than 90% rough, greater than 80% smooth, and greater than 90% smooth, respectively, consistent with prior experiments (18) (Fig. 1). Galactosyltransferase assay was performed by using uridine diphosphate [U-^{14}C]galactose (New England Nuclear; 302 mCi/mmol) and ovalbumin with a method modified slightly from that of Spiro and Spiro (20); the average activities per mg protein for the three interfaces noted above were 12, 36, and 68 nmol/h, respectively. Prior pulse-chase experiments (18) demonstrated that *de novo* labeled proteins moved from the heavy through the intermediate to the light density fraction. Thus, for present purposes, vesicles derived from interfaces 2.0 M/1.35 M, 1.35 M/0.86 M, and 0.86 M/0.6 M sucrose have been designated RER, pSER/G, and dSER/G, respectively.

TSH and free β-subunits were immunoprecipitated from detergent-treated homogenates and microsomal subfractions with rabbit antibovine TSHβ and Staphylococcus A (Calbiochem, La Jolla, CA), as described previously (11, 18). Free α-subunits remaining in supernatants were then immunoprecipitated with rabbit antibovine LHα. Finally, remaining TP in the supernatants were precipitated with trichloroacetic acid (TCA). This strategy enabled the [^{3}H]Man-labeled oligosaccharides on TSH and free β-subunits to be compared with those on free α-subunits as well as TP in every fraction.

TSH or subunits were eluted from Staphylococcus pellets by boiling for 3 min in 0.06 M NH_4HCO_3 buffer adjusted to pH 8.5 with NH_4OH. These supernatants as well as resuspended TCA precipitates were incubated with 100 μg/ml trypsin for 4 h at 37 C, lyophilized, and resuspended in 0.01 M Na citrate buffer with 0.1% sodium dodecyl sulfate (SDS) and 1% 2-mercaptoethanol, pH 5.5. After boiling for 3 min, each 50-μl specimen was incubated with 5 mIU endoglycosidase H (provided by Dr. Frank Maley, New York State Department of Health, Albany) at 37 C for 16 h. [^{14}C]Man-labeled standard oligosaccharides were then added to each [^{3}H]Man-labeled specimen as internal standards; these had been prepared from thyrotropic tumors by methods similar to those described above and had been characterized by comparing their chromatographic migration to that of fully characterized [^{3}H]Man-labeled standard oligosaccharides generously supplied by Drs. Stuart Kornfeld (Washington University, St. Louis, MO), Phillips Robbins (Massachusetts Institute of Technology, Cambridge), Sam Turco (University of Kentucky, Lexington), and Frank Maley. Each specimen was then spotted on Whatman no. 1 paper (Whatman, London, England) and subjected to descending chromatography using the buffer system l-propanol-nitromethane-water (5:2:4). After 30–48 h the paper was dried at room temperature, lanes were cut at 0.5-cm intervals, and radioactivity was eluted with 0.7 ml water in scintillation vials for 1 h at room temperature. After the addition of scintillant (Ultrafluor, National Diagnostics, Somerville, NJ), radioactivity was counted on a Beckman LS9000 counter (Beckman Instruments, Palo Alto, CA) with a program for double isotope analysis.

Results

Thyrotropic tumor homogenates were subfractionated by differential and discontinuous sucrose gradient centrifugation into three microsomal subfractions, designated RER, pSER/G, and dSER/G. Prior pulse-chase experiments which employed radioactive amino acids demonstrated that TSH subunits moved sequentially through the three fractions (18). Recently total labeled proteins were quantified in these fractions after cells were incubated for 1 h with [^{35}S]methionine, followed by chase incubations of varying length (data not shown). The RER contained the most labeled proteins at 0 h of chase, and the radioactivity in this fraction declined precipitously between 2 and 4 h of chase. The label reached maximal levels in pSER/G at about 2 h of chase and in dSER/G at about 4 h of chase. The degree of unavoidable cross-contamination between the fractions (at most 10% between RER and dSER/G), as judged by assay for galactosyltransferase activity and electron microscopy of vesicles from the interfaces (Fig. 1), as well as the sucrose gradient yield of immunoprecipitable TSH subunits (~10%) were comparable to those prior experiments (18). Purity of subfractions rather than full recovery was our aim in this study.

After a 3-h incubation with [^{3}H]Man, tumor minces were homogenized, TSH subunits were sequentially im-

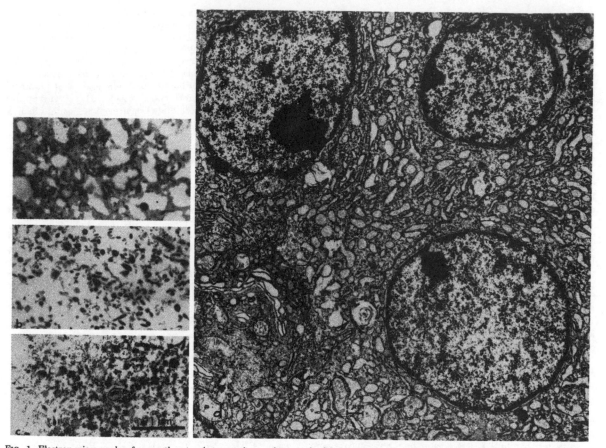

FIG. 1. Electron micrographs of mouse thyrotropic tumor tissue microsomal subfractions. Homogenates were centrifuged at 10,000 × g for 15 min at 4 C, and the supernatants were loaded onto discontinuous sucrose density gradients and centrifuged as described in *Materials and Methods*. a) Vesicles near interface 0.86 M/0.6 M sucrose, which were enriched in dSER/G, as determined by assay for galactosyltransferase activity and kinetic analysis of the movement of *de novo* labeled proteins through microsomal subfractions (18). b) Vesicles near interface 1.35 M/0.86 M sucrose enriched in pSER/G. c) Vesicles near interface 2.0 M/1.35 M sucrose enriched in RER. Magnification, ×17,000. *Bar* = 1 μm. d) Intact tumor cells with cytoplasm filled with hypertrophied RER with dilated cisternae. Few secretory granules are present. The appearance is similar to that of pituitary thyroidectomy cells (47, 49, 50). Magnification, ×5,000. *Bar* = 1 μm.

munoprecipitated, and endoglycosidase H-released carbohydrate units were analyzed by descending paper chromatography (Fig. 2a). Because endoglycosidase H cleaved oligosaccharides between the two proximal GlcNAc residues, units migrating on the chromatograms presumably contained only one proximal GlcNAc. Although further chemical characterization will ultimately be necessary to absolutely identify the [^{3}H]Man-labeled units, tentative structures were assigned with confidence because of the high specificity of endoglycosidase H as well as the comigration of radioactivity with well characterized standards. In fact, data obtained with alternate chromatographic methods, labeling with other radioactive precursors, and α-mannosidase treatment of selected species have supported the proposed structures (19).

Radioactivity at the origin represented units not cleaved from tryptic fragments by endoglycosidase H, predominantly units processed to complex forms. The types of carbohydrate units found in TSH and free β-subunits differed substantially from those found in free α-subunits (Fig. 2a). For TSH and free β-subunits, no $Glc_3Man_9GlcNAc_2$ was detected, $Glc_1Man_9GlcNAc_2$ predominated, and large amounts of $Man_9GlcNAc_2$ and $Man_8GlcNAc_2$ were detected along with smaller amounts of $Man_{7-5}GlcNAc_2$ and complex units. For free α-subunits, no $Glc_3Man_9GlcNAc_2$ was detected, small amounts of $Glc_1Man_9GlcNAc_2$ and $Man_9GlcNAc_2$ were found, $Man_8GlcNAc_2$ predominanted, and smaller amounts of $Man_{7-5}GlcNAc_2$ and complex units were present. Radioactivity in slices 80–95 formed a broad peak with a sharp

Free to Decide

1022 TSH OLIGOSACCHARIDE PROCESSING IN MICROSOMES Endo • 1984
Vol 115 • No 3

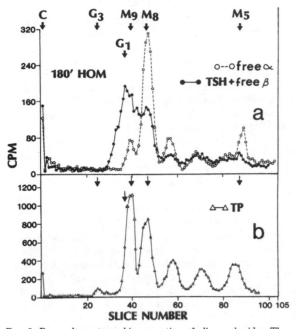

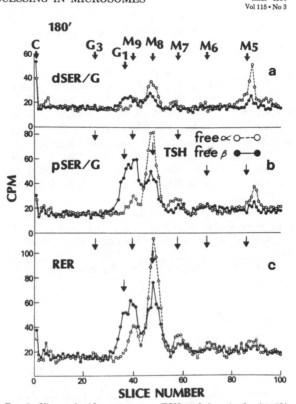

FIG. 2. Paper chromatographic separation of oligosaccharides. Thyrotropic tumor minces were incubated for 3 h with [2-³H]Man and then homogenized. TSH and free β-subunits were immunoprecipitated from homogenates first, then free α-subunits remaining in supernatants were immunoprecipitated, and finally TP remaining in supernatants were precipitated with TCA. Labeled oligosaccharides were released by endoglycosidase H and analyzed by descending paper chromatography. [¹⁴C]Mannose labeled internal standards (*arrows*) were included with each specimen and used to align figures. G_3, $Glc_3Man_9GlcNAc$; G_1, $Glc_1Man_9GlcNAc$; M_9, $Man_9GlcNAc$; M_8, $Man_8GlcNAc$; M_5, $Man_5GlcNAc$. Complex oligosaccharides (C) remained at the origin. The pattern of high Man oligosaccharides differed for TSH and free β-subunits, free α-subunits, and TP.

portion which migrated slightly faster than standard $Man_5GlcNAc$ on some chromatograms. This may represent a particular isomer containing five Man residues; a trace of this species was also present in TSH and free β-subunits.

After TSH subunits were immunoprecipitated from the homogenate, TP were precipitated with TCA, and oligosaccharides released by endoglycosidase H were analyzed (Fig. 2b). In contrast to TSH subunits, $Glc_3Man_9GlcNAc_2$ units were detected in TP. The predominant species in TP at 3 h was $Man_9GlcNAc_2$, with smaller amounts of $Man_{8-5}GlcNAc_2$ and complex units also present. The proportion of units processed to complex forms at 3 h was greatest for TSH and free β-subunits, and least for TP.

To learn the intracellular location of various processing steps, TSH subunits were immunoprecipitated from microsomal subfractions, and their labeled carbohydrate units were analyzed. In Fig. 3 chromatograms have

FIG. 3. Oligosaccharides present on TSH and free β-subunits (●) compared to those on free α-subunits (○) obtained from microsomal subfractions. Thyrotropic tumor tissue was incubated for 3 h with [2-³H]Man, homogenized, and subjected to differential and discontinuous sucrose gradient centrifugation to obtain microsomal subfractions enriched in RER, pSER/G, and dSER/G. First TSH and free β-subunits and then free α-subunits were immunoprecipitated from the three fractions. Labeled oligosaccharides were released by endoglycosidase H and analyzed by paper chromatography. The migration of [¹⁴C]Man-labeled internal standards of complex form (C) or high Man form containing Glc (G) and Man (M) is noted (*arrows*).

been aligned to facilitate comparison among the RER, pSER/G, and dSER/G. At 3 h, the RER still contained the largest quantity of radioactivity, reflecting in part the large volume of this compartment; electron micrographs of these stimulated cells showed the RER to be greatly hypertrophied and dilated (Fig. 1d). The majority of units in RER and pSER/G were sensitive to endoglycosidase H, whereas in the dSER/G, a sizable fraction was complex, especially if one considers that complex units may have only 3 mol Man/mol, whereas other species may have up to 9. After 3 h of continuous labeling, no $Glc_3Man_9GlcNAc_2$ was detected in the RER on TSH and free β-subunits or free α-subunits (Fig. 3c) even though nascent species were presumably enriched in this subfraction. Instead, TSH and free β-subunits had substantial amounts of $Glc_1Man_9GlcNAc_2$, $Man_9GlcNAc_2$, and $Man_8GlcNAc_2$, whereas free α-subunit oligosaccharides were predominantly $Man_8GlcNAc_2$, with little $Glc_1Man_9GlcNAc_2$ and only small amounts of $Man_9GlcNAc_2$. Trimming of $Man_9GlcNAc_2$ began in the RER. Substantial amounts of $Glc_1Man_9GlcNAc_2$ were retained by TSH and free β-subunits in pSER/G, whereas only trace amounts of this intermediate were detected in free α-subunits (Fig. 3b). TSH, free β-subunits, and free α-subunits had detectable $Man_9GlcNAc_2$ and $Man_8GlcNAc_2$ even in dSER/G (Fig. 3a). The progressive increase in $Man_5GlcNAc_2$ as free α-subunits translocated from the RER through pSER/G to dSER/G was striking.

The carbohydrate units of TP from these same fractions were also analyzed (Fig. 4). The proportion of complex units progressively increased from RER through

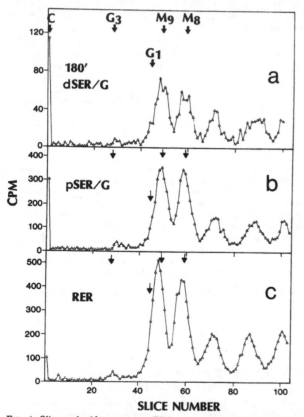

FIG. 4. Oligosaccharides present on TP in microsomal subfractions at 3 h. Thyrotropic tumor tissue was processed as described in Fig. 3. After immunoprecipitation of TSH and free β-subunits as well as free α-subunits (analyses shown in Fig. 3), the TP remaining in supernatants were precipitated with TCA. Labeled oligosaccharides were released by endoglycosidase H and analyzed by paper chromatography. The positions of [^{14}C]Man-labeled internal standards (*arrows*) are shown. See Fig. 3 for abbreviations.

pSER/G to dSER/G. In contrast to TSH subunits immunoprecipitated from the very same specimens, $Glc_3Man_9GlcNAc_2$ was detected in TP. Trimming of $Man_9GlcNAc_2$ to $Man_8GlcNAc_2$ in TP was relatively slow.

To better study the kinetics of oligosaccharide trimming, a pulse-chase design was employed. Tumor tissue minces were incubated for 60 min with [^{3}H]Man, followed by a 120-min chase incubation in the absence of radioactivity. TSH and free β-subunits, free α-subunits, and TP in homogenates were obtained sequentially, and endoglycosidase H-released units were analyzed (Fig. 5). At 60 min, $Man_9GlcNAc_2$ predominated in both TSH and free β-subunits (Fig. 5b) and TP (Fig. 5c), whereas $Man_8GlcNAc_2$ units were as prominent as $Man_9GlcNAc_2$ units in free α-subunits (Fig. 5a). After chase, the ratio of $Man_9GlcNAc_2$ to $Man_8GlcNAc_2$ units had decreased in TSH and free β-subunits (Fig. 5e) and TP (Fig. 5f), but decreased even more dramatically in free α-subunits (Fig. 5d). Except for a possibly spurious point in Fig. 5b, no $Glc_3Man_9GlcNAc_2$ was detected on TSH and free β-subunits or free α-subunits, whereas this species was present in TP at 60 min (Fig. 5c) and was long-lived (Fig. 5f). Accumulation of $Man_5GlcNAc_2$ in free α-subunits was noted after chase (Fig. 5d).

Analyses of microsomal subfractions demonstrated that at 60 min, the predominant oligosaccharides in free α-subunits, TSH, and free β-subunits were $Man_9GlcNAc_2$ and $Man_8GlcNAc_2$, with substantial amounts of $Glc_1Man_9GlcNAc_2$ present in TSH and free β-subunits (Fig. 6, a–c). Trimming of $Man_9GlcNAc_2$ to form $Man_8GlcNAc_2$ clearly began in RER before 60 min for TSH subunits (Fig. 6c) as well as for TP (Fig. 7c). After chase, $Man_8GlcNAc_2$ accumulated in free α-subunits of all compartments (Fig. 6, d–f), and accumulation of $Man_5GlcNAc_2$ in free α-subunits in pSER/G and dSER/G (Fig. 6, e and d) was marked. A species that comigrated with standard $Glc_1Man_9GlcNAc$ accumulated after chase in TSH and freeβ-subunits only and was detected in all three fractions (Fig. 6, d–f). $Glc_3Man_9GlcNAc_2$ was detected in all three fractions at 60 min in TP (Fig. 7, a–c) and persisted after chase (Fig. 7, d–f). Trimming of $Man_9GlcNAc_2$ to $Man_8GlcNAc_2$ in TP began in RER before 60 min (Fig. 7c) and proceeded in all fractions during the chase. Complex forms predominated in TP after chase in pSER/G and dSER/G (Fig. 7, e and d). In contrast to free α-subunits, no $Man_5GlcNAc_2$ was detected in TP.

Examining only figures of raw [^{3}H]Man disintegrations per min may be misleading, since the number of Man residues differs among oligosaccharide species. If one assumes that all Man residues were labeled to an equal specific activity at the long pulse time employed, then, for example, 900 dpm $Man_9GlcNAc$ and 500 dpm

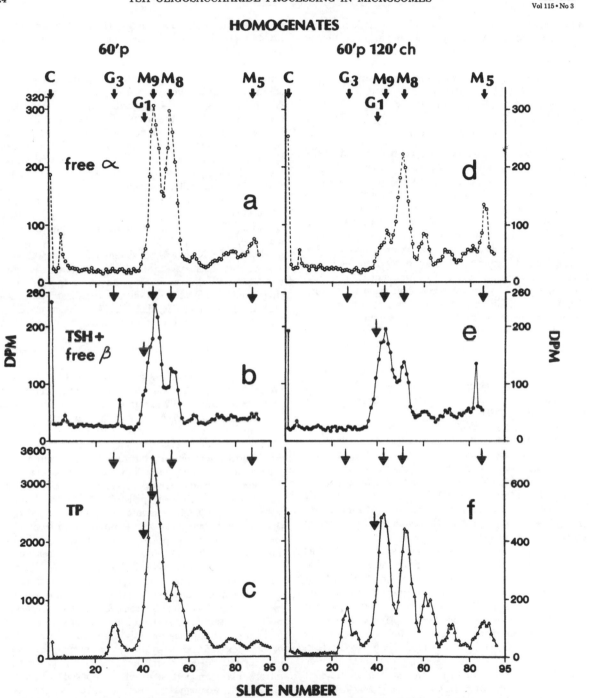

FIG. 5. Oligosaccharides present on TSH and free β-subunits (●), free α-subunits (○), and TP (△) in homogenates. Thyrotropic tumor tissue was pulse labeled with [2-³H]Man for 1 h, followed by a 2-h chase incubation in the absence of radioactive Man to study oligosaccharide precursor-product relationships. TSH and free β-subunits, free α-subunits, and TP were obtained, and endoglycosidase H-released oligosaccharides were analyzed as previously described. The *left panels* show oligosaccharides after the pulse labeling, and the *right panels* show oligosaccharides after the chase incubation. See Fig. 3 for abbreviations.

$Man_5GlcNAc$ would actually represent a 1:1 molar ratio of these two species. In Table 1, the molar percentage of oligosaccharide unit types observed under various circumstances has been calculated, as described.

Table 2 presents a summary of the differences in processing of the oligosaccharides of TSH and free β-subunits, free α-subunits, and TP.

Discussion

The mouse pituitary thyrotropic tumor is a useful model system for studying the biosynthesis of the glycoprotein hormone TSH (10). In the present studies, TSH subunits comprised about 15% of the protein synthesized (data not shown). The tumors have been shown to have morphological and biochemical features as well as endocrine responsiveness similar to nonneoplastic stimulated thyrotrophs (21). Our immunoprecipitation strategy was designed to separate excess free α-subunits from intact TSH, and thereby allowed a direct comparison of the high Man units in these species during various stages of biosynthesis in the microsomes. At the time points chosen, most β-subunits were combined with α-subunits (18), especially after 2-h chase. Moreover, every TSH molecule contributed three oligosaccharides, whereas any remaining free β-subunit contributed only one. Thus, although technically the immunoprecipitation with anti-β sera yielded TSH and free β-subunits, for practical purposes, one can consider the oligosaccharides as derived from TSH.

After cotranslational glycosylation of certain asparagine residues with high Man units, secretory glycoproteins and lysosomal enzymes follow a complicated three-dimensional path (22–25) through microsomes as sugar residues are first cleaved from and later added to the oligosaccharide units (26, 27). In only one recent study (28) have the oligosaccharide structures of a nonmembrane secretory glycoprotein, thyroglobulin, been directly analyzed in various subcellular fractions.

A striking finding of our present studies as well as other recent experiments from our laboratory (19) is that $Glc_3Man_9GlcNAc_2$ was not detected in TSH subunit precursors in the homogenates or any microsomal fraction, not even in RER presumably enriched in nascent forms. This is interesting because $Glc_3Man_9GlcNAc_2$ was found to be the primary precursor for units of various glycoproteins studied by others (26, 27) and was, in fact, a precursor for non-TSH-related glycoproteins in these cells. Instead, $Man_9GlcNAc_2$, and at certain times a species comigrating with the standard $Glc_1Man_9GlcNAc$, were the largest species found on TSH precursors. Prior control experiments using homogenates have excluded the possibilities of artifactitious removal of glucose from asparagine-linked oligosaccharides during incubations,

contamination of total proteins with oligosaccharide lipids, and selective immunoprecipitation of certain subunit forms (19). Possible explanations for the lack of $Glc_3Man_9GlcNAc_2$ in TSH subunits are 1) rapid trimming of glucose residues from a Glc_3-containing precursor, and 2) initial glycosylation with a unit other than a Glc_3-containing precursor, possibly $Man_9GlcNAc_2$. Because in other experiments (19), $Glc_3Man_9GlcNAc_2$ was not detected in α- or β-subunits in homogenates after 2-min pulses and was not detected in the RER fraction in the present studies, we currently favor the second explanation. Lack of a glucosylated precursor has been reported in whole cell homogenates of Leishmania (29), trypanosomatids (30, 31), and Concanavalin-A-resistant Chinese hamster ovary cells (32), and very little $Glc_3Man_9GlcNAc_2$ was detected on thyroglobulin precursors (28).

$Glc_3Man_9GlcNAc_2$ was consistently found in TP, suggesting that the majority of cell glycoproteins were glycosylated with this precursor. As in prior studies of thyrotropic tumor (19) as well as normal rat pituitaries (19), the half-life of $Glc_3Man_9GlcNAc_2$ was surprisingly long; substantial amounts were detected even after a 2-h chase and in distal microsomal compartments. After a 60-min pulse, 12% of the $Glc_3Man_9GlcNAc$ detected in the three microsomal fractions was present in dSER/G; after a 120-min chase, this percentage was 20%. Others have found that the half-life of $Glc_3Man_9GlcNAc_2$ on proteins was less than 2 min in chick embryo fibroblasts (33) and was about 15 min in calf thyroid (28).

A species that comigrated with authentic Glc_1-$Man_9GlcNAc$ was released in substantial amounts from TSH and free β-subunits, but only trace amounts were present in free α-subunits and TP. This species is a transient intermediate in other systems (26, 27), but was increased in both RER and pSER/G of thyrotrophs after a 2-h chase. At 3 h, it was more prominent in pSER/G than in RER (24% and 12% of units derived from TSH and free β-subunits in pSER/G and RER, respectively). This pattern suggests either that glucose was added posttranslationally to $Man_9GlcNAc_2$ units of TSH and free β-subunits or that glucose protected units from the action of mannosidase, making them appear more prominent during the chase as other forms were processed. Such a posttranslational addition was suspected in thyroid cells (34) and has recently been reported in trypanosomatids (35). Glucosylated oligosaccharides might interact with specific membrane receptors important for intracellular transport, as recently proposed by Parodi et al. (35). An analogous mechanism involving the phosphorylation of high Man units has been proposed for the sorting of lysosomal enzymes (36, 37). Glycosylation may play a role in the correct compartmentalization of mouse mammary tumor virus glycoproteins (38). However, in

1026   TSH OLIGOSACCHARIDE PROCESSING IN MICROSOMES   Endo • 1984
Vol 115 • No 3

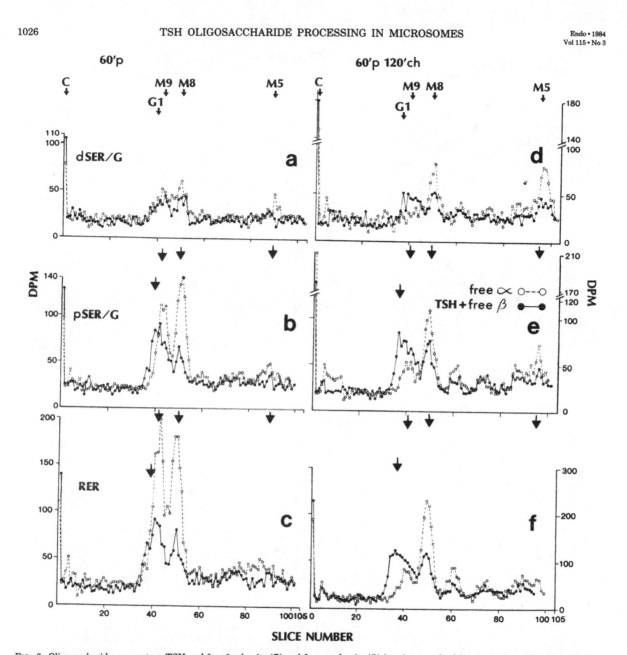

FIG. 6. Oligosaccharides present on TSH and free β-subunits (●) and free α-subunits (○) in microsomal subfractions after pulse-chase labeling. Thyrotropic tumor tissue was pulse labeled with [2-^{3}H]Man for 1 h, followed by a 2-h chase incubation. Homogenates (analyses shown in Fig. 5) were subfractionated into RER, pSER/G, and dSER/G. TSH with free β-subunits and free α-subunits were obtained sequentially, and endoglycosidase H-released oligosaccharides were analyzed by paper chromatography with the help of [^{14}C]Man-labeled internal standards (*arrows*). The *left panels* show oligosaccharides after the pulse labeling, and the *right panels* show oligosaccharides after the chase incubation. See Fig. 3 for abbreviations.

some model systems, oligosaccharides may be crucial to attain a proper glycoprotein conformation (39–42), but may not in themselves be the signal for sorting.

The pulse-chase study demonstrated differences in the rates of processing of high Man units on free α-subunits compared to those on TSH and free β-subunits, and TP. Man$_9$GlcNAc$_2$ units on free α-subunits were rapidly trimmed during the first hour to form Man$_8$GlcNAc$_2$,

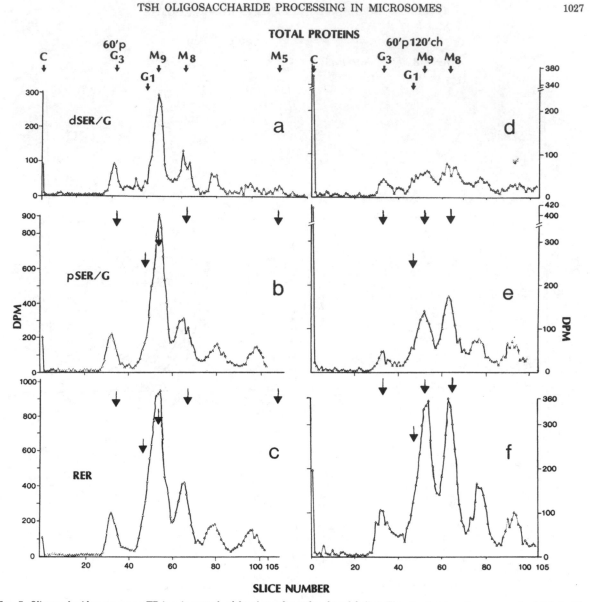

FIG. 7. Oligosaccharides present on TP in microsomal subfractions after pulse-chase labeling. Thyrotropic tumor tissue was pulse labeled with [2-³H]Man for 1 h, followed by a 2-h chase incubation. Homogenates were subfractionated as described in Fig. 6. After immunoprecipitation of TSH with free β-subunits and free α-subunits (analyses shown in Fig. 6), TP remaining in supernatants were precipitated with TCA. Endoglycosidase H-released oligosaccharides were analyzed by paper chromatography with the help of [¹⁴C]Man-labeled internal standards (*arrows*). The *left panels* show oligosaccharides after the pulse labeling, and the *right panels* show oligosaccharides after the chase incubation. See Fig. 3 for abbreviations.

but further trimming was slow, so that Man₈GlcNAc₂ accumulated during chase and was a prominent intermediate after 3 h of continuous labeling. In contrast, Man₉GlcNAc₂ units were common on TSH and free β-subunits as well as TP even after chase and at 3 h. Thus, we agree with Ruddon *et al.* (43, 44), who studied whole cell homogenates of trophoblastic tumor as well as normal placenta; they reported that the predominant units in hCG α-subunits were Man₉GlcNAc₂ and Man₈GlcNAc₂ at 2 h. More recently, in an elegant series of experiments, Peters *et al.* (45) analyzed the structures of carbohydrate units present on hCG and free α-sub-

Free to Decide

TABLE 1. Molar percentage of oligosaccharide unit types released from free α-subunits or TSH and free β-subunits isolated from microsomal subfractions

	Free α-subunits									TSH + free β-subunits								
	RER			pSER/G			dSER/G			RER			pSER/G			dSER/G		
	dpm	dpm%	mol%	dpm	dpm%	mol%	dpm	dpm%	mol%	dpm	dpm%	mol%	dpm	dpm%	mol%	dpm	dpm%	mol%
60-min pulse																		
Glc₁Man₉GlcNAc	44	2	2	22	1	1	36	5	4	124	10	8	286	31	23	32	5	3
Man₉GlcNAc	877	39	31	452	29	23	177	25	18	388	32	24	192	21	15	160	24	16
Man₈GlcNAc	828	37	33	608	39	34	217	30	24	270	22	19	184	20	16	148	23	17
Man₇GlcNAc	90	4	4	73	5	5	44	6	6	73	6	6	28	3	3	61	9	8
Man₆GlcNAc	138	6	7	123	8	9	64	9	10	142	12	13	69	7	8	75	11	12
Man₅GlcNAc	200	9	13	190	12	17	117	16	21	92	8	10	69	7	10	91	14	17
Endo H res	85	4	9	76	5	11	60	8	18	119	10	22	105	11	24	90	14	27
	2262			1544			715			1208			933			657		
60-min pulse, 120-min chase																		
Glc₁Man₉GlcNAc	33	1	1	17	1	1	15	1	1	490	23	17	314	22	15	75	8	5
Man₉GlcNAc	300	12	8	85	7	4	86	7	4	459	21	16	243	17	12	136	15	9
Man₈GlcNAc	1108	42	34	445	34	24	274	22	15	537	25	21	207	15	11	153	17	12
Man₇GlcNAc	332	13	12	85	7	5	111	9	7	130	6	6	86	6	5	100	11	9
Man₆GlcNAc	193	7	8	84	7	6	100	8	8	179	8	9	134	10	10	92	10	9
Man₅GlcNAc	483	19	24	393	30	33	509	42	46	175	8	11	265	19	23	205	22	25
Endo H res	168	6	14	191	15	27	128	11	19	204	9	21	156	11	23	161	18	32
	2617			1300			1223			2174			1415			922		

The disintegrations per minute in individual peaks in Fig. 6, and percent disintegrations per min within each set (dpm%) are tabulated. For example, the peak of Man₅GlcNAc in free α-subunits in dSER/G after 60-min pulse, 120-min chase (Fig. 6d) contained 509 dpm, 42% of the total disintegrations per min in free α-subunits in Fig. 6d. The molar percentage (mol%) was calculated based on the number of Man residues within each species type; uniform labeling of Man residues was assumed. Thus, 46% of the oligosaccharide units released from free α-subunits in dSER/G after the chase were of the form Man₅GlcNAc. Radioactivity at the origin (Endo H res) was assumed to represent complex units containing three Man residues each for purposes of this calculation.

TABLE 2. Summary of the differences in processing of units in TSH and free β-subunits, free α-subunits, and TP

	TSH and free β-subunits	Free α-subunits	TP
Glc₃Man₉GlcNAc detected			RER pSER/G dSER/G
Glc₁Man₉GlcNAc prominent	RER pSER/G		
Trimming Man₉GlcNAc to Man₈GlcNAc rapid		RER	
Major accumulation of Man₈GlcNAc		RER pSER/G	
Major accumulation of Man₅GlcNAc		dSER/G	

The microsomal subfraction(s) in which a given example was particularly prominent are noted.

units in unfractionated trophoblastic cell lysates and media. After an 8-h pulse with [2-³H]Man, intracellular hCG and free α-subunits had a similar array of asparagine-linked units, ranging from Man₉GlcNAc₂ to Man₅GlcNAc₂, with Man₈GlcNAc₂ especially prominent on free α-subunits. No major qualitative differences in oligosaccharide processing of units of hCG compared to that of free α-subunits were detected, unlike our findings for TSH and free β-subunits vs. free α-subunits.

We detected trimming of Man₉GlcNAc₂ to Man₈GlcNAc₂ before 1 h in the RER for free α-subunits, TSH, free β-subunits, and TP. This was also detected by Godelaine et al. (28) for thyroglobulin units; an α-mannosidase activity in RER different from previously described Golgi α-mannosidase activities has recently been reported (46).

In contrast to the thyroglobulin study (28), our detection of high Man units on TSH precursors in distal compartments has special implications, because all units in TSH ultimately achieve complex forms. Further investigation will be needed to determine whether TSH subunits with Man₈GlcNAc₂ units accumulate in Golgi elements transiently before further oligosaccharide processing resumes. Man₅GlcNAc₂ was a second major rate-limiting step in free α-subunit processing and accumulated in dSER/G, probably reflecting substrate-dependent differences in the kinetics of the action of N-acetylglucosaminyl transferase I.

In general, radioactivity at the origin was most prominent in dSER/G, but must be interpreted with caution. A better technique will be needed to determine whether subunits with complex forms actually exist in RER. Interestingly, autoradiographic studies have reported the uptake of fucose in RER of thyrotrophs (47) and gonadotrophs (48), but only when stimulated by the proper physiological environment.

Thus, we have identified the structures of high Man units in TSH precursors in various microsomal subfractions. The oligosaccharide processing of free α-subunits differs from that of TSH, free β-subunits, and TP. Selective processing mechanisms are at work within the thyrotroph during the biosynthesis of high Man precursors of TSH subunits.

References

1. Pierce JG 1971 Eli Lilly Lecture: The subunits of pituitary thyrotropin-their relationship to other glycoprotein hormones. Endocrinology 89:1331
2. Chin WW, Habener JF, Kieffer JD, Maloof F 1978 Cell-free translation of the messenger RNA coding for the α subunit of thyroid-stimulating hormone. J Biol Chem 253:7985
3. Kourides IA, Weintraub BD 1979 mRNA-directed biosynthesis of α subunit of thyrotropin: translation in cell-free and whole-cell systems. Proc Natl Acad Sci USA 76:298
4. Vamvakopoulos NC, Kourides IA 1979 Identification of separate mRNAs coding for the α and β subunits of thyrotropin. Proc Natl Acad Sci USA 76:3809
5. Guidice LC, Waxdal MJ, Weintraub BD 1979 Comparison of bovine and mouse pituitary glycoprotein hormone pre-α subunits synthesized in vitro. Proc Natl Acad Sci USA 76:4798
6. Guidice LC, Weintraub BD 1979 Evidence for conformational differences between precursor and processed forms of TSH-β subunit. J Biol Chem 254:12679
7. Pierce JG, Parsons TF 1981 Glycoprotein hormones: structure and function. Annu Rev Biochem 50:465
8. Kourides IA, Weintraub BD, Ridgway EC, Maloof F 1975 Pituitary secretion of free alpha and beta subunit of human thyrotropin in patients with thyroid disorders. J Clin Endocrinol Metab 40:872
9. Kourides IA, Weintraub BD, Rosen SW, Ridgway EC, Kliman B, Maloof F 1976 Secretion of alpha subunit of glycoprotein hormones by pituitary adenomas. J Clin Endocrinol Metab 43:97
10. Blackman MR, Gershengorn MC, Weintraub BD 1978 Excess production of free alpha subunits by mouse pituitary thyrotropic tumor cells in vitro. Endocrinology102:499
11. Weintraub BD, Stannard BS, Linnekin D, Marshall M 1980 Relationship of glycosylation to de novo thyroid-stimulating hormone biosynthesis and secretion by mouse pituitary tumor cells. J Biol Chem 255:5715
12. Chin WW, Maloof F, Habener JF 1981 Thyroid-stimulating hormone biosynthesis. J Biol Chem 256:3059
13. Strickland TW, Pierce JG 1983 The α subunit of pituitary glycoprotein hormones. Formation of three-dimensional structure during cell-free biosynthesis. J Biol Chem 258:5927
14. Weintraub BD, Stannard BS, Meyers L 1983 Glycosylation of thyroid-stimulating hormone in pituitary tumor cells: influence of high mannose oligosaccharide units on subunit aggregation, combination, and intracellular degradation. Endocrinology 112:1331
15. Magner JA, Weintraub BD, Thyroid-stimulating hormone biosynthesis. In: Ingbar S, Braverman L (eds) The Thyroid, S. Harper and Row, Hagerstown, in press
16. Chappel SC, Ulloa-Aquirre A, Coutifaris C 1983 Biosynthesis and secretion of follicle-stimulating hormone. Endocr Rev 4:179
17. Hussa RO 1980 Biosynthesis of human chorionic gonadotropin. Endocr Rev 1:268
18. Magner JA, Weintraub BD 1982 Thyroid-stimulating hormone subunit processing and combination in microsomal subfractions of mouse pituitary tumor. J Biol Chem 257:6709
19. Ronin C, Stanndard BS, Rosenbloom IL, Magner JA, Weintraub BD, Glycosylation and processing of high mannose oligosaccharides of thyroid stimulating hormone subunits: comparison to nonsecretory cell glycoproteins. Biochemistry, in press
20. Spiro MJ, Spiro RG 1968 Glycoprotein biosynthesis: studies on thyroglobulin. Thyroid galactosyltransferase. J Biol Chem 243:6529
21. Marshall MC, Williams D, Weintraub BD 1981 Regulation of de novo biosynthesis of thyrotropin in normal, hyperplastic and neoplastic thyrotrophs. Endocrinology 108:908
22. Claude A 1970 Growth and differentiation of cytoplasmic membranes in the course of lipoprotein granule synthesis in the hepatic cell. J Cell Biol 47:745
23. Schachter H 1974 Glycosylation of glycoproteins during intracellular transport of secretory products. Adv Cytopharmacol 2:207
24. Molnar J 1975 A proposed pathway of plasma glycoprotein synthesis. Mol Cell Biochem 6:3
25. Palade G 1975 Intracellular aspects of the process of protein synthesis. Science 189:347
26. Kornfeld R, Kornfeld S 1980 Structure of glycoproteins and their oligosaccharide units. In: Lennarz WJ (ed) The Biochemistry of Glycoproteins and Proteoglycans. Plenum Press, New York, p 1
27. Hubbard SC, Ivatt RJ 1981 Synthesis and processing of asparagine-linked oligosaccharides. Annu Rev Biochem 50:555
28. Goldelaine D, Spiro MJ, Spiro RG 1981 Processing of the carbohydrate units of thyroglobulin. J Biol Chem 256:10161
29. Parodi AJ, Martin-Barrientos J 1984 Glycoprotein assembly in Leishmania mexicana. Biochem Biophys Res Commun 118:1
30. Parodi AJ, Allue LAQ, Cazzulo JJ 1981 Pathway of protein glycosylation in the trypanosomatid Crithidia fasciculata. Proc Natl Acad Sci USA 78:6201
31. Parodi AJ, Cazzulo JJ 1982 Protein glycosylation in Trypanosoma cruzi. II. Partial characterization of protein-bound oligosaccharides labeled "in vivo." J Biol Chem 257:7641
32. Krag SS 1979 A Concanavalin-A-resistant Chinese hamster ovary cell line is deficient in the synthesis of [^{3}H] glucosyl oligosaccharide-lipid. J Biol Chem 254:9167
33. Hubbard SC, Robbins PW 1979 Synthesis and processing of protein-linked oligosaccharides in vivo. J Biol Chem 254:4568
34. Ronin C, Caseti C 1981 Transfer of glucose in the biosynthesis of thyroid glycoproteins. II. Possibility of a direct transfer of glucose from UDP-glucose to proteins. Biochim Biophys Acta 674:58
35. Parodi AJ, Mendelzon DH, Lederkremer GZ 1983 Transient glucosylation of protein-bound $Man_9GlcNAc_2$, $Man_8GlcNAc_2$, and $Man_7GlcNAc_2$ in calf thyroid cells. J Biol Chem 258:8260
36. Neufeld EF 1981 In: Callahan JW, Lowdn JA (eds) Lysosomes and Lysosomal Storage Diseases. Raven Press, New York, p 115
37. Rosenfeld MG, Kreibich G, Popov D, Kato K, Sabatini DD 1982 Biosynthesis of lysosomal hydrolases: their synthesis in bound polysomes and the role of co- and post-translational processing in determining their subcellular distribution. J Cell Biol 93:135
38. Firestone GL 1983 The role of protein glycosylation in the compartmentalization and processing of mouse mammary tumor virus glycoproteins in mouse mammary tumor virus-infected rat hepatoma cells. J Cell Biol 258:6155
39. Gibson R, Kornfeld S, Schlesinger S 1981 The effect of oligosaccharide chains of different sizes on the maturation and physical properties of the G protein of vesicular stomatitis virus. J Biol Chem 256:456
40. Fitting T, Kabat D 1982 Evidence for a glycoprotein "signal" involved in transport between subcellular organelles. J Biol Chem 257:14011
41. Polonoff E, Machida CA, Kabat D 1982 Glycosylation and intracellular transport of membrane glycoproteins encoded by murine leukemia viruses. J Biol Chem 257:14023
42. Zilberstein A, Snider MD, Porter, M, Lodish HF 1980 Mutants of vesicular stomatitis virus blocked at different stages in maturation of the viral glycoprotein. Cell 21:417
43. Ruddon RW, Bryan AH, Hanson CA, Perini F, Ceccorulli LM, Peters BP 1981 Characterization of the intracellular and secreted

forms of the glycoprotein hormone chorionic gonadotropin produced by human malignant cells. J Biol Chem 256:5189

44. Ruddon RW, Hartle RJ, Peters BP, Anderson C, Huot RI, Stromberg K 1981 Biosynthesis and secretion of chorionic gonadotropin subunits by organ cultures of first trimester human placenta. J Biol Chem 256:11389

45. Peters BP, Brooks M, Hartle R, Krzesicki RF, Perini R, Ruddon RW 1983 The use of drugs to dissect the pathway for secretion of the glycoprotein hormone chorionic gonadotropin by cultured human trophoblastic cells. J Biol Chem 258:14505

46. Bischoff J, Kornfeld R 1983 Evidence for an α-mannosidase in endoplasmic reticulum of rat liver. J Biol Chem 258:7907

47. Pelletier G, Puviani R 1973 Detection of glycoproteins and autoradiographic localization of [^{3}H] fucose in the thyroidectomy cells of rat anterior pituitary gland. J Cell Biol 56:600

48. Pelletier G 1974 Autoradiographic studies of synthesis and intracellular migration of glycoproteins in the rat anterior pituitary gland. J Cell Biol 62:185

49. Halmi NS, Gude WD 1954 The morphogenesis of pituitary tumors induced by radiothyroidectomy in the mouse and the effects of their transplantation on the pituitary body of the host. Am J Pathol 30:403

50. Furth J 1954 Morpholic changes associated with thyrotrophin-secreting pituitary tumors. Am J Pathol 30:421

Subcelluar Localization of Fucose Incorporation

Chance events can change a life. As a biologist I have been fascinated by the role of chance during evolution, and a few years ago I enjoyed reading the fascinating book by Nassim Taleb, *The Black Swan: The Impact of the Highly Improbable*. Recall that I met my future wife in a laundromat.

But now we must turn the clock back to about 1982 to see how chance enters into this research story. At NIH I had learned to use an ultracentrifuge to perform subcellular fractionation of thyrotrophs. While waiting in a small conference room at NIH for a meeting to start I absent-mindedly picked up a book off a shelf: a part of volume 78 of the J Cell Biol, 1973. As I flipped through the pages I stumbled across an article by Pelletier and Puviani entitled "Detection of glycoproteins and autoradiographic localization of [3H]fucose in the thyroidectomy cells of rat anterior pituitary gland." My mind snapped to attention. These authors seemed to find that in active pituitary thyrotrophs the fucose residues were binding to glycoproteins within the rough endoplasmic reticulum, whereas most textbooks stated that the sugar fucose was added at a late stage to glycoproteins, probably in the Golgi. They used autoradiography as their method, but I actually had the ability to study this unusual phenomenon in subcellular fractions of thyrotrophs. I also had antibody to bring down a key thyrotroph glycoprotein, TSH. I had within my reach the ability to shed substantial new information on an unusual phenomenon in cell biology, a phenomenon that could represent alteration of subcellular compartments for certain processing steps depending on the metabolic activation of the cells. Because I was finishing up my work in a few months at NIH with Dr. Weintraub, I thought that this fucose localization project could be my first major project in my new laboratory in Chicago. It could be the topic of my NIH application in 1983, and I had substantial experience with the required laboratory techniques.

In Chicago in mid-1983 I saw patients in the hospital and clinic, taught medical students and other trainees, wrote up my ^{3}H-mannose data from NIH, and started writing various research grant applications. I hired a skilled technician, Elaine Papagiannes, and began to set up my research laboratory. It was a hectic time for a young assistant professor who had a wife and sick toddler at home. Elaine and I used rabbits to raise a number of polyclonal antisera to TSH alpha- and also beta-subunits. Over many weeks we bled the rabbits using ear veins (which did not really hurt them), and we then characterized the antisera as possible tools in future experiments. Luckily, several antisera seemed to be perfect for purifying very specifically the separate TSH subunits. As my TSH-oriented laboratory was getting organized and equipped, I assisted colleagues by doing analyses for them on Apo E oligosaccharides, and also thyroxine binding globulin oligosaccharides, and those side-projects eventually resulted in nice publications in 1986. Elaine and I made steady progress on the fucose localization experiments in 1984 and 1985, and the project also provided some technical experience for a summer student, William Novak, who I included as a co-author on the fucose publication when it appeared in 1986.

The experiments were sophisticated and labor intensive, and were made possible by funding from an institutional grant, as well as my brand new NIH grant. I developed a new model for TSH biosynthesis, as shown in Figure 6 of the paper, in which the metabolic state of the thyrotrophs (euthyroid versus hypothyroid) altered the subcellular locations at which certain TSH processing steps were taking place. Biosynthetic steps were being regulated by physiology, presumably to make somewhat different isoforms of TSH in different physiologic conditions.

0013-7227/86/1193-1315$02.00/0
Endocrinology
Copyright © 1986 by The Endocrine Society

Vol. 119, No. 3
Printed in U.S.A.

Subcellular Localization of Fucose Incorporation into Mouse Thyrotropin and Free α-Subunits: Studies Employing Subcellular Fractionation and Inhibitors of the Intracellular Translocation of Proteins*

JAMES A. MAGNER, WILLIAM NOVAK, AND ELAINE PAPAGIANNES

Division of Endocrinology, Michael Reese Hospital, University of Chicago, Chicago, Illinois 60616

ABSTRACT. To determine the subcellular sites of fucose incorporation into TSH subunits, pituitaries from hypothyroid mice were incubated with [³H]fucose and fractionated by sucrose gradient centrifugation. To assess potential molecular cross-contamination between subcellular fractions enriched in rough endoplasmic reticulum (RER) or Golgi elements, trace amounts of exogenous [³⁵S]methionine-labeled proteins or [¹²⁵I]rat TSH were added before tissue homogenization. Particulate contamination of fractions was monitored by electron microscopy. TSH subunits were immunoprecipitated from fractions and analyzed by gel electrophoresis. After both a 2-h pulse incubation and a 2-h pulse, 3-h chase incubation, about half (range, 44–71%) of the [³H]fucose-labeled TSH subunit precursors present in microsomes were in the RER (amounts in excess of estimated contamination by nonspecific readsorption of molecules to vesicles or the presence of Golgi vesicles in the RER fractions); [³H]fucose-labeled free α-subunits were also detected in RER as well as in Golgi fractions. During chase incubations, both monensin and carboxyl cyanide *m*-chlorophenylhydrazone inhibited the appearance of [³⁵S]methionine- or [³H]fucose-labeled TSH subunits in medium in a dose-dependent manner, suggesting that [³H] fucose was added to subunits, in part, early in the secretory pathway. Free α-subunits were more fucosylated than was TSH; in TSH heterodimers, β-subunits were richer in fucose than were α-subunits. Thus, the fucosylation of TSH and free α-subunits in pituitaries of hypothyroid mice appears to begin at an unusually early stage of intracellular transport and may represent an adaptation to special posttranslational processing requirements. (*Endocrinology* **119:** 1315–1328, 1986)

TSH IS a glycoprotein hormone that consists of two noncovalently linked subunits, α and β, which are derived from separate mRNAs (1–4). Under certain conditions, thyrotrophs secrete excess α-subunits which are not combined with β-subunits and are termed free α-subunits. Mature α-subunits have two asparagine-linked oligosaccharides, whereas β-subunits have one; subunit species of 12,000, 18,000–19,000, and 21,000–22,000 mol wt have zero, one, and two asparagine-linked oligosaccharides, respectively (5).

The widely accepted scheme of glycoprotein biosynthesis (reviewed in Ref. 6) includes recent notions about the functional importance of the compartmentalized processing of oligosaccharides (7–10). We hoped that study of a physiologically regulated system might demonstrate how compartmentalized oligosaccharide processing has been adopted in the case of a particular differentiated cell type, the thyrotroph. Subcellular frac-

Received December 6, 1985.
Address all correspondence and requests for reprints to: Dr. James A. Magner, Division of Endocrinology, Michael Reese Hospital, Lake Shore Drive at 31st Street, Chicago, Illinois 60616.
* This work was supported in part by BRSG S07-RR-0576 and USPHS Grant AM-35619-01.

tionation studies (5, 11) of mouse thyrotropic tumor tissue have recently determined the sites of some TSH posttranslational processing steps. We sought to apply subcellular fractionation techniques to nontumorous mouse pituitary tissue. Although pituitary tissue from various species has been subjected to subcellular fractionation (12–18), biosynthetic labeling studies of pituitary tissue employing subcellular fractionation have not previously been performed for study of any of the glycoprotein hormones. Moreover, our study is the first to include exogenous radioactive proteins at the time of pituitary tissue homogenization, as described by Scheele *et al.* (19), to assess the cross-contamination of pituitary subcellular fractions by the nonspecific adsorption of labeled proteins to organelles.

The primary goal of this study was to learn whether [³H]fucose incorporation into TSH and free α-subunits begins in rough endoplasmic reticulum (RER) unlike the Golgi-associated fucosylation of other well studied glycoproteins (reviewed in Ref. 6). This unusual possibility was first considered because of a report that autoradiographs of stimulated rat thyrotrophs demonstrated acute uptake of [³H]fucose in RER as well as Golgi

1315

regions (20).

As an adjunct to direct analyses of subcellular fractions, we studied unfractionated thyrotrophs that had putatively become enriched in subunit precursors within certain subcellular compartments while being incubated with drugs that inhibited the intracellular translocation of newly synthesized proteins. In some cell types, monensin (Mon) blocks intracellular transport in middle Golgi elements (21), whereas carboxyl cyanide m-chlorophenyldrazone (CCCP) blocks transport from RER to proximal Golgi elements (22). These drugs have been used in dozens of recent studies in a wide variety of tissues (23–33), but have been used in only one other study of TSH biosynthesis (34).

By employing both methodological approaches, subcellular fractionation as well as use of translocation inhibitors, we have gained new insights into the subcellular sites of TSH and free α-subunit processing.

Materials and Methods

Thyrotropic tissues

Mouse pituitary tissue was obtained from LAF$_1$ female mice that had been radiothyroidectomized (35) 10–16 weeks before the experiment. Thirty to 80 pituitaries were minced and distributed into incubation tubes. Tissue minces were preincubated for 60 min at 37 C in a moist 5% CO_2-95% O_2 atmosphere within a shaking water bath in sterile tubes containing serum-free Dulbecco's Modified Eagle's Medium supplemented with 10 mM 4-(2-hydroxyethyl)1-piperazineethane-sulfonic acid, 2 mM glutamine, 1.2 mg/dl alanine, 1.4 mg/dl asparagine, 1.5 mg/dl aspartic acid, 4.0 mg/dl glutamic acid, and 2.0 mg/dl proline and specially constituted with 100 mg/dl glucose and methionine-free for [^{35}S]methionine incubations or 10 mg/dl glucose and 3.0 mg/dl methionine for [^{3}H]fucose incubations. Labeling was initiated by the addition of 500–800 μCi/ml L-[^{35}S]methionine (Amersham/Searle, Arlington Heights, IL; 800–1100 Ci/mmol) or 300–600 μCi/ml L-[6-^{3}H]fucose (New England Nuclear, Boston, MA; 84 Ci/mmol) (36). For chase incubations, labeling media were removed by centrifugation of minces at 100 × g at room temperature for 2 min, followed by one wash with PBS, pH 7.4. Complete medium containing 100 mg/dl glucose and 10 mg/dl methionine was then added to the minces, and the incubations were continued, with or without the addition of Mon or CCCP. To terminate incubations, minces were centrifuged at 500 × g for 5 min at 4 C and washed once with ice-cold PBS. Minces destined for subcellular fractionation were homogenized immediately and processed further without freezing, whereas other minces and media were quickly

frozen with dry ice and acetone, and stored at −20 C for a few days before analysis.

Preparation of [^{35}S]methionine-labeled secretory proteins (exogenous radioactivity)

Ten pituitaries from hypothyroid mice were minced, incubated with [^{35}S]methionine for 2 h, and then incubated in nonradioactive medium for 3 h, as described above. Sodium dodecyl sulfate (SDS)-gel electrophoresis of an aliquot of the medium showed that a wide variety of secretory proteins were present with mol wt of 12,000–100,000, with a prominent species of 29,000 mol wt. Some were glycoproteins, as shown in other experiments using [^{3}H]mannose incorporation. TSH constituted less than 1% of these ^{35}S-labeled proteins. Small amounts of this medium (10 μl, containing ~10,000 dpm) were later added to [^{3}H]fucose-incubated pituitary minces immediately before homogenization to assess the degree of nonspecific adsorption of labeled proteins to subcellular organelles.

Subcellular fractionation

Tissue minces were homogenized and fractionated as previously described (5, 11), except that an SW27.1 rotor was used rather than an SW27 rotor. Homogenates were centrifuged at 10,000 × g for 15 min at 4 C, and the resultant postmitochondrial supernatants were applied to sucrose step-gradients and centrifuged at 75,000 × g for 16 h at 4 C. Glass pipettes were used to obtain gradient fractions near the interfaces: 2.0 M/1.35 M, 1.35 M/0.86 M, and 0.86 M/0.6 M sucrose. These were designated the heavy, intermediate, and light density fractions and were putatively enriched in RER, heavy Golgi, and light Golgi elements, respectively. Both the top "load region" and bottom sucrose cushion were also collected from each gradient.

Subcellular fractions were assayed for galactosyltransferase activity, as described previously (11), with the use of uridine diphosphate [U-^{14}C]galactose (New England Nuclear; 302 mCi/mmol) and ovalbumin. Protein was determined by a method modified slightly from that of Lowry et al. (37), with ovalbumin as the standard. The galactosyltransferase specific activities in the 10,000 × g supernatant and heavy, intermediate, and light density fractions were 148, 257, 2259, and 73 μmol/h·mg protein × 10^{-6}, respectively, thus demonstrating a 15-fold enrichment in the intermediate density fraction.

Gradient fractions were examined by electron microscopy (Figs. 1 and 2), performed by Martha Newbill and Dr. Wellington Jao of Michael Reese Hospital, using fixation and staining techniques similar to those described previously (5, 11). Electron microscopy of the 10,000 × g pellet revealed unbroken cells, secretory granules (mean granule diameter, 191 nm; range, 100–350 nm), nuclei, and mitochondria.

FIG. 1. Electron micrographs of vesicles derived from sucrose step-gradient. Mouse pituitaries were homogenized and centrifuged at 10,000 × g for 15 min at 4 C. The postmitochondrial supernatants were loaded onto sucrose step-gradients (5, 11) and centrifuged at 75,000 × g for 16 h at 4 C. a) Vesicles near interface 0.6 M/0.86 M sucrose lacked ribosomes. b) Vesicles near interface 0.86 M/1.35 M sucrose were mostly lacking in ribosomes and were enriched in galactosyltransferase activity, consistent with Golgi-derived vesicles. c) Vesicles near interface 1.35 M/2.0 M sucrose were more than 95% rough vesicles. A few membrane-coated granules were present which seemed to be intimately associated with rough vesicles in many cases; these were 50–100 nm in diameter, similar to the intracisternal granules reported to be in the RER of stimulated thyrotrophs (20, 50–55). Bar = 1 μm.

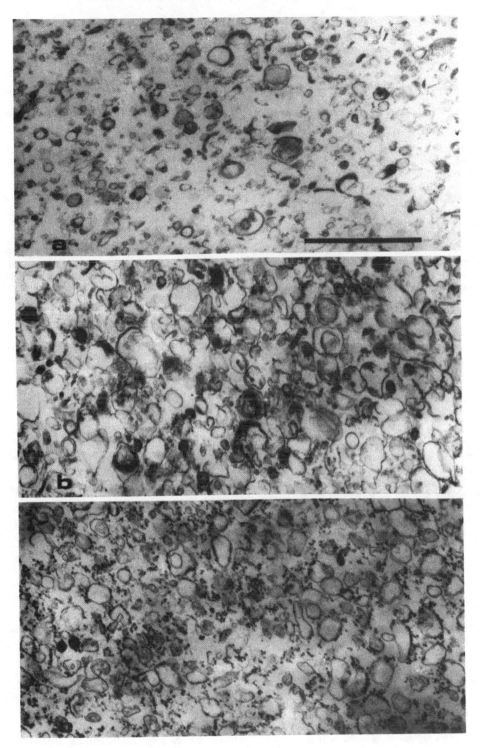

Immunoprecipitation of TSH and free α-subunits

Aliquots of specimens were added to small volumes of buffer containing 0.15 M sodium chloride, 0.02 M Tris-HCl, 0.01 M EDTA, 1% (wt/vol) Triton X-100, and 100 U/ml aprotinin, pH 7.6. The mixtures were vortexed vigorously, incubated at 4 C for 1–4 h, and then centrifuged at 10,000 × g for 15 min at 4 C. Solubilized radioactivity was immunoprecipitated by a sequential scheme employing specific antisera and *Staphylococcus A* (Pansorbin, Calbiochem, La Jolla, CA), as previously described (5). First, rabbit antirat TSHβ serum (J7) was used to obtain TSH and small amounts of free β-subunits. Antiovine LHα serum (J5) was then added to the poststaphylococcal supernatants to obtain residual free α-subunits and small amounts of LH and FSH in these eugonadal animals. (Only trace amounts of these labeled hormones were detected in other experiments using pituitaries from euthyroid mice.) The cross-reactivity of the anti-β serum for α-subunits was previously determined to be less than 4% (Table 1). The anti-β serum was shown to precipitate more than 99% of labeled TSH molecules, and the anti-α serum precipitated more than 86% of labeled free α-subunits from selected mouse pituitary lysates, as judged by subjecting poststaphylococcal supernatants to repeated immunoprecipitations. Radioactivity precipitated from specimens with nonimmune serum was analyzed by SDS-gel electrophoresis and was at background levels at all wt regions, except for a peak of radioactivity at 26,000 mol wt in [^{35}S]methionine-labeled pituitary lysates. This did not interfere with our analyses, since this nonspecific peak of radioactivity was well resolved from the TSH subunit precursors.

SDS-gel electrophoresis

Subunits were analyzed by electrophoresis in SDS-polyacrylamide slab gels with use of a 5% polyacrylamide stacking gel (1 cm) and a 12–20% linear gradient resolving gel (12 cm), as previously described (36). The following protein standards [2–5 μg each; obtained from Calbiochem or Sigma (St. Louis, MO)] were mixed with each sample immediately before gel electrophoresis to serve as internal mol wt markers: carbonic anhydrase (29,000), soybean trypsin inhibitor (20,000), myoglobin (17,000), and cytochrome *c* (12,000). Coomassie brilliant blue-stained gels were slices into 1- or 2-mm sections, solubilized, and counted in 10 ml of a xylene-based detergent-containing solution (Scint A, Packard, Downers Grove, IL).

Total [^{35}S]methionine- or [^{3}H]fucose-labeled protein

Aliquots of specimens were supplemented with 2 mg ovalbumin and precipitated with cold 10% trichloroacetic acid (TCA). Pellets obtained by centrifugation at 1000 × g for 10 min at 4 C were washed with 10% TCA, dissolved in 0.4 ml 0.2 M NaOH, and counted.

Inhibitors of intracellular translocation

Separate stock solutions of 0.02 M Mon (Sigma) and 0.05 M CCCP (Calbiochem) were prepared in 95% ethanol 24 h before an experiment, stored at −20 C, and diluted appropriately with 95% ethanol immediately before use. The drugs in volumes of

1 μl were added to tissue incubations with 1 ml medium, and 1 μl ethanol was added to control incubations.

Use of endoglycosidase H

For selected specimens, TSH subunits were eluted from *Staphylococcus* pellets by boiling for 3 min in 50 μl 0.01 M Na citrate buffer with 0.1% SDS and 1% 2-mercaptoethanol, pH 5.5. Each specimen was equally divided and incubated for 4–16 h at 37 C with or without 5 mIU endoglycosidase H (Miles Scientific, Naperville, IL). Before electrophoresis, 6 μl buffer containing 40% 2-mercaptoethanol and 15% SDS were added, and the specimens were boiled for 5 min. Finally, the mol wt markers and 12 μl loading buffer with 70% glycerol (wt/vol), 0.05% bromphenol blue, and 0.02 M Tris-HCl, pH 6.8, were added to each specimen before SDS-gel electrophoresis.

Calculation of leakage and adsorption by use of the double label protocol

The calculations for leakage and adsorption followed the method of Scheele *et al.* (19) and were based on the following premises: 1) endogenously labeled ([^{3}H]fucose-labeled) secretory proteins are restricted *in vivo* to the intracisternal space of the secretory compartments of the thyrotroph; 2) all endogenously labeled secretory proteins that remain in fraction 1 (the top load region) of the sucrose gradients represent nonvesicle-associated proteins leaked from secretory compartments; and 3) during tissue homogenization, exogenously labeled ([^{35}S] methionine-labeled) secretory proteins added as a tracer and endogenously labeled proteins that leak from intracellular compartments mix fully and subsequently are adsorbed at the same rate and with the same affinity to available surfaces. Thus,

$$\frac{([^{35}S]\text{methionine-labeled proteins})_{\text{fxn } 1}}{(\text{nonspecifically adsorbed } [^{35}S]\text{methionine-labeled proteins})_{\text{fxn } n}}$$

$$= \frac{([^{3}H]\text{fucose-labeled proteins})_{\text{fxn } 1}}{(\text{nonspecifically adsorbed } [^{3}H]\text{fucose-labeled proteins})_{\text{fxn } n}}$$

Note that fxn 1 indicates the first sucrose gradient fraction (the specimen load region), and fxn n indicates the nth gradient fraction.

Because the [^{35}S]methionine-labeled proteins in fractions 1 and n as well as the [^{3}H]fucose-labeled proteins in fraction 1 can be measured, the [^{3}H]fucose-labeled proteins nonspecifically adsorbed in fraction n can be calculated and compared to the total [^{3}H]fucose-labeled proteins measured in fraction n. Like Scheele *et al.*, we also calculated a primary location index, the ratio of endogenous radioactivity still in its primary location to total endogenous radioactivity measured in a gradient fraction. Because we were most concerned about TSH localization, we also performed experiments in which [^{125}I]rat TSH was added as a tracer to tissue minces just before homogenization and cell fractionation. As discussed in *Results*, very little of the exogenous TSH adsorbed to cell organelles.

Results

Subcellular fractionation of mouse pituitary tissue incubated with [^{35}S]methionine

We sought to establish that pituitary tissue from hypothyroid mice could be incubated with radioactive iso-

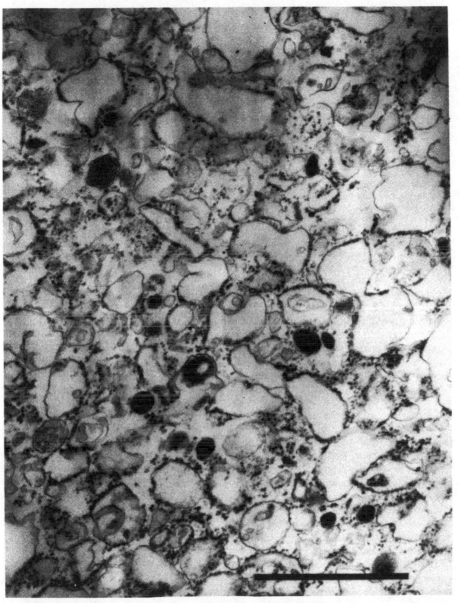

FIG. 2. Electron micrograph of a granule-rich region of a rough vesicle fraction. Material derived from the sucrose gradient in Fig. 1 near interface 1.35 M/2.0 M sucrose was predominantly rough vesicles, but selected regions were rich in granules. The granules were intimately associated with rough cisternae, and their mean diameter was approximately half that of secretory granules present in the 10,000 × g pellet. Many of these granules, however, may represent small secretory granules from a variety of pituitary cell types. *Bar* = 1 μm.

topes and subjected to subcellular fractionation, using techniques similar to our prior studies with thyrotropic tumor tissue (5, 11). We found it necessary to use pituitaries from 30–80 mice (10–16 weeks postthyroidectomy) to have an adequate amount of tissue (0.2–0.5 g). Pitui-

tary minces were incubated with [^{35}S]methionine for 20 or 120 min. Subsequently, TSH subunit precursors were immunoprecipitated from homogenates and subcellular fractions and analyzed by SDS-gel electrophoresis. Compared with the amount of TCA-precipitable radioactivity

SUBCELLULAR SITES OF TSH SUBUNIT PROCESSING Endo • 1986
Vol 119 • No 3

TABLE 1. Specificity of rabbit antisera in the precipitation of [^{125}I] iodo-TSH subunits

	[^{125}I]Ovine LHα^a	[^{125}I]Rat TSHβ
Anti-LHα (J5)[b]	79	2
Anti-TSHβ (J7)[c]	4	86
Nonimmune serum	<2	<2

Rat and ovine TSH subunits are chemically and immunologically similar to mouse forms (1, 7). Mouse TSH subunits are not available in pure form. Numbers represent the percentage of radioactivity immunoprecipitated by each serum at a final dilution of 1:10.

[a] Chemically identical with α prepared from TSH.

[b] Generated by immunization using ovine LHα provided by the National Hormone and Pituitary Agency.

[c] Generated by primary immunization using bovine TSHβ purified by Dr. J. G. Pierce, followed by injections of rat TSHβ provided by the National Hormone and Pituitary Agency.

present, TSH subunit precursors comprised only 0.01% of the labeled proteins in homogenates and fractions compared to about 15% in tumors (5).

Antisera were used sequentially in all experiments to allow TSH to be analyzed separately from residual free α-subunits. Thus, use of anti-TSHβ serum first resulted in gels with radioactivity at 21,000 mol wt (representing α-subunits that had bound noncovalently to β-subunits) and 19,000 mol wt (representing β-subunits; see Ref. 5 for illustrative gel pattern and discussion). Subsequent addition of anti-α serum to the poststaphylococcal supernatants resulted in gels with a peak of radioactivity at 21,000–23,000 mol wt (representing free α-subunits, which were consistently found to have a slightly higher mol wt than α-subunits derived from TSH heterodimers) and small peaks at 19,000 and 16,000 mol wt. In the homogenates at 20 and 120 min, there were 1,716 and 11,997 dpm free α-subunits, respectively, and 468 and 3,927 dpm TSH, respectively, demonstrating that incorporation of [^{35}S]methionine into subunits was approximately linear with time. Processing of α-subunit precursors from the 19,000 to the 21,000–23,000 mol wt forms was evident in homogenates with time, as previously demonstrated in tumor tissue (5, 36); at 20 min, the 19,000 and 21,000–23,000 mol wt forms constituted 26% and 74%, respectively, of the free α-subunits, whereas at 120 min, they were 7% and 93%, respectively.

TSH subunit precursors were immunoprecipitated from heavy, intermediate, and light density microsomes derived from the discontinuous sucrose gradients, and analyzed by SDS-gel electrophoresis. Radioactivity in the pertinent gel regions noted above was integrated, and the results are summarized in Fig. 3. At 20 min, the majority of subunit precursors were present in heavy density microsomes, which were enriched in RER, whereas by 120 min, subunits were detected in all three microsomal fractions. Combination of α- and β-subunits

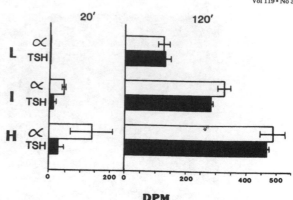

FIG. 3. The distribution of TSH and free α-subunits within microsomal fractions of mouse pituitary tissue. Pituitaries were incubated with [^{35}S]methionine for 20 or 120 min and fractionated into heavy (H), intermediate (I), and light (L) density microsomes enriched in RER, heavy Golgi, and light Golgi elements, respectively. TSH (■) and free α-subunits (□) were immunoprecipitated from fractions and analyzed by gel electrophoresis, and the radioactivity in appropriate gel regions was summed (mean ± range). Subunits predominated in RER at 20 min, but were distributed in all fractions, including light Golgi, by 120 min.

into TSH was detectable in heavy and intermediate density microsomes at 20 min and in all fractions at 120 min. The molar ratios of free α-subunits to TSH at 120 min in the heavy, intermediate, and light density fractions were 1.8, 1.8, and 1.5, respectively. The amounts of radioactive subunits immunoprecipitated from sucrose gradient fractions were summed and compared to the amounts of subunits in the homogenates to calculate an overall yield of subunits of 14% (range, 8–22%; n = 4). This is comparable to yields obtained in our prior studies of tumor tissue (5); relative purity of cell fractions rather than full recovery was our prime concern. Thus, the scheme of TSH biosynthesis postulated from studies of tumor tissue fractions seemed generally to be true in hypothyroid pituitary tissue as well.

Subcellular fractionation of mouse pituitary tissue incubated with [^{3}H]fucose

We next prepared subcellular fractions of pituitary tissue in an attempt to learn the subcellular compartment(s) in which [^{3}H]fucose was incorporated into TSH subunit precursors. Unlike the [^{35}S]methionine studies, comparable [^{3}H]fucose incorporation experiments employing subcellular fractionation had not been performed using the thyrotropic tumor model and have not been performed in studies of any glycoprotein hormone. Pituitaries from 40 thyroidectomized mice were minced and incubated with [^{3}H]fucose for 2 h, followed by 3-h chase incubations in nonradioactive medium containing no drug, 2 μM Mon, or 10 μM CCCP. Although shorter pulse incubations were preferred, only trace labeling of subunits occurred after a 20-min incubation (data not shown). To assess possible molecular cross-contamination of cell fractions, [35S]methionine-labeled proteins (see *Materials and Methods*) were added to the [3H]fucose-labeled tissue immediately before tissue homogenization.

[3H]Fucose-labeled TSH and free α-subunits were immunoprecipitated from homogenates and media and examined by gel electrophoresis. Radioactivity in the pertinent gel regions was integrated and is summarized in Table 2. TSH and free α-subunits constituted 0.59% (range, 0.35–0.86%) and 0.87% (range, 0.76–0.99%), respectively, of the total [3H]fucose-labeled glycoproteins present in the homogenates; after the 3-h chase incubation, TSH and free α-subunits constituted 2.5% and 5.5%, respectively, of the total [3H]fucose-labeled glycoproteins in the medium.

After a 2-h pulse incubation with [3H]fucose, substantial labeling continued during a 3-h chase incubation (Table 2), in spite of the fact that the radioactive medium had been physically removed. For example, the homogenates contained 5,760 dpm TSH at 2 h, but 15,605 dpm after the 3-h chase, with an additional 12,155 dpm present in the medium. The continued incorporation of [3H]fucose possibly reflected intracellular pools of accumulated [3H]fucose. Total (homogenate plus medium) labeled TSH, free α-subunits, and total proteins increased during the chase incubations by 480%, 306%, and 174%, respectively. This pattern of high continuing fucosylation of TSH and free α-subunits compared to total fucose-containing proteins was noted in multiple tubes in three separate labeling experiments. It may be that different pools of [3H]fucose with differing specific activities (perhaps even located in different types of pituitary cells) were available for the fucosylation of different glycoproteins. The presence of Mon or CCCP during the 3-h chase incubations appeared to diminish the ongoing fucose incorporation into TSH and free α-subunits more markedly than that of total proteins. Mon also inhibited the appearance of TSH and free α-subunits in the medium by 78% and 74%, respectively, whereas CCCP inhibited these by 83% and 78%, respectively. Most of the [3H]fucose-labeled total proteins were not secretory proteins, since the 537,000 dpm present in the medium after 3-h chase represented only 18% of the radioactivity in homogenate plus medium.

The postmitochondrial supernatants contained 58% (range, 56–60%) of the TCA-precipitable 3H radioactivity and 75% (range, 52–95%) of the labeled TSH subunit precursors originally present in the homogenates. Aliquots of these postmitochondrial supernatants were applied to discontinuous sucrose gradients. After centrifugation, each gradient was divided into six fractions, and TCA-precipitable 3H and 35S radioactivity were determined in each fraction using a dual isotope-counting program (Table 3). Most of the [35S]methionine-labeled proteins added as tracer remained at the top of each gradient (fraction 1), indicating that few proteins had adsorbed nonspecifically to the vesicles that had migrated into the gradients. Endogenous ([3H]fucose) radioactivity that remained in fraction 1 presumably represented glycoproteins that had leaked from vesicles during homogenization, but had not adsorbed to vesicles. The fraction 1 endogenous radioactivity was high for the 2-h pulse specimen, where it constituted 54% of the endogenous radioactivity of the gradient, but was only 23%, 26%, and 24% of the total gradient endogenous radioactivity for 3-h chase specimens incubated with no drug, Mon, and CCCP, respectively. The calculated primary location index for each fraction is shown in Table 4; the relatively high values indicate that little cross-contamination of the gradient fractions had occurred as a result of nonspecific adsorption of proteins to vesicles. In a separate experiment we also determined that [125I] rat TSH added to pituitary tissue immediately before homogenization did not readily adsorb to microsomal vesicles (Table 5).

TSH and free α-subunits were immunoprecipitated from the sucrose gradient fractions (Table 6). The yield of labeled subunits was similar to that of the [35S]methionine experiments; 18% of labeled subunits originally present in homogenates were recovered in gradient fractions. Only trace amounts of [35S]methionine-labeled TSH and free α-subunits were detected, contributed by the exogenous 35S-labeled proteins (data not shown). Substantial amounts of [3H]fucose-labeled TSH and free α-subunits were detected in the sample load region, heavy Golgi-containing, and RER-containing fractions of all gradients. If one considers the microsome-associated ra-

TABLE 2. Distribution in homogenates and media of [3H]fucose-labeled TSH, free α-subunits, and total proteins

	2-h pulse	2-h pulse, 3-h chase, control	2-h pulse, 3-h chase, 2 μM Mon	2-h pulse, 3-h chase, 10 μM CCCP
Homogenates				
TSH	5,760	15,605	12,127	14,957
Free α-subunits	14,859	18,281	19,594	14,281
Total proteins	1,638,000	2,394,000	1,974,000	1,743,000
Media				
TSH		12,155	2,695	2,052
Free α-subunits		27,263	7,203	5,908
Total proteins		537,000	379,000	564,000

Pituitaries from 40 hypothyroid mice were minced and incubated with [3H]fucose in pulse-chase fashion, as indicated. TSH and free α-subunits were immunoprecipitated from homogenates and media with specific antisera and analyzed by SDS-gel electrophoresis. Total labeled proteins were determined by precipitation using TCA. Values are expressed as disintegrations per min.

TABLE 3. Distribution among sucrose gradient fractions of endogenous [³H]fucose-labeled proteins and exogenous [³⁵S]methionine-labeled proteins

FXN[a]	2-h pulse		2-h pulse, 3-h chase, control		2-h pulse, 3-h chase, 2 μM Mon		2-h pulse, 3-h chase, 10 μM CCCP	
	³H (dpm)	³⁵S (dpm)	³H (dpm)	³⁵S (dpm)	³H (dpm)	³⁵S (dpm)	³H (dpm)	³⁵S (dpm)
1	214,400	6,825	176,650	5,300	170,950	6,825	161,975	5,450
2A	10,900	65	39,360	625	23,780	270	22,310	175
2B	17,040	70	47,330	270	28,450	130	35,120	190
3	107,080	100	349,740	100	325,100	180	290,520	480
4	35,055	180	155,182	225	103,567	315	143,100	135
5	8,958	36	16,602	84	15,840	18	25,470	72
Total	393,433		784,864		667,687		678,495	

Hypothyroid mouse pituitary minces were incubated with [³H]fucose in pulse-chase fashion, as indicated by the column headings. An aliquot of [³⁵S]methionine-labeled proteins was added to each tube of minces immediately before homogenization to test whether the exogenous radioactivity would absorb to microsomal vesicles and subsequently migrate from the load area (fraction 1) of the sucrose gradients during centrifugation. Precipitable radioactivity in gradient fractions was determined with TCA.

[a] Gradient fraction: 1, top load area; 2A and 2B, fractions at and slightly below, respectively, the 0.6 M/0.86 M sucrose interface; 3, fraction enriched in Golgi elements; 4, fraction enriched in RER; 5, sucrose cushion at bottom of the gradient.

TABLE 4. Calculated primary location indices for TCA-precipitable proteins in the gradient fractions displayed in Table 3

Gradient fraction	2-h pulse	2-h pulse, 3-h chase, control	2-h pulse, 3-h chase, 2 μM Mon	2-h pulse, 3-h chase, 10 μM CCCP
2A	0.813	0.471	0.716	0.767
2B	0.871	0.810	0.886	0.839
3	0.971	0.990	0.986	0.951
4	0.839	0.952	0.924	0.972
5	0.874	0.831	0.972	0.916

Indices were calculated by the method of Scheele et al. (19). A fraction with an index near 1.0 has most of the endogenous label (in this case [³H]fucose-labeled proteins) still in its primary location. Pituitary minces were incubated with [³H]fucose in pulse-chase fashion, as indicated by the column headings, before cells were fractionated. See Table 3 for abbreviations.

TABLE 5. Distribution of exogenous [¹²⁵I]rat TSH in sucrose gradient fractions

Fraction no.	[¹²⁵I]rat TSH (cpm)	Fraction no.	[¹²⁵I]rat TSH (cpm)
1 (top)	49,978	10	1511
2	52,813	11	950
3	54,789	12 (heavy Golgi)	590
4	50,180	13	353
5	39,779	14	275
6	24,240	15	339
7 (light Golgi)	9,128	16 (RER)	432
8	3,820	17	373
9	2,839	18 (bottom)	713

Pituitaries from euthyroid and hypothyroid mice were mixed and minced, and an aliquot of [¹²⁵I]rat TSH solution was added to the minces immediately before homogenization. The postmitochondrial supernatant (volume, 5 ml) was loaded onto a discontinuous sucrose gradient, which was later fractionated into 18 1-ml fractions. The pattern of radioactivity indicated that most of the exogenous TSH remained at the top of the gradient; very little absorbed to microsomes that migrated into the gradient.

dioactivity, then 51% of [³H]fucose-labeled free α-subunits were in the RER at 2 h, 44% after the 3-h chase, 22% after the 3-h chase in the presence of Mon, and 30% after the 3-h chase in the presence of CCCP. Similar surprisingly large amounts of [³H]fucose-labeled TSH were also present in RER fractions. There was a slight accumulation of labeled precursors in Golgi elements in the presence of Mon or CCCP. Primary location indices were calculated for fractions 3 and 4 from each gradient using [³H]TSH or [³H]free α-subunits and [³⁵S]methionine-labeled total proteins, and varied from 0.948–0.984, indicating that few of the ³H-labeled species in the fractions had been contributed by nonspecific adsorption.

Qualitative analyses of [³H]fucose-labeled TSH and free α-subunits

In every case, radioactivity eluted from *Staphylococcus* pellets was subjected to gel electrophoresis. Radioactivity was not detectable in any of the regions of the gels except in the 18,000–19,000 and 20,000–24,000 mol wt regions, where it was expected. Regarding the electrophoretic profile of [³H]fucose-labeled TSH, the ratio of 21,000 to 18,000 mol wt radioactivity in homogenates averaged 0.520 (range, 0.384–0.729), and that in media averaged 0.634 (range, 0.461–0.785) under a variety of pulse-chase conditions, suggesting that the β-subunit of the TSH heterodimer is normally richer in fucose than is the α-subunit. Mon and CCCP induced no consistent changes in the electrophoretic profile of TSH. [³H]Fucose-labeled free α-subunits migrated primarily at 22,000–24,000 mol wt, a slightly higher mol wt than that of α-subunits derived from TSH heterodimers. At 2 h, free α-subunits incorporated more [³H]fucose than did TSH. If the molar

TABLE 6. Distribution of [³H]fucose-labeled free α-subunits and TSH in sucrose gradient fractions

Gradient fraction	2-h pulse		2-h pulse, 3-h chase, control		2-h pulse, 3-h chase, 2 μM Mon		2-h pulse, 3-h chase, 10 μM CCCP	
	α	TSH	α	TSH	α	TSH	α	TSH
1 (load region)	1454	737	879	945	322	460	479	279
2B (light Golgi)	59	7	39	96	33	40	140	146
3 (heavy Golgi)	414	181	1093	819	1380	945	1717	953
4 (RER)	486	464	881	831	398	352	769	462
Total	2413	1389	2892	2691	2133	1797	3105	1840

Forty pituitaries from hypothyroid mice were minced, incubated with [³H]fucose in pulse-chase fashion as indicated, homogenized, and centrifuged at 10,000 × g. Aliquots of these postmitochondrial supernatants were loaded onto discontinuous sucrose gradients, and later, TSH and free α-subunits were immunoprecipitated from the gradient fractions and analyzed by SDS-gel electrophoresis. Values are expressed as disintegrations per min.

ratio of free α-subunits to TSH is assumed to be approximately 2, as determined in the [³⁵S]methionine experiments, then intracellular free α-subunits were somewhat richer in fucose than was TSH at 2 h.

Additional studies employing Mon and CCCP

Pituitaries from 30–35 previously thyroidectomized mice were minced and incubated with [³⁵S]methionine or [³H]fucose for 2 h. The minces were then washed and resuspended in chase medium lacking the radioactive precursors, and the incubations were continued for 3 h in the presence of no drug, 0.2 or 2 μM Mon, or 5 or 50 μM CCCP. TSH and free α-subunits were immunoprecipitated from cell lysates and chase media and analyzed by SDS-gel electrophoresis.

[³⁵S]Methionine-labeled free α-subunits were detectable in the lysate after the 2-h labeling period (Fig. 4, line 1, □) and were partially secreted into the medium during the 3-h chase period (Fig. 4, line 2, □); total free α-subunit radioactivity in lysate and medium increased by 63% during the chase incubation, a phenomenon commonly seen in the past (5, 36) and attributed to slow equilibration of the intracellular pools of precursors. Mon at 0.2 and 2 μM and CCCP at 5 and 50 μM inhibited the appearance of free α-subunits in medium by 24%, 74%, 56%, and 79%, respectively, compared to the control value. The drugs also caused free α-subunits to accumulate within the cells. Fewer total free α-subunits (lysate plus medium) were seen in the presence of 50 μM CCCP than in the other chase incubations, reflecting either decreased synthesis or increased degradation of free α-subunits. Similar effects on the distribution of [³⁵S]methionine-labeled TSH were noted. All subunits in medium were resistant to endoglycosidase H. Similarly, as illustrated in the *lower portion* of Fig. 4, the appearance in the medium of [³H]fucose-labeled free α-subunits was inhibited by Mon at 0.2 and 2 μM and by CCCP at

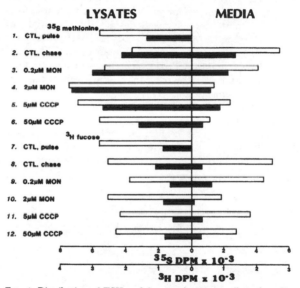

FIG. 4. Distribution of TSH and free α-subunits in cells and media after short chase incubations with Mon or CCCP. Pituitaries were incubated with [³⁵S]methionine or [³H]fucose for 2 h, followed by 3-h chase incubations with or without Mon or CCCP. TSH (■) and then free α-subunits (□) were sequentially immunoprecipitated from lysates or media and analyzed by SDS-gel electrophoresis, and radioactivity in the pertinent gel regions was summed. Mon and CCCP inhibited the appearance of [³H]fucose-labeled subunits in medium in a pattern similar to that of [³⁵S]methionine-labeled subunits. CTL, Control.

5 and 50 μM by 11%, 63%, 28%, and 44%, respectively. A dose-dependent inhibition of [³H]fucose-labeled TSH secretion may have occurred, but was less well demonstrated.

In a separate experiment, pituitaries were minced and incubated with [³⁵S]methionine or [³H]fucose for 2 h, and then resuspended in chase medium containing no drug, 2 μM Mon, or 10 μM CCCP. The incubations were continued for 18 h, and TSH and free α-subunits were then immunoprecipitated from lysates and media and analyzed by SDS-gel electrophoresis. The results are summarized in Fig. 5. As in the prior experiment, Mon and CCCP inhibited the appearance of the [³H]fucose-labeled precursors in medium, and the distribution of the [³H]fucose-labeled precursors between media and lysates was similar to that of the [³⁵S]methionine-labeled precursors.

Discussion

As an extension of prior studies of TSH processing by thyrotrophs (5, 11, 35, 36, 38–42) and in light of an interesting recent study of hCG which employed ionophore drugs (30), we chose to investigate the subcellular sites of TSH processing in the stimulated thyrotrophs of hypothyroid mice. Our goal was to study a more physiological nontumorous model despite the potential difficulties of detecting small amounts of TSH precursors in cell fractions. In early experiments using [³⁵S]methionine, we found that TSH precursors were about 3 orders of magnitude less prevalent in pituitary minces compared to thyrotropic tumors. However, the immunoprecipitation and electrophoretic techniques used here allowed these small amounts of labeled precursors to be analyzed. Processing of free α-subunits from 19,000 to 21,000–23,000 mol wt was detected; β-subunits of TSH were of 19,000 mol wt. TSH and free α-subunits were largely

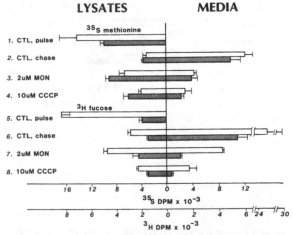

LYSATES   **MEDIA**

FIG. 5. Distribution of TSH and free α-subunits in cells and media after long chase incubations with Mon or CCCP. Pituitaries were incubated with [³⁵S]methionine or [³H]fucose for 2 h, followed by 18-h chase incubations with or without Mon or CCCP. TSH (■) and then free α-subunits (□) were sequentially immunoprecipitated from lysates or media and analyzed by SDS-gel electrophoresis, and radioactivity in the pertinent gel regions was summed (mean ± SEM; n = 2). CTL, Control. Mon and CCCP inhibited the secretion of [³H]fucose-labeled precursors in a pattern similar to that of [³⁵S]methionine-labeled precursors.

present in heavy density microsomes (enriched in RER) at 20 min and translocated in part to the Golgi apparatus by 120 min. Combination of α- and β-subunits began in the RER. The molar ratio of free α-subunits to TSH was lower in homogenates and cell fractions derived from the pituitary than in the tumor tissue (5), consistent with the known excess synthesis of free α-subunits by tumors (35, 36, 40, 41). The galactosyltransferase activity of the pituitary tissue predominated in Golgi elements that were somewhat denser than those of the tumor tissue (11).

We also sought to learn the subcellular site(s) of fucose incorporation into TSH precursors. Although the general scheme of glycoprotein biosynthesis has been established in a variety of systems (reviewed in Ref. 6), we considered that carbohydrate addition to TSH might involve novel features, because the processing of its oligosaccharides is apparently modulated by endocrine and other factors (43–46). The final carbohydrate composition of TSH may influence its rate of metabolic clearance as well as the intrinsic activity of the hormone (34, 47, 48). [³H]Fucose was chosen as the carbohydrate precursor in these studies because it is rarely converted to other sugars during short incubations (49) and because of an intriguing report that, unlike most cells, thyrotrophs may acutely concentrate fucose in the RER as well as Golgi elements under some conditions (20). Moreover, we have previously reported (11) that 9–22% of the carbohydrate units of free α-subunits and TSH isolated from the RER of thyrotropic tumor cells were resistant to endoglycosidase H, and that considerable amounts of these species are retained in the RER after chase incubations.

To determine the subcellular sites of [³H]fucose incorporation into TSH and free α-subunits, we employed a dual approach: studies of subcellular fractions and studies employing inhibitors of the intracellular translocation of newly synthesized proteins. When the first approach was used, labeled subunit precursors were immunoprecipitated from subcellular fractions and analyzed by gel electrophoresis; provisions were made to assess the degree of cross-contamination of subcellular fractions by 1) examining the degree of leakage and relocation of labeled TSH subunits by the tracer method of Scheele et al. (19) and 2) electron microscopy of the subcellular fractions to evaluate particulate contamination. With 2-h pulse and 2-h pulse, 3-h chase, roughly half of the microsome-associated [³H]fucose-labeled TSH and free α-subunits were present in the RER; we estimated that nonspecific leakage and readsorption of labeled subunits could have contributed only about 1–5%. We also estimated that less than 5% of the vesicles in the RER-enriched fractions were Golgi-derived smooth vesicles, but a potentially more serious type of particulate contamination was the presence of small 50- to 100-nm diameter granules. The interpretation of our detection of [³H] fucose-labeled TSH subunit precursors in RER depends on whether 1) the small granules are from late in the secretory pathway and are contaminating the RER-enriched fractions, or 2) some of these granules are so-called intracisternal granules (50–55), normally associated with RER *in vivo* in stimulated thyrotrophs, and may in fact represent the structural correlate for the RER-associated fucosylation. Of note, by 10 days post-thyroidectomy, rat thyrotrophs contained few or no secretory granules, and in subsequent days, the quantity of intracisternal RER-localized granules increased (50). Because our studies used mice thyroidectomized 10–16 weeks previously, few TSH-containing secretory granules should have been present in the thyrotrophs. Electron micrographs of RER-enriched fractions from euthyroid mouse pituitaries also showed similar granules (not shown), suggesting that most of these granules were secretory granules from a variety of pituitary cell types. However, after 20- and 90-min incubations of euthyroid mouse pituitaries with [³H]fucose (55a) only 5% and 20%, respectively, of microsome-associated labeled free α-subunits were detected in the RER fractions, with the remainder in the Golgi-enriched fractions. Because significant labeling of secretory granules under euthyroid conditions apparently required longer incubations with isotope and because few secretory granules are present in thyroidectomy cells, at present we believe that the RER-associated labeled TSH and free α-subunits found in the present experiments using hypothyroid mice may have been contributed in large part by the vesicles of hypertrophied RER, rather than solely by putative thyrotroph secretory granules contaminating the subcellular fraction. Clearly, however, another methodological approach not involving subcellular fractionation was necessary to complement our direct studies of cell fractions.

Our second approach was to study thyrotrophs incubated with [³H]fucose and then incubated without radioactivity in the presence of Mon or CCCP. We expected to enrich unfractionated cells with labeled precursors putatively within certain cell compartments proximal to the sites of the drug-induced blocks in the secretory pathway, whereas labeled subunits distal to those sites might be released into the medium. This approach, while avoiding concerns about the purity of subcellular fractions, engenders other concerns about inhibitor toxicity, precise site of action of the drugs, and unforeseen effects. For example, Mon may or may not prevent the acquisition of endoglycosidase H resistance by particular glycoproteins in various model systems (23–33); in Mon-treated hepatoma cells, for example, the vesicular stomatitis virus G protein became endoglycosidase H resistant, while transferrin remained endoglycosidase H sensitive (27). Thus, this drug may not provide an en-

tirely satisfactory means for localization of the sites of oligosaccharide-processing reactions. However, experiments in which mouse pituitaries were incubated with [³⁵S]methionine and then chase incubated in the presence of CCCP or Mon indicated that subunits accumulated in RER- or Golgi-enriched cell fractions, respectively (55a).

As an important control, we demonstrated that the release into medium of [³⁵S]methionine-labeled free α-subunits and TSH was blocked in a dose-dependent manner by both drugs. In general, the patterns of release

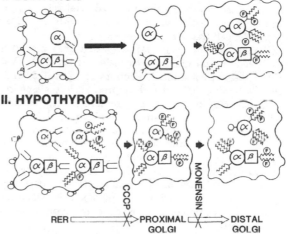

I. EUTHYROID

II. HYPOTHYROID

FIG. 6. Model of TSH biosynthesis. The autoradiographic observations made by Pelletier and Puviani (20) of thyrotrophs from euthyroid and hypothyroid rats have been interpreted in light of our present studies of thyrotrophs from hypothyroid mice and unpublished studies of euthyroid mice. The subcellular compartments in which certain TSH-processing steps occur apparently change under differing physiological conditions. The RER, proximal Golgi, and distal Golgi compartments are depicted, and the postulated sites of blockade of the secretory pathway by CCCP and Mon are indicated. *Large circles* represent the protein cores of α-subunits, *squares* indicate the protein cores of β-subunits, Y represents precursor high mannose oligosaccharides which are processed to zig-zag forms representing complex oligosaccharides, a *circled F* represents a fucose residue, and *small open circles* represent O-linked oligosaccharides of free α-subunits (68). In the euthyroid animal, the RER of thyrotrophs contains TSH subunit precursors with high mannose oligosaccharides, which are trimmed and processed to complex oligosaccharides with addition of fucose in a Golgi compartment. In the hypothyroid animal, the thyrotrophs enlarge, and the RER becomes hypertrophic. Subunit precursors with high mannose forms probably still predominate in this hypertrophied RER (5), but now some oligosaccharides are processed to complex forms in this compartment. Additional processing probably continues in Golgi compartments, so that β-subunits become richer in fucose than α-subunits of TSH heterodimers, and free α-subunits become more fucosylated than the hormone. The molar contents of fucose depicted are illustrative only. Thus, the thyrotroph responds to the physiological milieu by modulating the oligosaccharide processing of TSH in part by shifting the compartmental sites of certain processing steps.

into medium of [³H]fucose-labeled free α-subunits and TSH in the presence of the drugs were similar to those of the [³⁵S]methionine-labeled species. This is surprising, since methionine incorporation into proteins occurs in the RER (proximal to the sites of inhibition by the drugs), whereas fucose incorporation is generally believed to occur late in the secretory pathway of most cell types. However, the patterns of drug-induced accumulation of [³H]fucose-labeled species within the cell lysates were different from the patterns of [³⁵S]methionine-labeled species, suggesting that the intracellular handling of [³H] fucose-labeled species may be complex. Overall, the findings of the inhibitor studies supported the notion that some fucose was being incorporated relatively early in the secretory pathway, in agreement with our direct studies of cell fractions.

Ponsin and Mornex (34) suggested that monensin inhibited the terminal glycosylation of rat TSH. Yet, they detected substantial amounts of labeled TSH in cells, a finding difficult to interpret, since their chosen precursor may be added early or late in the secretory pathway. In view of our studies employing [³H]fucose, it may be that Mon did not inhibit terminal glycosylation in their studies, but inhibited the release into the medium of a portion of the terminally glycosylated TSH. In contrast, Mon did not slow the secretion of [³H]galactose- or [³H]fucose-labeled immunoglobulin (62), suggesting that the subcellular compartment in which terminal glycosylation occurs may differ in thyrotrophs and plasma cells.

Classic autoradiographic studies (56) of hepatocytes, duodenal cells, and other cell types have demonstrated fucose incorporation into glycoproteins in the Golgi apparatus. Yet, studies over the past 30 yr have suggested that terminal glycosylation of TSH, including addition of fucose, may occur in RER in addition to the Golgi elements of thyrotrophs stimulated by a hypothyroid milieu. In early light microscopic studies (57–59), glycoprotein stains suggested that TSH was being stored in granules in cisternae of hypertrophied RER. In an early electron microscopic study, Farquhar and Rinehart (50) demonstrated that the cisternae were RER and that the aldehyde fuchsin-positive granules were dense intracisternal inclusions. The intracisternal granules became more numerous with increasing time after thyroidectomy, and their existence was confirmed by other investigators (51–55). Autoradiographic studies have demonstrated that thyrotrophs (20), gonadotrophs (60), and placental tissue (61) may acutely concentrate [³H]fucose or [³H]galactose in RER, suggesting that the glycoprotein hormones (TSH, LH, FSH, and hCG) may be synthesized in cells with atypical compartmentalization of oligosaccharide-processing enzymes.

Of note, Pelletier and Puviani (20) reported [³H]fucose

uptake into the Golgi apparatus of thyrotrophs from euthyroid rats, but uptake into both RER and Golgi apparatus of thyrotrophs from hypothyroid rats. Although our studies have dealt only with pituitary tissue from hypothyroid animals, in light of their data we speculate that a balance between alternative posttranslational pathways (i.e. RER vs. Golgi sites of fucosylation) may be regulated in the thyrotroph by TRH, thyroid hormones, or other physiological factors (Fig. 6). This may be analogous to the reversibly altered distribution among Golgi cisternae of thiamine pyrophosphatase activity in vasopressin-synthesizing neurons when mice are exposed to osmotic stress (63). Other examples of apparent modulation of the sites of secretory product processing among Golgi cisternae, revealed by changing histochemical staining patterns, include estrogen-stimulated rat mammotrophs (64), differentiating polymorphonuclear leukocytes (65, 66), and regressing corpus luteum cells of the guinea pig (67). Apparently, the thyrotroph has evolved the differentiated ability to respond to the endocrine milieu of the organism by altering the compartmentalization of oligosaccharide processing and, perhaps, may thereby modulate the posttranslational processing of TSH. This may allow the qualitative nature of the final secreted hormone to be regulated to optimize its metabolic clearance or other biological properties.

Acknowledgment

Jan Smith provided expert secretarial assistance.

References

1. Pierce JG, Parsons TF 1981 Glycoprotein hormones: structure and function. Annu Rev Biochem 50:465
2. Chin WW, Habener JF, Kieffer JD, Maloof F 1978 Cell-free translation of the messenger RNA coding for the α-subunit of thyroid-stimulating hormone. J Biol Chem 253:7985
3. Kourides IA, Weintraub BD 1979 mRNA-directed biosynthesis of α-subunit of thyrotropin:translation in cell-free and whole-cell systems. Proc Natl Acad Sci USA 76:298
4. Vamvakopoulos NC, Kourides IA 1979 Identification of separate mRNAs coding for the α and β subunits of thyrotropin. Proc Natl Acad Sci USA 76:3809
5. Magner JA, Weintraub BD 1982 Thyroid-stimulating hormone subunit processing and combination in microsomal subfractions of mouse pituitary tumor. J Biol Chem 257:6709
6. Kornfeld R, Kornfeld S 1985 Assembly of asparagine-linked oligosaccharides. Annu Rev Biochem 54:631
7. Goldberg DE, Kornfeld S 1983 Evidence for extensive subcellular organization of asparagine-linked oligosaccharide processing and lysosomal enzyme phosphorylation. J Biol Chem 258:3159
8. Rothman JE, Miller RL, Urbani LJ 1984 Intercompartmental transport in the Golgi is a dissociative process: facile transfer of membrane protein between two Golgi populations. J Cell Biol 99:260
9. Dunphy WG, Brands R, Rothman JE 1985 Attachment of terminal N-acetylglucosamine to asparagine-linked oligosaccharides occurs in central cisternae of the Golgi stack. Cell 40:463
10. Dunphy WG, Rothman JE 1985 Compartmental organization of the Golgi stack. Cell 42:13

11. Magner JA, Ronin C, Weintraub BD 1984 Carbohydrate processing of thyrotropin differs from that of free α-subunit and total glycoproteins in microsomal subfractions of mouse pituitary tumor. Endocrinology 115:1019

12. Kwa HG, Van Der Bent EM, Feltkamp CA, Rumke PH, Bloemendal H 1965 Studies on hormones from the anterior pituitary gland. I. Identification and isolation of growth hormone and prolactin from the "granular" fraction of bovine pituitary. Biochim Biophys Acta 111:447

13. Jacobs LS, McKeel DW, Jarett L, Daughaday WH 1973 The distribution of growth hormone and prolactin in subcellular fractions of porcine adenohypophysis. Endocrinology 92:477

14. McKeel DW, Jarett L 1974 The enrichment of adenylate cyclase in the plasma membrane and Golgi subcellular fractions of porcine Relationship of glycosylation. J Cell Biol 62:231

15. DeMarco L, Mashiter K, Peters TJ 1981 Analytical subcellular fractionation of rat pituitary homogenates, with special reference to prolactin proteolysis by lysosomes. Biochim Biophys Acta 677:489

16. Caughey B, DeMarco L, Peters TJ, Mashiter K, Gibbons WA 1983 Analytical subcellular fractionation of rat pituitary homogenates with special reference to the subcellular localization and properties of alkaline phosphatases. Biochim Biophys Acta 757:296

17. Moriarty CM, Dowd F, Fontaine M 1983 Isolation and characteristics of bovine pituitary secretory granules. Biochim Biophys Acta 797:209

18. DeMarco L, Mashiter K, Peters TJ 1984 The levels and subcellular distribution of hormones and marker enzymes in pituitaries from control subjects and patients with prolactinomas, acromegaly or functionless pituitary tumours. Clin Endocrinol (Oxf) 21:515

19. Scheele GA, Palade GE, Tartakoff AM 1978 Cell fractionation studies on the guinea pig pancreas. Redistribution of exocrine proteins during tissue homogenization. J Cell Biol 78:110

20. Pelletier G, Puviani R 1973 Detection of gycoproteins and autoradiographic localization of [³H]fucose in the thyroidectomy cells of rat anterior pituitary gland. J Cell Biol 56:600

21. Griffiths G, Quinn P, Warren G 1983 Dissection of the Golgi complex. I. Monensin inhibits the transport of viral membrane proteins from medial to trans Golgi cisternae in baby hamster kidney cells infected with Semliki Forest virus. J Cell Biol 96:835

22. Tartakoff AM, Vassali P, Detraz M 1977 Plasma cell immunoglobulin secretion. Arrest is accompanied by alterations of the Golgi complex. J Exp Med 146:1332

23. Moore C, Pressman BC 1964 Mechanism of action of valinomycin on mitochondria. Biochem Biophys Res Commun 15:562

24. Uchida N, Smilowitz H, Ledger PW, Tanzer ML 1980 Kinetic studies of the intracellular transport of procollagen and fibronectin in human fibroblasts. J Biol Chem 255:8638

25. Johnson DC, Schlesinger MJ 1980 Vesicular stomatitis virus and sindbis virus glycoprotein transport to the cell surface is inhibited by ionophores. Virology 103:407

26. Alonso FV, Compans RW 1981 Differential effect of monensin on enveloped viruses that form at distinct plasma membrane domains. J Cell Biol 89:700

27. Strous GJ, Willemsen R, Van Kerkhof P, Slot JW, Geuze HJ, Lodish HF 1983 VSV glycoprotein, albumin, and transferrin are transported to the cell surface via the same Golgi vesicles. J Cell Biol 97:1815

28. Ledger PW, Nishimoto SK, Hayashi S, Tanzer ML 1983 Abnormal glycosylation of human fibronectin secreted in the presence of monensin. J Biol Chem 258:547

29. Goldberg RL, Toole BP 1983 Monensin inhibition of hyaluronate synthesis in rat fibrosarcoma cells. J Biol Chem 258:7041

30. Peters BP, Brooks M, Hartle RJ, Krzesicki RF, Perini F, Ruddon RW 1983 The use of drugs to dissect the pathway for secretion of the glycoprotein hormone chorionic gonadotropin by cultured human trophoblastic cells. J Biol Chem 258:14505

31. Devault A, Zollingr M, Crine P 1984 Effects of the monovalent ionophore monensin on the intracellular transport and processing of pro-opiomelanocortin in culture intermediate lobe cells of the rat pituitary. J Biol Chem 259:5146

32. Hickman S, Theodorakis JL, Greco JM, Brown PH 1984 Processing of MOPC 315 immunoglobulin A oligosaccharides: evidence for endoplasmic reticulum and trans Golgi α 1,2-mannosidase activity. J Cell Biol 98:407

33. Strous GJ, Van Kerkhof P, Williamsen R, Slot JW, Geuze HJ 1985 Effect of monensin on the metabolism, localization, and biosynthesis of N- and O-linked oligosaccharides of galactosyltransferase. Eur J Cell Biol 36:256

34. Ponsin G, Mornex R 1983 Control of thyrotropin glycosylation in normal rat pituitary cells in culture: effect of thyrotropin-releasing hormone. Endocrinology 113:549

35. Blackman MR, Gershengorn MC, Weintraub BD 1978 Excess production of free alpha subunits by mouse pituitary thyrotropic tumor cells in vitro. Endocrinology 102:499

36. Weintraub BD, Stannard BS, Linnekin D, and Marshall M 1980 Relationship of glycosylation to de novo thyroid-stimulating hormone biosynthesis and secretion by mouse pituitary tumor cells. J Biol Chem 255:5715

37. Lowry OH, Rosenbrough NJ, Farr AL, Randall RJ 1951 Protein measurement with the Folin phenol reagent. J Biol Chem 193:265

38. Weintraub BD, Stannard BS 1978 Precursor-product relationships in the biosynthesis and secretion of thyrotropin and its subunits by mouse thyrotropic tumor cells. FEBS Lett 92:303

39. Weintraub BD, Stannard BS, Meyers L 1983 Glycosylation of thyroid-stimulating hormone in pituitary tumor cells: influence of high mannose oligosaccharide units on subunit aggregation, combination, and intracellular degradation. Endocrinology 112:1331

40. Chin WW, Maloof F, Habener JF 1981 Thyroid-stimulating hormone biosynthesis. J Biol Chem 256:3059

41. Chin WW, Habener JF 1981 Thyroid-stimulating hormone subunits: evidence from endoglycosidase-H cleavage for late presecretory glycosylation. Endocrinology 108:1628

42. Ronin C, Stannard BS, Rosenbloom IL, Magner JA, Weintraub BD 1984 Glycosylation and processing of high-mannose oligosaccharides of thyroid-stimulating hormone subunits: Comparison to nonsecretory cell glycoproteins. Biochemistry 23:4503

43. Wilber JF, Utiger RD 1969 Thyrotropin incorporation of ¹⁴C-glucosamine by the isolated rat adenohypophysis. Endocrinology 84:1316

44. Wilber JF 1971 Stimulation of ¹⁴C-glucosamine and ¹⁴C-alanine incorporation into thyrotropin by synthetic thyrotropin-releasing hormone. Endocrinology 89:873

45. Taylor T, Weintraub BD 1985 Differential regulation of thyrotropin subunit apoprotein and carbohydrate biosynthesis by thyroid hormone. Endocrinology 116:1535

46. Taylor T, Weintraub BD 1985 Thyrotropin (TSH)-releasing hormone regulation of TSH subunit biosynthesis and glycosylation in normal and hypothyroid rat pituitaries. Endocrinology 116:1968

47. Chappel SC, Ullos-Aquirre A, Coutifaris C 1983 Biosynthesis and secretion of follicle-stimulating hormone. Endocr Rev 4:179

48. Joshi LR, Weintraub BD 1983 Naturally occurring forms of thyrotropin with low bioactivity and altered carbohydrate content act as competitive antagonists to more bioactive forms. Endocrinology 113:2145

49. Schachter H 1978 In: Horowitz MI, Pigman W (eds) The Glycoconjugates. Academic Press, New York, vol 2:91

50. Farquhar MG, Rinehart JF 1954 Cytologic alterations in the anterior pituitary gland following thyroidectomy: an electron microscope study. Endocrinology 55:857

51. Kamat VB, Hoelzl Wallach DF, Crigler JF, Ladman AJ 1960 The intracellular localization of hormonal activity in transplantable thyrotropin-secreting pituitary tumors in mice. J Biophys Biochem Cytol 7:219

52. Farquhar MG 1971 In: Heller H, Lederis K (eds) Subcellular Organization and Function in Endocrine Tissues. Cambridge University Press, London, vol 1:79

53. Cuerdo-Rocha S, Zambrano D 1974 The action of protein synthesis inhibitors and thyrotropin releasing factor on the ultrastructure of rat thyrotrophs. J Ultrastruct Res 48:1

54. Cuerdo-Rocha S, Zambrano D 1974 Thyrotrophs of the rat anterior pituitary after different periods of thyroidectomy. A conventional and histochemical electron microscope study. J Ultrastruct Res 49:312

55. Moriarty GC, Tobin RB 1976 An immunocytochemical study of TSH storage in rat thyroidectomy cells with and without D or L thyroxine treatment. J Histochem Cytochem 24:1140

55a. Magner JA, Papagiannes E, Effects of CCCP and monensin on mouse thyrotropin biosynthesis: direct analyses of subcellular fractions. Program of the 68th Annual Meeting of The Endocrine Society, Anaheim, CA, 1986 (Abstract 791)

56. Farquhar MG, Palade GE 1981 The Golgi apparatus (complex)—(1954–1981)—from artifact to center stage. J Cell Biol 91:77s

57. Purves HD, Griesbach WE 1951 The site of thyrotrophin and gonadotrophin production in the rat pituitary studied by McManus-Hotchkiss staining for glycoprotein. Endocrinology 49:244

58. Halmi NS 1952 Two types of basophils in the rat pituitary: thyrotrophs and gonadotrophs vs. beta and delta cells. Endocrinology 50:140

59. Halmi NS, Gude WD 1954 The morphogenesis of pituitary tumors induced by radiothyroidectomy in the mouse and the effects of their transplantation on the pituitary body of the host. Am J Pathol 30:403

60. Pelletier G 1974 Autoradiographic studies of synthesis and intracellular migration of glycoproteins in the rat anterior pituitary gland. J Cell Biol 62:185

61. Nelson DM, Enders AC, King BF 1978 Cytological events involved in glycoprotein synthesis in cellular and syncytial trophoblast of human placenta. J Cell Biol 76:418

62. Tartakoff A, Vassali P 1979 Plasma cell immunoglobulin M molecules. Their biosynthesis, assembly, and intracellular transport. J Cell Biol 83:284

63. Broadwell RD, Oliver C 1981 Golgi apparatus, GERL, and secretory granule formation within neurons of the hypothalamo-neurohypophysial system of control and hyperosmotically stressed mice. J Cell Biol 90:474

64. Smith RE, Farquhar MG 1970 Modulation in nucleoside diphosphatase activity of mammatrophic cells of the rat adenohypophysis during secretion. J Histochem Cytochem 18:237

65. Bainton DF, Farquhar MG 1966 Origin of granules in polymorphonuclear leukocytes. Two types derived from opposite faces of the Golgi complex in developing granulocytes. J Cell Biol 28:277

66. Bainton DF, Farquhar MG 1968 Differences in enzyme content of azurophil and specific granules of polymorphonuclear leukocytes. J Cell Biol 39:299

67. Paavola LG 1978 The corpus luteum of the guinea pig. III. Cytochemical studies on the Golgi complex and GERL during normal postpartum regression of luteal cells, emphasizing the origin of lysosomes and autophagic vacuoles. J Cell Biol 79:59

68. Parsons TF, Bloomfield GA, Pierce JG 1983 Purification of an alternative form of the α subunit of the glycoprotein hormones from bovine pituitaries and identification of its 0-linked oligosaccharide. J Biol Chem 258:240

Miura et al. Study of Human TSH Oligosaccharides

The pituitary hormone thyrotropin (TSH) is a major regulator of thyroid function in humans and many "higher" animals, and is first found in the animal kingdom with this function in the lampreys and other jawless fishes. Thus, from an evolutionary perspective the molecule has had that basic physiologic role for at least 360 million years! TSH was actually present in cells even millions of years before that but had other signaling functions. The TSH molecule has two protein subunits (alpha and beta) that are non-covalently bound together, and over eons the precise protein sequences of these subunits have gradually changed in different species. Each subunit also has branched chains of sugars attached, two chains on alpha and one on beta. Thus, TSH is not just a protein – it is a glycoprotein. The protein surfaces are very important for binding to and activating the hormone's specific cell surface receptor (most significantly on cells of the thyroid gland), but the functions of the sugar chains (oligosaccharides) have been less well understood. It turns out that one role of oligosaccharides on some glycoproteins is to adjust the amount of time the molecule circulates in the blood before being removed by the liver or kidney.

Near the ends of the branched sugar chains the oligosaccharides may have in some cases a certain type of charged sugar called sialic acid. That sugar is essentially always sitting on top of a foundation one link earlier in the sugar chain, and that supporting sugar is nearly always galactose. If a glycoprotein has several sialic acid sugars decorating its chains, then the clearance of the glycoprotein from the circulating blood is slowed. Alternatively, if a glycoprotein has no or very few sialic acids, then the galactose sugars are exposed, which enhances the removal of the circulating glycoprotein from the blood. Note that the circulation time of a hormone is related to how much response the tissues will have to that hormone.

Another concept is that in an individual person, the amino acid sequence of a protein very rarely changes within that person's lifetime, whereas it had been thought that the sugar chains of some glycoproteins might change somewhat from hour to hour or day to day. A theory our group had was that physiologic means of regulating sugar chain structure had evolved over eons, and that such normal regulation of oligosaccharides might be part of a mechanism to allow adjustment of the activity of

certain glycoproteins, especially hormones. In the experiments described in the Miura et al. paper we wanted to determine if the oligosaccharides of human TSH were structurally different in each of three specific physiologic states: euthyroidism, primary hypothyroidism (caused by failure of thyroid tissue), and central hypothyroidism (caused by disease in the brain or pituitary rather than in the thyroid gland, and often associated with much lower amounts of TSH in the blood than what might be otherwise expected in a hypothyroid clinical state). We suspected that in primary hypothyroidism the body would be producing not only quantitatively more TSH to try to stimulate thyroid tissue, but also the structure of the TSH oligosaccharides might become sculpted to have a bigger positive impact on thyroid tissue. This sculpting might include changes that would increase the circulation time of TSH molecules in the blood. Thus, we would look for increased sialylation of the sugar chains of TSH in patients with primary hypothyroidism as compared with the amount of TSH sialylation seen in normal euthyroid subjects. We planned to look for increased sialylation by seeing how well TSH molecules bound to certain lectins, which are substances that have more or less specific binding to certain sugars. A caveat is that there can be technical issues when trying to use a lectin to detect the amount of sialic acid directly, so we used an indirect approach because we had access to a pure enzyme that very specifically could remove just the sialic acid sugars from glycoproteins. That enzyme would expose more underlying galactose residues. So the method was to divide a given patient's TSH sample into two parts, and treat one half with the enzyme to remove sialic acid residues. We then could run the non-treated part of the sample over a lectin column that bound galactose and measure what percentage of the TSH had exposed galactose resides. Later we could run the enzyme-treated TSH over an identical lectin column and see how many more galactose resides had become exposed by the enzyme treatment. This indirect method was analogous in some respects to determining the weight of library books in a backpack by having a child wear the full back pack and stepping onto a scale, followed by emptying the back pack and then having the child step back onto the scale. So subtraction was involved, although in the TSH experiment the enzyme treatment might make the lectin binding increase, whereas in the library book example emptying the backpack would make the weight decrease.

This was an important and quite novel project for Dr. Miura and Dr. Perkel, who were young trainees (from Japan and South Africa, respectively) gaining research experience in my laboratory. Kim Papenberg, a bright college student who assisted me for a few weeks in the summer, also learned a lot from the project, while Melanie Johnson, my laboratory technician, provided some logistical support. I always made a point of trying to give co-authorship to trainees, summer students, and also my technician if they played a meaningful role in completing the project and interpreting the results. This was grateful payback for the help I had received years before when I did experiments at Woods Hole and wrote my first scientific abstract with the help of Dr. Eberhard and Dr. Nealson.

The TSH sialic acid results were presented as an abstract at a scientific meeting, and then appeared as a full publication.

It turns out that human TSH normally is secreted as a heterogeneous mix of isoforms all having the same amino acid sequence but with varying oligosaccharides that normally contain just a bit of sulfate and sialic acid. Our experiments proved that circulating TSH from patients with primary hypothyroidism is more highly sialylated than is the TSH of normal persons. The extra sialic acid residues cover galactose residues and thereby hide them from liver receptors, and that likely is responsible for the longer TSH circulating half-time seen in patients with primary hypothyroidism. The average half-life for elimination of forms of TSH in a normal person is about an hour, whereas the high TSH in a hypothyroid person has a longer half-life of several hours. When recombinant human TSH (rhTSH) was first manufactured in the 1990s, eukaryotic cells were required (Chinese Hamster Ovary cells) because addition of oligosaccharides to the TSH subunits was mandatory for optimal hormonal activity. Also, the manufacturing of rhTSH was set so that a highly sialylated form of TSH was produced to be used clinically as a drug, since when highly sialylated the molecule has a half-life of about 20 hours, which is 20-fold longer than minimally sialylated TSH. That long half-life increased the potency of the drug, and made commercial use of Thyrogen (rhTSH) feasible with one intramuscular injection on each of two consecutive days. When I designed and performed the Miura et al. experiments in Chicago I had no idea that someday I would become a Genzyme employee with the role of key company medical expert to design Thyrogen clinical studies, and assist with getting regulatory approvals for Thyrogen.

0021-972X/89/6905-0985$02.00/0
Journal of Clinical Endocrinology and Metabolism
Copyright © 1989 by The Endocrine Society

Vol. 69, No. 5
Printed in U.S.A.

Concanavalin-A, Lentil, and Ricin Lectin Affinity Binding Characteristics of Human Thyrotropin: Differences in the Sialylation of Thyrotropin in Sera of Euthyroid, Primary, and Central Hypothyroid Patients*

YOSHITAKA MIURA†, VICTOR S. PERKEL‡, KIMBERLY A. PAPENBERG, MELANIE J. JOHNSON, AND JAMES A. MAGNER§

Division of Endocrinology, Michael Reese Hospital and Medical Center, University of Illinois, Chicago, Illinois 60616

ABSTRACT. TSH from human serum was separated into classes by serial lectin affinity chromatography using Concanavalin-A (ConA), lentil, and ricin lectins. TSH from 10 euthyroid subjects, 40 patients with primary hypothyroidism, and 1 patient with central hypothyroidism was studied. The patterns of ConA and lentil affinity binding were similar for diverse patients; forms of TSH that bound firmly to ConA also tended to bind firmly to lentil. Differences in TSH-ricin binding suggested that there were differences in the sialylation of TSH in sera of euthyroid, primary, and central hypothyroidism patients. For euthyroid subjects, $16.1 \pm 5.4\%$ (mean ± SD) of the TSH bound to ricin, while after neuraminidase treatment, $38.4 \pm 5.4\%$ bound. For patients with primary hypothyroidism, $23.6 \pm 6.0\%$ of the TSH bound to the ricin, while after neuraminidase treatment, $65.7 \pm 8.8\%$ bound. The increase in ricin binding induced by neuraminidase treatment was significantly higher for TSH from patients with primary hypothyroidism than in that from euthyroid subjects ($42.3 \pm 7.6\%$ vs. $22.3 \pm 4.4\%$; $P < 0.01$) and

was greater for long term than for short term hypothyroid patients ($49.5 \pm 5.0\%$ vs. $36.5 \pm 6.5\%$; $P < 0.01$). While 30% of native TSH from the serum of the patient with central hypothyroidism bound to ricin, the amount bound increased only 17.6% after neuraminidase treatment. McKenzie bioassay of pituitary-derived TSH that was similarly fractionated using ricin failed to show detectable differences in bioactivity among the lectin column fractions.

Thus, 1) circulating human TSH can be consistently separated into discrete classes using serial lectin affinity chromatography; 2) there is relatively more core fucosylation of the less processed high mannose and hybrid forms of TSH and less core fucosylation of more processed complex forms; 3) ConA and lentil binding of TSH in primary and central hypothyroidism is similar to that in the euthyroid state; 4) patients with primary hypothyroidism have more sialylated TSH than a patient with central hypothyroidism or euthyroid subjects; and 5) the degree of TSH sialylation increases with prolonged primary hypothyroidism. (J Clin Endocrinol Metab 69: 985, 1989)

T SH IS a glycoprotein composed of two noncovalently linked subunits that are synthesized from separate mRNAs (1–6). The α-subunit has two asparagine-linked oligosaccharide units, whereas the β-subunit has one. Deglycosylation studies (7–9) have suggested that the peptide portion of TSH is essential for its binding to the receptor, while the oligosaccharides influence the hormone's MCR and intrinsic biological activity. Heterogeneity of TSH molecular size, isoelectric point, and biological activity (10–12) has been attributed to the oligosaccharide units. The oligosaccharide structures are modulated during TSH biosynthesis when thyrotropic tissues are incubated with TRH and thyroid hormones (13–15). However, the physiological significance of the heterogeneity of TSH has not been adequately investigated.

Lectins are compounds that bind specific carbohydrate groups. Affinity chromatography of glycopeptides on immobilized lectins is a powerful method for oligosaccharide fractionation. The oligosaccharide structures that interact with Concanavalin-A (ConA) have the following characteristics (Fig. 1): triantennary, tetraantennary, and bisecting oligosaccharides do not bind (Fig. 1a); biantennary and truncated hybrid oligosaccharides bind weakly (Fig. 1b); and high mannose and hybrid oligosaccharides bind firmly to ConA (Fig. 1c). In attempting to fractionate intact TSH heterodimers instead of the more

---

Received March 8, 1989.

Address all correspondence and requests for reprints to: Dr. James A. Magner, Division of Endocrinology, Michael Reese Hospital, Lake Shore Drive at 31st Street, Chicago, Illinois 60616.

* Both Y.M. and V.S.P. contributed equally, and each should be considered first author.

† Present address: First Department of Internal Medicine, Nagoya University School of Medicine, Nagoya 466, Japan.

‡ Supported by a fellowship award from the Michael Reese Medical Center Research Institute Council. Present address: Division of Mineral Metabolism (151), Jerry Pettis Veterans Administration Hospital, 11201 Benton Street, Loma Linda, California 92357.

§ Supported by USPHS Grant DK-38835.

985

usual glycopeptides, Lee *et al.* (16) demonstrated decreased binding of the TSH heterodimers to a ConA slurry in hospitalized subjects with the euthyroid sick syndrome. Lectins were employed in a study of another glycoprotein by Ain and Refetoff (17) who fractionated T₄-binding globulin (TBG) on ConA. They showed an increase in multiantennary structures in intact TBG in the serum of hyperestrogenic female subjects. Lentil lectin-Sepharose (lentil) binds oligosaccharides that contain core fucose residues linked α1,6 to an asparagine-linked *N*-acetylglucosamine residue (Fig. 2a, position 1) whereas oligosaccharides that contain peripheral fucose linked α1,3 to outer chain *N*-acetylglucosamine (Fig. 2a, position 2) or linked α1,2 to outer chain galactose (Fig. 2a, position 3), on the other hand, do not bind to lentil (18, 19). In addition, two α-mannosyl residues are required for binding to lentil. This binding to lentil is further enhanced by the presence of exposed *N*-acetylglucosamine residues (*i.e.* those that lack peripheral galactose and sialic residues) (19). The presence of an α-mannose substituted at both carbon positions C-2 and C-4 inhibits binding of oligosaccharides to lentil (Fig. 2b) (19).

Serial lectin affinity chromatography has been used to separate glycopeptides into various subclasses (18, 19),

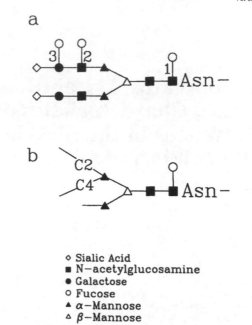

FIG. 2. Representative structures of theoretical fucosylated oligosaccharides that bind (a) and fail to bind (b) to lentil lectin Sepharose 4B. The oligosaccharides that bind to lentil and are eluted with 500 mM α-methylmannopyranoside (a) contain core fucose residues at position 1; oligosaccharides with fucose residues at positions 2 and 3 do not bind to lentil. The two α-mannosyl residues are also necessary for binding, and binding is enhanced by exposed terminal *N*-acetylglucosamine residues, although binding still occurs in the presence of a terminal galactose or galactose-sialic acid residue. Most of the oligosaccharides that do not bind to lentil lack core fucose residues at position 1. Core fucosylated oligosaccharides that do not bind to lentil (b) are substituted at carbons C-2 and C-4 on an α-mannose.

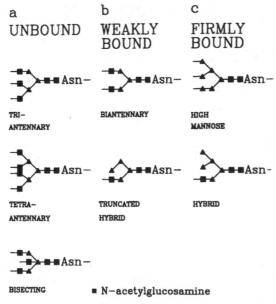

FIG. 1. Representative structures of TSH oligosaccharides based on ConA affinity chromatography. a, Tris-buffered saline eluted the unbound triantennary, tetraantennary, and bisecting oligosaccharide structures; b, 10 mM α-methylglucopyranoside eluted weakly bound biantennary and truncated hybrid oligosaccharide structures; c, 500 mM α-methylmannopyranoside eluted firmly bound high mannose and hybrid structures. [Figure adapted with permission from ref. 48 by V. S. Perkel].

but has not been used previously to separate intact TSH heterodimers. Gesundheit *et al.* (20) used these techniques to study the glycopeptides of murine TSH. They showed that TRH increased biantennary or truncated hybrid structures in secreted TSH. Intact TSH has three oligosaccharides and, in theory, might bind to a lectin if only one of the three oligosaccharides has appropriate characteristics.

Sialic acid, a negatively charged terminal sugar that covers penultimate galactose residues, is known to influence the MCRs of several circulating glycoproteins by protecting them from hepatic galactose receptors (21–23). In addition, sialic acid has been reported to be very important for receptor binding and ligand-receptor coupling (24), although cleavage of sialic acid from glycoprotein hormones may increase binding to the receptor (25). Recently, DeCherney *et al.* (26) reported that mouse TSH becomes more sialylated and less sulfated during prolonged hypothyroidism of up to 12 months. Variation in the sialylation of human serum TSH, however, has not been previously studied. Using the β-galactose-specific lectin *Ricinus communis* (RCA$_{120}$) in the present study, we compared the sialylation of TSH in sera of 10 euthyroid subjects, 40 patients with primary hypothyroidism, and a patient with central hypothyroidism. We are able to estimate the degree of sialylation of TSH by comparing the ricin binding of TSH with or without prior neuraminidase digestion, because glycoproteins with β-galactose covered by sialic acid fail to bind to the ricin. Our data demonstrate that while fucosylation and branching of TSH oligosaccharides are not modulated by the physiological state, the degree of TSH sialylation varies with the physiological state and increases with the duration of hypothyroidism.

Materials and Methods

Subjects

Serum samples for TSH analysis were obtained from 10 normal volunteers (5 men and 5 women, aged 28–38 yr) and 40 patients with primary hypothyroidism (5 men and 35 women, aged 21–91 yr) and 1 patient with central hypothyroidism (female, aged 40 yr). The diagnoses of primary hypothyroidism were based on laboratory data and clinical assessment. Seven of the 40 patients with primary hypothyroidism had a duration of hypothyroidism of less than 3 months and generally had received radioiodine therapy or thyroid surgery for hyperthyroidism. Eleven of the 40 patients apparently had been hypothyroid for more than 1 yr, generally due to noncompliance with medications in the setting of Hashimoto's disease or after radioiodine therapy. TSH concentrations in serum from patients with primary hypothyroidism ranged from 22.3–937 μU/mL (normal range, 0.3–6.0 μU/mL). The patient with central hypothyroidism had a TSH value of 13.6 μU/mL caused by sarcoidosis of the hypothalamus. Euthyroid subjects had no symptoms or signs of thyroid disease, were not taking thyroid medications, and had serum TSH levels within the normal range. All serum samples were stored at −20 C until analysis.

Immunoradiometric assay (IRMA) of TSH

TSH in each serum specimen or column fraction was measured in duplicate using a commercial TSH IRMA kit (Bio-Rad, Hercules, CA). The minimum detectable dose was 0.02 μU/mL. To exclude the possibility that the kit's monoclonal antibody was reporting only a selected population of TSH molecules, some specimens were remeasured using another TSH IRMA kit with a different monoclonal antibody (Diagnostic Product Corp., Los Angeles, CA). The minimum detectable dose was 0.03 μU/mL. In these assays the presence or absence of sugar in specimens, as occurred in some lectin column fractions, did not change the TSH values.

ConA and lentil lectin affinity chromatography

Each sample was centrifuged at 10,000 × g at 4 C for 4 min, and a 100-μL aliquot of clear serum was removed. The serum sample was diluted in 900 μL column buffer containing 0.01 M Tris-HCl (pH 8.0), 0.15 M sodium chloride, and 1 mM each of

magnesium chloride, manganese chloride, calcium chloride, 0.1% sodium azide, and 0.1% BSA (all from Sigma Chemical Co., St. Louis, MO). After prewashing each lectin column with 20 mL column buffer, each serum specimen (diluted 1:10 in 1 mL column buffer) was loaded onto a column containing either 3 mL fresh ConA-Sepharose 4B or 2 mL fresh lentil lectin-Sepharose 4B (Pharmacia Fine Chemicals, Piscataway, NJ) and allowed to equilibrate for 30 min. Chromatography was performed at 22 C at a flow rate of 10–20 mL/h, and 20-mL fractions were collected. Unbound TSH was eluted with 20 mL column buffer. Weakly bound TSH was eluted from the ConA columns with 20 mL of the same buffer containing 10 mM α-methylglucopyranoside (Sigma). Firmly bound TSH was subsequently eluted from both the lentil and ConA columns with 20 ml of column buffer containing 500 mM α-methylmannopyranoside (Sigma). Approximately 90% of the TSH that had been applied to a column was recovered in the fractions. Immunoaffinity-concentrated TSH (see below) was chromatographed on 1-mL lectin columns, and 7-mL fractions were collected.

A serum sample from each subject was first separated on a ConA column; the fractions were dialyzed against column buffer to remove eluting sugars and then applied to a lentil column. Chromatography of serum from each subject was also performed in the reverse order; *i.e.* each serum sample was first separated on lentil, then the fractions were dialyzed and applied to ConA.

Validation of ConA and lentil lectin chromatography

TSH fractions eluted from the ConA column (unbound, weakly bound, and firmly bound) were reapplied to another ConA column to demonstrate that, on rechromatography, each fraction again eluted in the expected position. Fractions already containing the eluting sugars α-methylglucopyranoside and α-methylmannopyranoside were first dialyzed before reapplication to ConA. TSH fractions eluted from the lentil column (unbound and bound) were also reapplied to another lentil column to validate this technique. As above, fractions already containing the eluting sugar, α-methylmannopyranoside, were first dialyzed before reapplication to lentil.

Immunoaffinity concentration of TSH

TSH in serum was concentrated using antihuman (anti-hTSH) monoclonal antibody-coated polystyrene tubes (Bio-Rad). Aliquots (500 μL) of each serum sample were incubated at room temperature for 3 h in tubes with gentle shaking. Serum was then aspirated, and each tube was washed with 1 mL phosphate-buffered saline (PBS), pH 7.4, twice. Then, 400 μL 0.2 M glycine-HCl, pH 2.2, were added to each tube and allowed to incubate at room temperature for 30 min with gentle shaking. After incubation, aliquots were immediately collected, and two to four drops of 1 N sodium hydroxide were added to adjust the pH to neutral. These aliquots were dialyzed against 0.1 M ammonium bicarbonate buffer, pH 8.0, divided into two portions, and then lyophilized.

Because we used a monoclonal antibody to concentrate TSH, it was theoretically possible that only some subpopulations of the heterogeneous molecules bound to the antibody. This possibility was ruled out by repeating portions of the ricin affinity studies using a different monoclonal antibody. There was little dissociation of TSH heterodimers during the 30-min elution with glycine-HCl buffer because the recovery of this step was 90%. The overall recovery of the whole immunoaffinity procedure was greater than 60%.

Neuraminidase treatment

Lyophilized specimens were resuspended in 20 μL 0.1 M citrate buffer, pH 6.6, then a portion of each specimen was incubated with or without 10 mU neuraminidase from *Clostridium perfringens* (type X, Sigma) for 4 h at 37 C. Prior experiments (27) demonstrated that under these conditions almost all of the sialic acid residues were cleaved from TSH.

Ricinus communis affinity column chromatography

Specimens with or without neuraminidase treatment were loaded onto a column containing 0.7 mL *Ricinus communis* (RCA$_{120}$) insolubilized on beaded agrose (Sigma). After equilibration for 60 min, each column was washed with 5 mL PBS-0.1% BSA, then 5 mL PBS-0.1% BSA containing 0.2 M galactose (Sigma) to elute bound TSH. All elutions were performed at room temperature at a flow rate of 2.5 mL/h. The recovery of TSH was greater than 90%. When the same sample was analyzed four times, the interassay coefficient of variation was 4.6%. This technique was validated by reapplication of fractionated TSH molecules to ricin columns.

β-Galactosidase treatment

As a control to check the specificity of the lectin affinity binding, fractions containing bound TSH were dialyzed and lyophylized, then resuspended in 20 μL 50 mM Tris-HCl buffer, pH 7.4, containing 50 mM magnesium sulfate. Then, 40 U β-galactosidase (Sigma) were added and incubated for 16 h at 37 C. After digestion, these specimens were reapplied to the ricin.

McKenzie bioassay

TSH from human pituitaries (Sigma) was treated with or without neuraminidase, then samples were applied to the ricin and fractionated as described above. After dialysis and lyophilization, the TSH of each fraction was resuspended in normal saline-1% human serum albumin, and the TSH concentrations were measured by IRMA. Each specimen was then diluted to a final TSH concentration of 600 μU/300 μL for McKenzie bioassay (28–30).

Swiss-Webster female mice (Charles River, Wilmington, MA; 13–15 g) that had been receiving a Remington low iodine diet (Teklad, Madison, WI) for about 4 days were injected with 4–5 μCi ^{131}I, ip, and then given L-T$_4$ in water (sodium salt; 6 μg/ml: Sigma) for a 3-day period. The mice were bled by retroorbital sinus puncture for the baseline sample. After bleeding each animal was injected into a tail vein with 300 μL of the appropriate TSH sample or standard amounts of hTSH. Generally, three mice were included in each test group, and a typical assay used about 20 mice. After 2 h a second blood sample was

taken. The radioactivity of a 50- or 100-μL aliquot of serum was counted for 10 min. The blood radioactivity 2 h after each injection was expressed as a percentage of the baseline radioactivity for each animal.

Statistical analysis

Classes of TSH defined by ConA and lentil serial lectin affinity chromatography were compared by χ^2 analysis combined with Yates continuity correction (31). The ricin lectin column data were analyzed by Student's t test. The McKenzie assay data were evaluated by analysis of variance.

Results

ConA and lentil analyses of TSH from primary hypothyroid subjects

The results of initial ConA lectin chromatography for each subject with primary hypothyroidism are shown in Fig. 3a. In summary, 10.8 ± 0.6% (mean ± SEM) of the TSH did not bind to ConA (ConA Fx 1), 37.3 ± 1% of the TSH bound weakly (ConA Fx 2) and was eluted with 10 mM α-methylglucopyranoside, and 52 ± 1.2% of the TSH bound firmly to ConA (ConA Fx 3) and was eluted with 500 mM α-methylmannopyranoside. The initial lentil lectin binding of TSH for each hypothyroidism subject is shown in Fig. 3b. In summary, 48 ± 1.6% of the TSH did not bind to lentil (lentil Fx 1). The remaining 52 ± 1.6% of the TSH bound to lentil (lentil Fx 2) and eluted

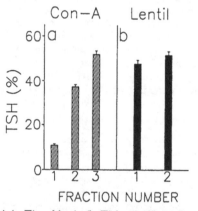

FIG. 3. ConA (a, ▨) and lectin (b; ■) lentil affinity chromatographic analysis of circulating hTSH from 29 subjects with primary hypothyroidism. a, One hundred microliters of each patient's serum were diluted in 900 μL Tris-buffered saline and loaded onto a 3-mL ConA column. Unbound TSH was removed with Tris-buffered saline (1). Weakly bound TSH was eluted with 10 mM α-methylglucopyranoside (2). Firmly bound TSH was then eluted with 500 mM α-methylmannopyranoside (3). b, Another aliquot of serum from each subject was loaded onto a 2-mL lentil column. Unbound TSH was removed with Tris-buffered saline (1). Bound TSH was then eluted with 500 mM α-methylmannopyranoside (2). TSH was measured in each column fraction using an IRMA method. Values shown are percentages of TSH (mean ± SEM) in each column fraction. Note that ConA Fx 1 + Fx 2 + Fx 3 = 100%, and lentil Fx 1 + Fx 2 = 100%.

with 500 mM α-methylmannopyranoside.

Serial lectin chromatography was performed by applying TSH eluted from one lectin to a different lectin. When lentil Fx 1 was rechromatographed on fresh ConA (Fig. 4a), 24.9 ± 1.1% of the TSH from lentil Fx 1 appeared in ConA Fx 1, 46.4 ± 1% appeared in ConA Fx 2, and 28.7 ± 0.8% appeared in ConA Fx 3. Lentil Fx 2 from each serum was redialyzed against column buffer, and when rechromatographed on fresh ConA, 18.6 ± 1% and 20.9 ± 0.9% of the TSH appeared in ConA Fx 1 and 2, respectively (Fig. 4a). In contrast to TSH from lentil Fx 1, 60.5 ± 1.4% of the TSH from lentil Fx 2 appeared in ConA Fx 3.

Serial lectin chromatography was also performed for each of the samples in the reverse order. When ConA Fx 2 was rechromatographed on fresh lentil (Fig. 4b), 72.8 ± 1.4% of the TSH appeared in lentil Fx 1, whereas only 27.2 ± 1.4% appeared in lentil Fx 2. ConA Fx 3 from each sample was dialyzed against column buffer and was rechromatographed on fresh lentil (Fig. 4b); 46.9 ± 1.5% of the TSH from ConA Fx 3 appeared in lentil Fx 1, whereas 53.1 ± 1.5% appeared in lentil Fx 2. Because of

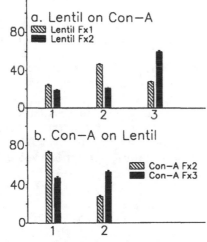

FIG. 4. Serial lectin chromatography of hypothyroid sera. Lentil Fx 1 and Fx 2 (Fig. 3b) were rechromatographed on ConA, and ConA Fx 2 and Fx 3 (Fig. 3a) were rechromatographed on lentil. a, Lentil Fx 1 (▨) and lentil Fx 2 (■), after dialysis to remove the eluting sugar α-methylmannopyranoside, were rechromatographed on ConA. Unbound TSH was removed with Tris-buffered saline (1). Weakly bound TSH was eluted with 10 mM α-methylglucopyranoside (2). Firmly bound TSH was then eluted with 500 mM α-methylmannopyranoside (3). b, After dialysis to remove eluting sugars, ConA Fx 2 (▨) and ConA Fx 3 (■) were rechromatographed on lentil. Unbound TSH was removed with Tris-buffered saline (1). Bound TSH was then eluted with 500 mM α-methylmannopyranoside (2). TSH was measured in each column fraction using an IRMA method. Values shown are percentages of TSH (mean ± SEM) in each column fraction. Note that ConA Fx 1 + Fx 2 + Fx 3 = 100%, and lentil Fx 1 + Fx 2 = 100%.

the low TSH content, ConA Fx 1 was not rechromatographed on lentil.

When we rechromatographed ConA Fx 2 and Fx 3 on lentil, we sorted five classes of TSH molecules according to their extent of binding to both ConA and lentil (Table 1). TSH molecules, although heterogeneous, must share certain structures within each class. The classes were as follows: class I (27.6 ± 1.1%), TSH that bound firmly to both ConA and lentil; class II (24.4 ± 0.9%), TSH that bound firmly to ConA but did not bind to lentil; class III (10.1 ± 0.6%), TSH that bound weakly to ConA and firmly to lentil; class IV (27.2 ± 1%), TSH that bound weakly to ConA but did not bind to lentil; and class V (10.8 ± 0.6%), TSH that did not bind to ConA. χ^2 analysis combined with Yates continuity correction, using classes I–IV (89% of the TSH) showed that TSH that bound firmly to ConA (ConA Fx 3) was more likely than TSH that bound weakly to ConA (ConA Fx 2) to bind to lentil (lentil Fx 2; $P = 0.025$). When we rechromatographed lentil fractions on ConA, we again sorted TSH into classes (Table 1). Class I comprised 31.2 ± 1.2% of the TSH; class II comprised 13.7 ± 0.6%; class III comprised 11 ± 0.5%; class IV comprised 22.5 ± 1.1%; class Va comprised 9.8 ± 0.6%; and class Vb comprised 11.9 ± 0.6%. Classes Va and Vb contained TSH that did not bind to ConA, and either bound firmly to lentil (Va) or did not bind (Vb). Using classes I–Vb (100% of the TSH), we demonstrated that the TSH that bound firmly to lentil (lentil Fx 2) was more likely to bind to ConA (ConA Fx 3), and the TSH that did not bind to lentil (lentil Fx 1) was less likely to bind firmly to ConA (ConA) Fx 1 and 2, $P = 0.005$).

ConA and lentil analyses of TSH from euthyroid subjects and the central hypothyroid subject

Immunoaffinity-concentrated TSH from sera of nine euthyroid subjects and one central hypothyroid subject

TABLE 1. TSH classes obtained after serial lectin affinity chromatography on ConA and lentil

Class	ConA binding	Lentil binding	ConA on lentil (%)	Lentil on ConA (%)
I	++	++	27.6 ± 1.1	31.2 ± 1.2
II	++	−	24.4 ± 0.9	13.7 ± 0.6
III	+	++	10.1 ± 0.6	11.0 ± 0.5
IV	+	−	27.2 ± 1.0	22.5 ± 1.1
Va	−	++	(10.8 ± 0.6)[a]	9.8 ± 0.6
Vb	−	−		11.9 ± 0.6

ConA Fx 2 and ConA Fx 3 (after dialysis) were rechromatographed on lentil, and lentil Fx 1 and lentil Fx 2 (after dialysis) were rechromatographed on ConA. Fx 1 was collected, and then glycoproteins were eluted as described in *Materials and Methods*. TSH was measured in each column fraction using IRMA. The binding characteristics and the proportion of TSH present in each class are shown. All values are the mean ± SEM. ++, Firmly bound; +, weakly bound; −, unbound.

[a] Class V not subfractionated into Va and Vb due to low amount of TSH.

990   MIURA *ET AL.* JCE & M • 1989
Vol 69 • No 5

(two sera) was studied using ConA and lentil (Fig. 5a). TSH (3–5 μU for euthyroid subjects; 13 and 18 μU for the central hypothyroid subject) was loaded onto a ConA column and eluted as described above. The amount of TSH per fraction from the sera of the euthyroid subjects was as follows: 13.7 ± 1.7% of the TSH did not bind to ConA (ConA Fx 1), 28.4 ± 2.6% of the TSH bound weakly (ConA Fx 2), and 57.7 ± 3.2% of the TSH bound firmly to ConA (ConA Fx 3). The amount of TSH per fraction for each of the two sera from the central hypothyroid subject was as follows: 2% and 4%, respectively, of the TSH did not bind to ConA (ConA Fx 1), 22% and 27% of the TSH bound weakly (ConA Fx 2), and 76% and 69% of the TSH bound firmly to ConA (ConA Fx 3). A similar amount of TSH from each subject was also initially loaded onto a lentil column and eluted as described above (Fig. 5b). The amount of TSH per fraction for the euthyroid subjects was as follows: 38 ± 2.7% of the TSH did not bind to lentil (lentil Fx 1), whereas 62 ± 2.7% bound firmly (lentil Fx 2). The amount of TSH per fraction from each of the two sera from the central hypothyroid subject was as follows: 40% and 41%, re-

spectively, of the TSH did not bind to lentil (lentil Fx 1), whereas 60% and 59% bound firmly (lentil Fx 2).

As this technique differed slightly from the chromatographic technique employed for the primary hypothyroid subjects, a direct statistical comparison was not possible. Therefore, we analyzed pooled sera from 62 hypothyroid subjects (TSH, >25 μU/mL) after immunoaffinity concentration. TSH (90 μU) from these hypothyroid subjects was processed in a manner similar to that described for euthyroid and central hypothyroid sera (Fig. 5a); 8% of the TSH did not bind to ConA (ConA Fx 1), 28% of the TSH bound weakly (ConA Fx 2), and 64% of the TSH bound firmly to ConA (ConA Fx 3). A similar amount of TSH was also initially separated on a lentil column and eluted as described above (Fig. 5b). The amount of TSH per fraction was as follows: 39% of the TSH did not bind to lentil (lentil Fx 1), whereas 61% bound (lentil Fx 2).

Ricin analyses of TSH from euthyroid, primary, and central hypothyroid subjects

After immunoaffinity concentration, TSH specimens were treated with or without neuraminidase, then loaded on ricin columns. Figure 6 shows a typical pattern of TSH elution from the ricin. This particular TSH specimen was from serum of a patient with primary hypothyroidism and the TSH had been pretreated with neuraminidase. As a control, TSH from the second fraction was dialyzed and treated with β-galactosidase to remove exposed β-galactose residues and was then reloaded onto the ricin. More than 75% of the TSH failed to bind to the ricin, while without treatment with β-galactosidase this TSH had fully bound to the ricin. This indicated that the ricin was relatively specific for exposed β-galactose residues.

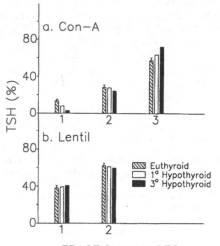

FIG. 5. ConA (a) and lentil (b) lectin affinity chromatographic analysis of circulating hTSH from euthyroid subjects (▨), pooled sera from 62 primary hypothyroid subjects (□), and 2 serum samples from a subject with central hypothyroidism (■). a, TSH from sera was enriched using monoclonal antibody-coated tubes, dialyzed against column buffer, and loaded onto a 1-mL ConA column. Unbound TSH was removed with Tris-buffered saline (1). Weakly bound TSH was eluted with 10 mM α-methylglucopyranoside (2). Firmly bound TSH was then eluted with 500 mM α-methylmannopyranoside (3). b, Another aliquot of enriched TSH from serum was loaded onto a 1-mL lectin column. Unbound TSH was removed with Tris-buffered saline (1). Bound TSH was then eluted with 500 mM α-methylmannopyranoside (2). TSH was measured in each column fraction using an IRMA method. Values shown are mean percentage of TSH in each column fraction (values for euthyroid sera, mean ± SEM). Note that ConA Fx 1 + Fx 2 + Fx 3 = 100%, and lentil Fx 1 + Fx 2 = 100%.

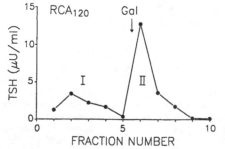

FIG. 6. Example of *Ricinus communis* (RCA$_{120}$)-agarose affinity column chromatography of TSH. Immunopurified TSH from serum of a patient with primary hypothyroidism was treated with neuraminidase and then applied to a 0.7-mL RCA$_{120}$ column. After equilibration for 60 min, the column was washed with 5 mL PBS, then 5 mL PBS containing 0.2 M galactose (Gal). Fractions of 1 mL were collected, and TSH was measured by IRMA in each fraction. The *arrow* indicates the addition of 0.2 M galactose to elute TSH bound to the RCA$_{120}$ (fraction II). Fraction I represents TSH that did not bind to RCA$_{120}$.

For euthyroid subjects, 16.1 ± 5.4% (mean ± SD) of the native TSH bound to the ricin, while after neuraminidase treatment, 38.4 ± 5.4% bound. For patients with primary hypothyroidism, 23.5 ± 6.0% of the native TSH bound to the ricin, while after neuraminidase treatment, 65.7 ± 8.8% bound (Fig. 7). The increase in ricin binding induced by neuraminidase treatment was significantly higher for TSH from patients with primary hypothyroidism than for that from euthyroid subjects (42.3 ± 7.6% vs. 22.3 ± 4.4%; $P < 0.01$). There was no correlation of the degree of ricin binding with age, sex, or serum TSH level. The ricin binding of neuraminidase-treated TSH was higher for patients with long term (>1 yr) than short term (<3 months) hypothyroidism (72.4 ± 6.6% vs. 64.2 ± 8.6%; Fig. 8), and the increase in the ricin binding induced by neuraminidase treatment was greater for long term than short term patients (49.5 ± 5.0% vs. 36.5 ± 6.5%; $P < 0.01$). These data indicated that patients with primary hypothyroidism had more sialylated TSH than did euthyroid subjects, and the degree of sialylation increased with the duration of hypothyroidism. Serum from a single patient with central hypothyroidism was analyzed; 30.0% of the TSH bound to the ricin without neuraminidase treatment (Fig. 7), and this increased 17.6% after neuraminidase treatment.

To measure the bioactivity of TSH, we employed the McKenzie bioassay with minor modifications. Because the amounts of TSH obtainable from human serum samples were insufficient for multiple bioassay measurements, we employed commercially available pituitary-

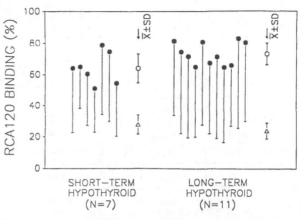

FIG. 8. Percentage of TSH bound to RCA$_{120}$ for individual patients with short or long term primary hypothyroidism. Immunopurified TSH from 7 patients with short term primary hypothyroidism (<3 months) and 11 patients with long term primary hypothyroidism (>1 yr) was treated with or without neuraminidase and applied to the RCA$_{120}$. The percentage of TSH bound to RCA$_{120}$ was calculated for each specimen. *Vertical lines* connect values with (●) or without (——) neuraminidase treatment for each individual. Shown to the *right* of each set of patients are the mean values of RCA$_{120}$ binding with (○) and without (△) prior neuraminidase treatment of TSH; *error bars* attached to those symbols represent ±SD.

derived hTSH for this purpose. The pituitary-derived TSH was fractionated using the ricin lectin column in a manner analogous to the serum-derived TSH. Only 16.1% and 10.3% of the pituitary-derived TSH bound to the ricin after prior incubation with or without neuraminidase, respectively, suggesting that the oligosaccharides of this TSH differed from those of the serum-derived TSH. No significant differences in bioactivity were observed among the fractions (Table 2).

Discussion

We have employed lectins to probe whether the oligosaccharides of hTSH differ in various physiological states. As part of this study we employed a simple technique to enrich hTSH by making use of monoclonal antibody-coated tubes, analogous to the studies of LH performed by Gospdarowicz (32). Pekonen *et al.* (33) and Dahlberg *et al.* (34) also employed immunoaffinity techniques to concentrate TSH, but their elution conditions were relatively harsh.

Lectins are carbohydrate-binding proteins and have been used widely as analytical tools (18). The lectin ConA was chosen because its binding properties are well characterized and because of its ability to separate glycopeptides and glycoproteins according to the extent of their oligosaccharide branching (equivalent to the degree of processing). Lentil was chosen because of its ability to bind core fucose residues. *Ricinus communis* (RCA$_{120}$) is a lectin isolated from *Ricinus communis* beans that binds

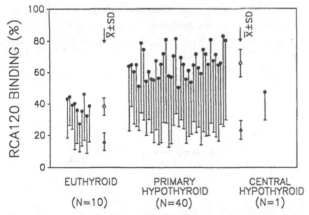

FIG. 7. Percentage of TSH bound to RCA$_{120}$ after prior treatment with or without neuraminidase. Immunopurified TSH from 10 euthyroid subjects, 40 patients with primary hypothyroidism, and 1 patient with central hypothyroidism was treated with or without neuraminidase and then applied to the RCA$_{120}$. The percentage of TSH that bound to RCA$_{120}$ was calculated for each specimen. *Vertical lines* connect values with (●) or without (——) neuraminidase treatment for each individual. Shown to the *right* of each set of patients are the mean values of RCA$_{120}$ binding with (○) and without (△) prior neuraminidase treatment of TSH: *error bars* attached to those symbols represent ±SD.

MIURA *ET AL.* JCE & M • 1989
Vol 69 • No 5

TABLE 2. Typical McKenzie *in vivo* bioassay of TSH subtypes fractionated by RCA$_{120}$

Test group	n	Blood radioactivity[a]
I. Saline, 1% HSA	3	99 ± 20[b]
II. +Neu Fx I (600 μU/mouse)	2	159 ± 86
III. +Neu Fx II (600 μU/mouse)	2	173 ± 46
IV. −Neu Fx I (600 μU/mouse)	2	187 ± 24
V. −Neu Fx II (600 μU/mouse)	3	188 ± 55
VI. TSH STD (600 μU/mouse)	3	175 ± 35

Five separate McKenzie assays testing RCA$_{120}$ fractions, each using about 20 mice, gave similar results. Mice were injected with ^{131}I to label the thyroid. Three days later, test substances were injected iv. See *Materials and Methods.* HSA, Human serum albumin; +Neu, TSH preincubated with neuraminidase; −Neu, TSH not treated with neuraminidase; Fx I, TSH that failed to bind to RCA$_{120}$; Fx II, TSH that bound to RCA$_{120}$ and eluted with galactose.

[a] Fifty or 100 μL serum were counted for each animal at 0 and 2 h. Blood radioactivity is reported as a percentage of baseline (mean ± SD).

[b] By analysis of variance, saline control was significantly different from all test substances ($P < 0.05$); differences among test substances were not significant.

specifically to Galβ1,4GlcNAc moieties. The presence of sialic acid substitution on those galactose residues markedly reduces the association constant (35). We estimated the degree of sialylation of TSH by noting the increase in binding of TSH to ricin after treatment with neuraminidase.

Serial lectin chromatography of ConA fractions on lentil (and lentil fractions on ConA) allowed the separation of TSH into classes (Table 1). Class I consisted of TSH that bound firmly to both ConA and lentil, indicating that these molecules contained at least one high mannose or hybrid oligosaccharide and an oligosaccharide with a core fucose residue. Class II consisted of TSH that bound firmly to ConA, but did not bind to lentil, indicating that these molecules contained at least one high mannose or hybrid oligosaccharide and lacked core fucose residues. Class III consisted of TSH that bound weakly to ConA and firmly to lentil, indicating that these molecules lacked high mannose or hybrid oligosaccharides; they contained at least one biantennary or truncated hybrid oligosaccharide as well as a core fucose residue. Class IV consisted of TSH that bound weakly to ConA but did not bind to lentil, indicating that these molecules contained at least one biantennary or truncated hybrid oligosaccharide and lacked high mannose and hybrid oligosaccharides and core fucose residues. Class Va consisted of TSH that did not bind to ConA, but bound firmly to lentil, indicating that these molecules contained in addition to an oligosaccharide with a core fucose residue, multiantennary oligosaccharides at all three glycosylation sites. Class Vb consisted of TSH that bound to neither ConA nor lentil, indicating

that these molecules contained multiantennary oligosaccharides at all three glycosylation sites and lacked core fucose residues. Although these discrete classes of TSH were identifiable using ConA and lentil, the proportion of TSH molecules in each class did not vary markedly as a function of the physiological state of the patient.

We demonstrated a strong inverse relationship between the degree of fucosylation and the extent of processing of TSH. More processed TSH (*i.e.* TSH containing mainly complex branched oligosaccharides) also tended to lack core fucose residues [classes IV and Vb], whereas less processed TSH (*i.e.* TSH containing at least one high mannose or hybrid oligosaccharide) also tended to contain core fucose residues (class I). Hybrid oligosaccharides may contain core fucose and would then bind firmly to both ConA and lentil, but core fucose is generally thought to be absent from high mannose oligosaccharides. Because intact TSH heterodimers containing three oligosaccharides, rather than glycopeptides, were analyzed, it was not possible to determine unambiguously to which oligosaccharide the fucose is bound. We have devised a putative TSH molecule to explain the properties of lentil binding and firm ConA binding in the same molecule (Fig. 9). Theoretically, the presence of a high mannose or hybrid oligosaccharide at one site (Fig. 9, position 1), a core fucose residue on a second oligosaccharide (Fig. 9, position 2), and any oligosaccharide at the third site (Fig. 9, position 3) would have allowed binding to both ConA and lentil to occur.

The trend favoring increased core fucosylation of less processed TSH molecules has not been described previously. It is known that in intestinal and hepatic cells, the addition of core fucose by 6α-fucosyltransferase to an asparagine-linked *N*-acetylglucosamine occurs in the

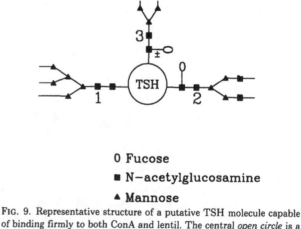

0 Fucose

■ N−acetylglucosamine

▲ Mannose

FIG. 9. Representative structure of a putative TSH molecule capable of binding firmly to both ConA and lentil. The *central open circle* is a schematic representation of the TSH α-β heterodimer with three oligosaccharide residues: 1, a high mannose or hybrid structure; 2, a fucosylated oligosaccharide as in Fig. 2a; and 3, any oligosaccharide structure from Fig. 1.

Golgi apparatus after the addition of a peripheral N-acetylglucosamine by the enzyme N-acetylglucosamine transferase I (36). The 6α-fucosyltransferase enzyme does not act on substrate carrying bisecting N-acetylglucosamine residues or after the addition of Galβ1,4 or sialic acid-Galβ1,4 sequences (37, 38). Thus, more processed structures on TSH may inhibit core fucosylation.

Sialic acid is widely distributed in the glycoprotein hormones of several mammalian species (39) and is believed to influence the biological properties of these molecules (21, 40, 41). In the present study we demonstrated that the degree of sialylation of human serum TSH varied with the physiological state. The degree of sialylation was significantly higher for TSH from sera of patients with primary hypothyroidism than for euthyroid subjects and increased with the duration of hypothyroidism. Of note, the binding of TSH to ricin even without prior neuraminidase treatment was not due to hydrophobic or other nonspecific interactions, because the TSH was eluted using 0.2 M galactose; some TSH molecules may have naturally contained peripheral galactose residues not covered by sialic acid.

Dimond and Rosen (42) demonstrated that human serum TSH displayed both charge and size heterogeneity in primary hypothyroidism, and that there were chromatographic differences between circulating and pituitary TSH. Constant and Weintraub (22) compared the MCRs of TSH from normal or hypothyroid rat pituitaries and TSH from hypothyroid rat serum and showed that the MCRs of TSH from hypothyroid serum and hypothyroid pituitaries were decreased. Recently, De-Cherney et al. (26) used anion exchange HPLC to determine that mouse TSH became more sialylated and less sulfated during prolonged hypothyroidism. This may explain why the MCR of TSH may decrease in hypothyroidism. Mori et al. (13) showed in the rat that after thyroidectomy TSH components became more variegated, and TSH components with more acidic isoelectric points became more evident using isoelectric focusing. This might have reflected an increase in sialic acid. Thus, our finding of increased TSH sialylation in humans with primary hypothyroidism is compatible with these findings. Unfortunately, we did not assess whether other circulating glycoproteins in hypothyroid serum, such as TBG, were overly sialylated. Because the TSH of our patient with central hypothyroidism did not have increased sialylation in spite of the clinical and biochemical state of hypothyroidism, we speculate that hypothalamic factors such as TRH may influence the sialylation of secreted TSH.

Structural changes in the carbohydrate units of TSH have been observed in a variety of pathological or physiological states. Gyves et al. (43) showed that during rat postnatal ontogenesis more multiantennary and/or bi-

sected biantennary complex carbohydrate structures appeared. Lee et al. (16) showed that TSH from sera of patients with severe nonthyroidal illness had altered glycosylation associated with reduced biological activity. They studied TSH binding to ConA, but did not assess the sialylation of TSH. Several studies of patients with central hypothyroidism suggested that secreted TSH had altered biological activity (44, 45). Beck-Peccoz et al. (46) showed that secreted TSH had impaired binding to its receptor, and this was corrected by chronic TRH treatment. The effects of TRH on the carbohydrate structure of mouse TSH in vitro were investigated by Taylor et al. (47) and Gesundheit et al. (20). They showed that TRH promoted the secretion of specific TSH molecules enriched in biantennary complex or unusual hybrid oligosaccharides (20) and less sulfated and less sialylated TSH molecules (27). Taylor et al. (48), using ConA affinity chromatography, demonstrated that hypothalamus-lesioned rats secreted TSH with altered carbohydrate structures compared to sham or hypothyroid rats. This qualitative change in TSH carbohydrate structure could be attributed to impaired TRH or other hypothalamic factors. Our patient with central hypothyroidism (who presumably has diminished central TRH) has a low degree of sialylation of TSH compared to that from sera of patients with primary hypothyroidism. Future studies of these uncommon patients will be required to better define the sialylation of TSH in central hypothyroidism.

A number of TSH bioassays have been developed in recent decades. McKenzie et al. (28) first developed an in vivo bioassay employing mice to measure the percent increase in blood ^{131}I after iv administration of TSH samples. Webster et al. (49) separated isoforms of human pituitary TSH by isoelectric focusing, tested them in a McKenzie bioassay, and found isoforms of TSH with varying ratios of immunoreactivity/bioactivity. TSH bioassays have been reported by a number of workers (49–53), and their findings have recently been summarized (6). Liu et al. (54) reported that deglycosylated hCG was a full agonist at the LH/CG receptor in the primate in vivo, despite having minimal intrinsic activity in the rat Leydig cell adenylate cyclase assay; desialylated hCG and deglycosylated hCG were full agonists in the monkey in vivo, capable of stimulating a full testicular response over 6 h despite very short MCRs. Thus, assessment of glycoprotein hormone bioactivity is a complex enterprise and may be very assay dependent. Because we wished to learn about the in vivo bioactivity of heterogeneous forms of TSH, we employed a McKenzie-type bioassay to assess the bioactivity of each ricin fraction, but we failed to show any significant differences between fractions. Further studies will be required to clarify these issues.

In conclusion, we have used ConA, lentil, and ricin lectin affinity chromatography to analyze intact hTSH molecules in serum from a variety of types of patients. We showed that TSH can be consistently separated into discrete subclasses using serial lectin affinity chromatography. There is relatively more core fucosylation of TSH molecules that also have less processed high mannose and hybrid oligosaccharides. Different degrees of sialylation of TSH occur in various physiological states. This variability of TSH sialylation is one possible mechanism for adjusting the biological properties of TSH to different physiological states.

Acknowledgments

We thank Drs. J. Michael McMillin, Stuart P. Bownes, and Ms. Helen Jackson from the Michael Reese Health Plan for supplying patient information, and Leonida Sinio, Josè Zapata, and Neil Staib for collecting sera and retrieving patient data. We also thank Drs. Arthur B. Schneider, Leon Fogelfeld, and Marta Nakao for useful discussions.

References

1. Pierce JG. Eli Lilly Lecture; The subunits of pituitary thyrotropin—their relationship to glycoprotein hormones. Endocrinology. 1971;89:1331–44.
2. Chin WW, Habener JF, Kieffer JD, Maloof F. Cell-free translation of the messenger RNA coding for the α-subunit of thyroid-stimulating hormone. J Biol Chem. 1978;253:7985.
3. Kourides IA, Weintraub BD. mRNA-directed biosynthesis of α-subunits of thyrotropin: translation in cell free and whole-cell systems. Proc Natl Acad Sci USA. 1979;76:298.
4. Pierce JG, Parsons TF. Glycoprotein hormones: structure and function. Annu Rev Biochem. 1981;50:465.
5. Magner JA, Weintraub BD. Thyroid-stimulating hormone biosynthesis. In: Ingbar S, Braverman L, eds. The thyroid. Philadelphia; Lippincott; 1986;271–87.
6. Magner JA. Thyroid-stimulating hormone: Structure and function. In: Ekholm R, Kohn L, Wolman S, eds. Control of the thyroid gland. New York; Plenum Press; In Press.
7. Berman MI, Thomas Jr CG, Manjunath P, Sairam MR, Nayfeh SN. The role of the carbohydrate moiety in thyrotropin action. Biochem Biophys Res Commun. 1985;133:680–7.
8. Amr S, Menezes-Ferreira MM, Shimohigashi Y, Chen HC, Nisula B, Weintraub BD. Activities of deglycosylated thyrotropin at the thyroid membrane receptor-adenylate cyclase system. J Endocrinol Invest. 1985;8:537–41.
9. Amir SM, Kubota K, Tramontano D, Ingbar SH, Keutmann HT. The carbohydrate moiety of bovine thyrotropin is essential for full bioactivity but not for receptor recognition. Endocrinology. 1987;120:345–52.
10. Goetinck PF, Pierce JG. A study of the polymorphism of bovine thyrotropin preparations by immunochemistry and peptide mapping. Arch Biochem Biophys. 1966;115:277–90.
11. Vanhaelst L, Goldstein-Golaire J. Gel filtration profile of immunoreactive thyrotropin and subunits of human pituitaries. J Clin Endocrinol Metab. 1976;43:836–41.
12. Yora T, Matsuzaki S, Kondo Y, Ui N. Changes in the contents of multiple components of rat pituitary thyrotropin in altered thyroid states. Endocrinology. 1979;104:1682–5.
13. Mori M, Ohshima K, Fukuda H, Kobayashi I, Wakabayashi K. Changes in the multiple components of rat pituitary TSH and TSHβ subunit following thyroidectomy. Acta Endocrinol (Copenh). 1984;105:49–56.
14. Taylor T, Weintraub BD. Thyrotropin (TSH)-releasing hormone regulation of TSH subunit biosynthesis and glycosylation in normal and hypothyroid rat pituitaries. Endocrinology. 1985;116:1968–76.
15. Menezes-Ferreira MM, Petrick PA, Weintraub BD. Regulation of thyrotropin (TSH) bioactivity by TSH-releasing hormone and thyroid hormone. Endocrinology. 1986;118:2125–30.
16. Lee HY, Suhl J, Pekary AE, Hershman JM. Secretion of thyrotropin with reduced concanavalin-A-binding activity in patients with severe nonthyroidal illness. J Clin Endocrinol Metab. 1987;65:942–5.
17. Ain KB, Refetoff S. Relationship of oligosaccharide modification to the cause of serum thyroxine-binding globulin excess. J Clin Endocrinol Metab. 1988;66:1037–43.
18. Cummings RD, Kornfeld S. Fractionation of asparagine-linked oligosaccharides by serial lectin-agarose affinity chromatography: a rapid, sensitive, and specific technique. J Biol Chem. 1982;257:11235–40.
19. Kornfeld K, Reitman HL, Kornfeld R. The carbohydrate-binding specificity of pea and lentil lectins: fucose is an important determinant. J Biol Chem. 1981;256:6633–40.
20. Gesundheit N, Fink DL, Silverman LA, Weintraub BD. Effect of thyrotropin releasing hormone on the carbohydrate structure of secreted mouse thyrotropin: analysis by lectin affinity chromatography. J Biol Chem. 1987;262:5197–5203.
21. Ashwell G, Harford J. Carbohydrate-specific receptors of the liver. Annu Rev Biochem. 1982;51:531–54.
22. Constant RB, Weintraub BD. Differences in the metabolic clearance of pituitary and serum thyrotropin (TSH) derived from euthyroid and hypothyroid rats: effects of chemical deglycosylation of pituitary TSH. Endocrinology. 1986;119:2720–7.
23. Morell AG, Gregoriadis G, Scheinberg IH, Hickman J, Ashwell G. The role of sialic acid in determining the survival of glycoproteins in the circulation. J Biol Chem. 1971;246:1461–7.
24. Amr S, Shimohigashi Y, Carayon P, Chen HC, Nisula B. Sialic acid residues of the α-subunit are required for the thyrotropic activity of hCG. Biochem Biophys Res Commun. 1982;109:146–51.
25. Channing CP, Sakai CN, Bahl OP. Role of the carbohydrate residues of human chorionic gonadotropin in binding and stimulation of adenosine 3′,5′-monophosphate accumulation by porcine granulosa cells. Endocrinology. 1978;103:341–8.
26. DeCherney GS, Gesundheit N, Gyves PW, Showalter CR, Weintraub BD. Alterations in the sialylation and sulfation of secreted mouse thyrotropin in primary hypothyroidism. Biochem Biophys Res Commun. 1989;159:755–62.
27. Gesundheit N, Magner JA, Chen T, Weintraub BD. Differential sulfation and sialylation of secreted mouse thyrotropin (TSH) subunits: regulation by TSH-releasing hormone. Endocrinology. 1986;119:455–63.
28. McKenzie JM. The bioassay of thyrotropin in serum. Endocrinology. 1958;63:372–82.
29. Florsheim WH, Williams AD, Schoenbaum E. On the mechanism of the McKenzie bioassay. Endocrinology. 1970;87:881–8.
30. Good BF, Stenhouse NS. An improved bio-assay for TSH by modification of the method of McKenzie. Endocrinology. 1966;78:429–39.
31. Matthews DE, Farewell VT. Using and understanding medical statistics. Basel: Karger; 1988;39–57.
32. Gospodarowicz D. Single step purification of ovine luteinizing hormone by affinity chromatography. J Biol Chem. 1972;247:6491–8.
33. Pekonen F, Williams DM, Weintraub BD. Purification of thyrotropin and other glycoprotein hormones by immunoaffinity chromatography. Endocrinology. 1980;106:1327–32.
34. Dahlberg PA, Petrick PA, Nissim M, Menezes-Ferreira MM, Weintraub BD. Intrinsic bioactivity of thyrotropin in human serum is inversely correlated with thyroid hormone concentrations: application of a new bioassay using the FRTL-5 rat thyroid cell strain. J Clin Invest. 1987;79:1388–94.
35. Baenziger JU, Fiete D. Structural determinations of *Ricinus communis* agglutinin and toxin specificity for oligosaccharides. J Biol Chem. 1979;254:9795–9.
36. Ellinger A, Pavelka M. Localization of fucosyl residues in cellular compartments of rat duodenal absorptive enterocytes and goblet cells. Eur J Cell Biol. 1988;47:62–71.
37. Longmore GD, Schachter H. Product identification and substrate-

specificity studies of GDP-L-fucose: 2-acetamide-2-deoxy-β-D-glucoside(fuc→Asn-linked GlcNAc) 6α-L-fucosyltransferase in a Golgi-rich fraction for porcine liver. Carbohydr Res. 1982;100:365–92.

38. Schachter H. Coordination between enzyme specificity and intracellular compartmentation in the control of protein-bound oligosaccharide biosynthesis. Biol Cell. 1984;51:133–45.

39. Green ED, Baenziger JU. Asparagine linked oligosaccharides on lutropin, follitropin and thyrotropin: distribution of sulfated and sialylated oligosaccharides on bovine, ovine and human pituitary glycoprotein hormones. J Biol Chem. 1988;263:36–44.

40. Rosa C, Amr S, Birken S, Wehmann R, Nisula B. Effect of desialylation of human chorionic gonadotropin on its metabolic clearance rate in humans. J Clin Endocrinol Metab. 1984;59:1215–9.

41. Baenziger JU, Green ED. Pituitary glycoprotein hormone oligosaccharides: structure, synthesis and function of the asparagine-linked oligosaccharides on lutropin, follitropin and thyrotropin. Biochim Biophys Acta. 1988;947:287–306.

42. Dimond RC, Rosen SW. Chromatographic differences between circulating and pituitary thyrotropins. J Clin Endocrinol Metab. 1974;39:316–25.

43. Gyves PW, Gesundheit N, Taylor T, Bulter LB, Weintraub BD. Changes in thyrotropin (TSH) carbohydrate structure and response to TSH-releasing hormone during postnatal ontogeny: analysis by concanavalin-A chromatography. Endocrinology. 1987;121:133–40.

44. Faglia G, Bitensky L, Pinchera A, et al. Thyrotropin secretion in patients with central hypothyroidism: evidence for reduced biological activity of immunoreactive thyrotropin. J Clin Endocrinol Metab. 1979;48:989–98.

45. Faglia G, Beck-Peccoz P, Ballabio M, Nara C. Excess of β-subunit of thyrotropin (TSH) in patients with idiopathic central hypothyroidism due to the secretion of TSH with reduced biological activity. J Clin Endocrinol Metab. 1983;56:908–14.

46. Beck-Peccoz P, Amr S, Menezes-Ferreira MM, Faglia G, Weintraub BD. Decreased receptor binding of biologically inactive thyrotropin in central hypothyroidism: effect of treatment with thyrotropin-releasing hormone. N Engl J Med. 1985;312:1085–90.

47. Taylor T, Gesundheit N, Weintraub BD. Effects of in vivo bolus versus continuous TRH administration on TSH secretion, biosynthesis, and glycosylation in normal and hypothyroid rats. Mol Cell Endocrinol. 1986;46:253–61.

48. Taylor T, Gesundheit N, Gyves PW, Jacobowitz DM, Weintraub BD. Hypothalamic hypothyroidism caused by lesions in rat paraventricular nuclei alters the carbohydrate structure of secreted thyrotropin. Endocrinology. 1988;122:283–90.

49. Webster BR, Hummel BCW, McKenzie JM, Brown GM, Paice JC. Isoelectric focusing of human thyrotropin identification of multiple components with dissociation of biological and immunological activities. Structure-activity relationships of protein and polypeptide hormones. Proc of the 2nd International Symp., Excerpta Medica, Inter. Congr. Series, 1972; No. 241:369–78.

50. Peterson V, Smith BR, Hall R. A study of thyroid stimulating activity in human serum with the highly sensitive cytochemical bioassay. J Clin Endocrinol Metab. 1975;41:199–202.

51. Rapaport B, Adams J. Bioassay using dog thyroid cells in monolayer culture. Metabolism. 1978;27:1732–42.

52. Ambesi-Impiombato FS, Parks LAM, Coon HG. Culture of hormone-dependent functional epithelial cells from rat thyroids. Proc Natl Acad Sci USA. 1980;77:3455–9.

53. Nissim M, Lee KO, Petrick PA, Dahlberg PA, Weintraub BD. A sensitive thyrotropin (TSH) bioassay based on iodide uptake in rat FRTL-5 thyroid cells: comparison with the adenosine 3',5'-monophosphate response to human serum TSH and enzymatically deglycosylated bovine and human TSH. Endocrinology. 1987;121:1278–87.

54. Liu L, Southers JL, Banks SM, et al. Stimulation of testosterone production in the cynomolgus monkey in vivo by deglycosylated and desialylated human choriogonadotropin. Endocrinology. 1989;124:175–80.

Modulation of Sialyltransferase In Thyrotrophs

A key theme of my bench research through the years was that the oligosaccharides of TSH are important, and might perform useful roles. Those sugars might protect against enzyme degradation of TSH, for example. They also potentially might alter the intrinsic bioactivity of a TSH molecule, such as by altering the charge or shape of the TSH molecule causing its receptor affinity to increase or decrease. The oligosaccharides might also lengthen or shorten the circulation time of a TSH molecule in a living animal, which would change its effective bioactivity (even if its intrinsic bioactivity in a test tube was not changed).

Sialic acid is a type of sugar that sits at the periphery of oligosaccharides. The amount of sialic acid seemed to be associated with the amount of bioactivity or metabolic clearance of a number of glycoproteins, and perhaps this might be true for TSH. Perhaps having more or less sialic acid on TSH was actually physiologically regulated, such that the optimal qualitative type of TSH could be secreted in certain physiologic conditions. In the Muira et al. paper included in this collection my laboratory in Chicago showed in 1989 that the TSH circulating in the blood of hypothyroid patients had more sialic acid residues than did TSH in the blood of euthyroid subjects. Perhaps during primary hypothyroidsm the cells in the pituitary caused the enzyme that adds sialic acid to TSH during biosynthesis to be up-regulated. This idea could be tested directly in mice.

Todd Helton was a bright graduate student on track to become a newly-minted PhD when I hired him in 1992 to be my lab technician and partner in my new laboratory at East Carolina University. He knew biochemistry, and he knew how to do in situ hybridization, a technique by which up- or down-regulation of specific genes could be measured. Of course, I hired him to show me how we could use his technical knowledge to learn about the possible up-regulation of certain genes in hypothyroidism versus euthyroidism, using mice as a model system. Of several candidate genes of interest, a type of sialyltransferase was high on my list for investigation, and the publication that follows was a unique and interesting report. We showed that a type of sialyltransferase mRNA increased in the thyrotrophs of hypothyroid mice, and an important control was that this same mRNA did not increase in anterior pituitary cells of other types that were adjacent to the thyrotrophs. This was a sign of the specific regulation of sialyltransferase in thyrotrophs in the hypothyroid milieu. We later applied this technique to study two other thyrotroph enzymes.

My experiments at East Carolina University were quite successful, but the funding pay-line for NIH grants was so competitive that I still could not get funding. After five years in North Carolina, I had to close my lab and make some sort of change. I elected for my future work to do clinical research within large pharmaceutical companies. I secured a position in 1997 doing clinical research studies related to type 2 diabetes at Bayer in Connecticut, and I stayed more than six years. But when I got a phone call from Genzyme in 2003 asking if I would consider moving to Cambridge to help them with some clinical TSH projects, I could not pass up the opportunity to move back into the TSH field.

0013-7227/94/1346-2347$03.00/0
Endocrinology
Copyright © 1994 by The Endocrine Society

Vol. 134, No. 6
Printed in U.S.A.

Sialyltransferase Messenger Ribonucleic Acid Increases in Thyrotrophs of Hypothyroid Mice: An *in Situ* Hybridization Study*

TODD E. HELTON AND JAMES A. MAGNER

Department of Medicine, Section of Endocrinology, East Carolina University School of Medicine, Greenville, North Carolina 27858–4354

ABSTRACT

Hypothyroid patients and mice have been shown to have circulating TSH that is more highly sialylated than their euthyroid counterparts. To learn about the underlying cellular mechanisms responsible for this increased sialylation of TSH, we used *in situ* hybridization to examine the β-galactoside α-2,6-sialyltransferase (STase) mRNA content in thyrotrophs and corticotrophs of euthyroid and hypothyroid mice. Mice were treated with or without 0.05% propylthiouracil for 1, 2, 3, 4, or 6 weeks, then pituitaries were removed, and 5-μm slices were immunocytochemically stained for TSH and ACTH. Adjacent sections were used for *in situ* hybridization. A 48-mer deoxynucleotide probe to rat STase and two control probes were labeled with ^{35}S, and autoradiog-

raphy was performed. There was an approximately 140% increase in STase mRNA in hypothyroid thyrotrophs compared to euthyroid thyrotrophs by the first week, with a mean increase of 170% in weeks 1–6, whereas corticotrophs exhibited no change in STase mRNA. The increase in hybridization of the STase probe in hypothyroid thyrotrophs may be due to an increased transcription of the STase gene, stabilization of the STase mRNA, or both. Thus, modulation of the STase mRNA levels occurs in thyrotrophs and represents one important mechanism by which the oligosaccharides of TSH are altered under different physiological conditions. (*Endocrinology* **134**: 2347–2353, 1994)

TSH IS A pituitary glycoprotein hormone made up of α-and β-subunits that are noncovalently linked. The α-subunit of TSH contains two asparagine (Asn)-linked oligosaccharides, whereas the β-subunit has one (1–5). Considerable heterogeneity of the oligosaccharides has been noted in numerous studies (reviewed in Ref. 2), in part due to variable sulfation and sialylation (Fig. 1). These complex oligosaccharides affect the MCR of the circulating hormone (6–10), its intrinsic biopotency (11–22), and its immunological properties (23, 24). The complex structures of the oligosaccharides of TSH may be modulated in different physiological or pathological states, perhaps tailoring the metabolic clearance and/or biopotency properties of the hormone (2, 25–35).

Sialic acid is a negatively charged sugar, often present in TSH oligosaccharides; other oligosaccharides may be sulfated or uncharged (Fig. 1). Desialylation is known to dramatically decrease the circulating time of glycoprotein hormones (6, 10), presumably by exposing the underlying galactose residue, which becomes a target for clearance by a hepatic galactose receptor and perhaps by a renal receptor. The biological importance of sialylated glycoproteins is currently being studied with several hormones. Amano and Kobata (36), for example, recently demonstrated that desialylated hLH and hCG still will bind to the LH/CG receptor, but the

production of cAMP induced by asialo-LH and asialo-CG was much lower. More recently, Szkudlinski *et al.* (37) tested two recombinant forms of TSH, rhTSH-G and rhTSH-N. rhTSH-G was shown to be highly sialylated, whereas rhTSH-N had less sialic acid and was structurally more similar to pituitary-derived TSH. rhTSH-G was shown to have a prolonged MCR and increased biopotency, presumably due to the sialic acid residues, compared to rhTSH-N and pituitary-derived TSH. TSH from hypothyroid patients is more highly sialylated than TSH from euthyroid individuals (34), and TSH sialylation is also increased in hypothyroid rodents (31, 33). The molecular mechanisms responsible for the increased sialylation of TSH during hypothyroid states are unclear. Both an α-2,6- and an α-2,3-sialyltransferase (STase) may be active in pituitary tissue (46, 47). We tested the hypothesis that the mRNA levels of β-galactoside α-2,6-STase, an enzyme that adds sialic acid to TSH, increases in thyrotrophs of hypothyroid mice. To serve as an internal control, the STase mRNA levels in corticotrophs were assessed simultaneously in the same euthyroid or hypothyroid tissue.

Materials and Methods

Animal procedures

Male CD-1 mice (n = 8, preliminary experiment; n = 40, kinetic experiment), weighing 16–18 g (Charles River, Raleigh, NC), were housed in groups of 4–10 in clear plastic cages and maintained under standard light-dark cycles, with water and food *ad libitum*. Half of the mice received water containing 0.05% propylthiouracil (PTU), and the other half received untreated water. In a preliminary experiment, mice were treated with or without PTU for 6 weeks. In a kinetic experiment, mice were treated with or without PTU for 1, 2, 3, 4, and 6 weeks. At each of these time points, four euthyroid and four hypothyroid mice

Received January 6, 1994.

Address all correspondence and requests for reprints to: Dr. James Magner, Endocrinology, Brody Building, Room 2N-72, East Carolina University School of Medicine, Greenville, North Carolina 27858–4354.

* This work was supported by the Boots Pharmaceutical Corp., the East Carolina University Department of Medicine, and a starter grant from the East Carolina University Medical Foundation.

2347

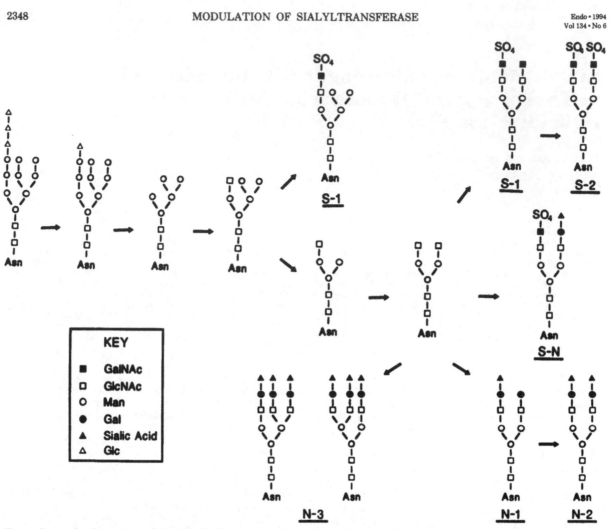

FIG. 1. Proposed pathway for synthesis of sulfated and sialylated Asn-linked oligosaccharides of the pituitary glycoprotein hormones. A key branch point in the pathway is the addition of GalNAc *vs.* Gal to peripheral GlcNAc residues. Sialic acid residues may then be added to Gal. This figure is reproduced with permission from Magner *et al.* (45).

were killed using CO_2, and pituitaries were removed. The pituitaries were immediately frozen on dry ice and stored at −70 C. Once all of the pituitaries had been collected, they were fixed in 4% phosphate-buffered paraformaldehyde for 24 h. The pituitaries were embedded in paraffin to be sectioned. Serial thin sections (5 μm) were collected (one section per glass microscope slide) and stored at −20 C. In the kinetic study, blood samples were taken from each mouse at the time of death and stored at −20 C. Serum T_4 levels were determined using a kit from Diagnostic Products Corp. (Los Angeles, CA). The T_4 assay was generously provided by Dr. Ralph Cooper (U.S. Environmental Protection Agency, Research Triangle Park, NC).

Immunocytochemistry

The pituitary sections were deparaffinized in xylene (30 min) and rehydrated in a descending alcohol series. The sections were allowed to equilibrate in PBS for 5 min before adding the blocking serum (1% normal goat serum) for 20 min. After removal of the blocking serum, the primary antibodies to TSH β-subunit (1:5000) (43) or ACTH (1:10,000; a gift from J. F. McGinty, Department of Anatomy, East Carolina University) were incubated with the tissue slices for 2 h at

room temperature. After washing, the tissue slices then were reacted with avidin-biotin-peroxidase reagents (Elite Vectastain kit, Vector Laboratories, Burlingame, CA), followed by 0.001% H_2O_2 and 0.5% 3,3′-diaminobenzidine HCl as a chromagen. The slides were counterstained with 0.1% thionin, coverslipped, evaluated for qualitative changes in immunoreactivity, and photographed on an Olympus Vanox microscope (Olympus Corp., New Hyde Park, NY) using Kodak Kodacolor film (Eastman Kodak, Rochester, NY). The use of color rather than black and white film allowed easy unambiguous identification of the chromagen.

In situ hybridization histochemistry

Sections immediately adjacent to those used for immunocytochemistry were deparaffinized in xylene (30 min), rehydrated in a descending alcohol series, pretreated with 0.25% acetic anhydride in sterile 0.1 M triethanolamine-0.9% NaCl, washed in alcohol and sterile water, and dried. The 48-mer deoxyoligonucleotide probe to STase (the antisense probe, synthesized in the DNA Synthesis Core Laboratory at East Carolina University) was chosen from the cDNA sequence (38) and was complementary to bases 901–949 within exon 6. Exon 6 is in the globular head of the enzyme, far from domains (such as the transmembrane domain) that might be less specific for the STase. This sequence was searched in the GenBank/EMBL Data Bank and was found specifically to recognize only the STase gene sequence. The sense probe (cDNA sequence, bases 901–949) and a randomized probe made of the same basepair composition as the sense probe were searched on the GenBank/EMBL Data Bank and synthesized, and no unanticipated sequence matches were found. Each probe was labeled at the 3'-end using [α-^{35}S] deoxy-ATP (1075 Ci/mmol; New England Nuclear Corp., Boston, MA) and terminal deoxynucleotidyltransferase (Boehringer Mannheim, Indianapolis, IN), as previously described (39). Probes were incubated with tissue at an annealing temperature of 40 C (39). Slides were dipped in Kodak NTB-3 photographic emulsion and stored at 4 C for 3 weeks before being developed in Dektol and fixed in Kodak fixer. Sections were counterstained with 0.1% thionin, coverslipped, and photographed on an Olympus Vanox microscope using Kodak TMAX black and white film.

Quantitative analysis

Color photographs were taken of microscopic fields of pituitary tissue with either immunostained thyrotrophs or corticotrophs (Fig. 2). Black and white darkfield photomicrographs were taken at the same magnification of the corresponding microscopic field of adjacent tissue sections that had been incubated with DNA probes and subjected to autoradiography (Fig. 3). Immunostained corticotrophs and thyrotrophs were outlined on tracing paper, and then each tracing was overlain with its corresponding darkfield photomicrograph from the *in situ* hybridization. Using a needle, the relevant silver grains were marked, the photograph and tracing paper were placed on a light box, and the silver grains were recorded (Fig. 4). To avoid bias, the photographs were numbered, and the identity of the cells as thyrotrophs or corticotrophs was not revealed until all of the photographs had been scored. In the preliminary experiment, a χ^2 analysis was performed, whereas in the kinetic experiment, an analysis of variance was performed to test significance.

To assess thyrotroph size at different durations of hypothyroidism, immunostained thyrotroph tracings from the kinetic experiment were chosen at random from each PTU treatment time point (weeks 0–6; ~140 cells from each treatment group), and the cell outlines were photocopied. Two separate methods to estimate cell sizes were used. First, each outlined thyrotroph was cut out, and groups of cell cut-outs were weighed to determine if there was an increase in the size of hypothyroid thyrotrophs. A magnification factor was calculated, and the mean cut surface area of the cells was calculated. In the second method, the cell cut-outs were hand-sorted and ranked by cell size, and each cell cut-out was assigned a percentile ranking within its treatment group. Multiple circular cut-outs of standard sizes were constructed, and the irregularly shaped thyrotrophs were matched by eye to the standard

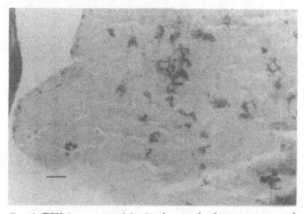

FIG. 2. TSH immunoreactivity in thyrotrophs from a mouse made hypothyroid for 4 weeks. This is a black and white print, and the dark cells are positive for chromagen. The use of color prints for the actual study allowed easy identification of the chromagen. *Bar* = 20 μm.

FIG. 3. *In situ* hybridization for STase mRNA. This pituitary tissue section was adjacent to that used for TSH immunostaining shown in Fig. 2. This is a darkfield photomicrograph, and the white dots indicate silver grains. Quantitative analysis of changes in the levels of STase mRNA was performed by tracing the immunostained thyrotrophs and then overlaying the tracing on this darkfield photograph of the STase *in situ* hybridization. *Bar* = 20 μm.

circles to estimate each cell's surface area. We judge that the first method, based on the weight of the paper cut-outs, is the more accurate, but only provided information about the mean cell size. The second method, based on estimating individual cell sizes, seemed to have a systematic error causing overestimation of cell size by 10–20%, but was useful to assess the distribution of thyrotroph size within each treatment group.

Results

Preliminary experiment

The purpose of the preliminary experiment was to determine whether hybridization of the STase probe increased in hypothyroid compared to euthyroid thyrotrophs. Corticotrophs present in the same tissue served as a useful internal control, because no change in probe hybridization was expected in corticotrophs. A simple comparison of pituitary tissue from euthyroid mice *vs.* that of mice hypothyroid for 6 weeks was performed. The corticotrophs and thyrotrophs were identified immunocytochemically by a dark brown precipitate within the cells (Fig. 2). In general, the thyrotrophs from the hypothyroid mice appeared larger than the thyrotrophs from euthyroid mice. However, the size of the corticotrophs did not change. A total of 2033 cells and 985 silver grains were recorded (Fig. 5). The number of silver grains per cell in euthyroid thyrotrophs and euthyroid corticotrophs (0.47 *vs.* 0.43 silver grains/cell) did not differ significantly. Using χ^2 analysis, there was a significant increase in the number of silver grains per cell in the hypothyroid thyrotrophs compared to hypothyroid corticotrophs (0.61 *vs.* 0.38 silver grains/cell), and the increased number of silver grains in hypothyroid thyrotrophs compared to euthyroid thyrotrophs also was significant. This increase in STase mRNA was statistically significant even though no measurement of nonspecific probe binding was made at this time; as can be imagined when viewing the raw data depicted in Fig. 5, subtraction of nonspecific background from each bar in

2350 MODULATION OF SIALYLTRANSFERASE Endo • 1994
Vol 134 • No 6

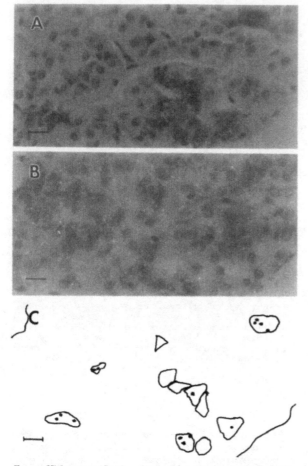

FIG. 4. Higher magnification views of thyrotrophs, *in situ* hybridization, and tracing of thyrotrophs with relevant grains marked. A, Immunostained thyrotrophs in pituitary tissue of a mouse treated with PTU for 3 weeks. B, Adjacent pituitary tissue section subjected to *in situ* hybridization. C, Thyrotrophs were traced by hand from A; grains in thyrotrophs in B were pierced using a needle, then the tracing was placed on a light box over B, and the pierced grains were marked on the tracing using a pen to create a permanent record for analysis. Magnification, ×800. *Bar at lower left* = 10 μm.

that graph would enhance the relative differences. Use of sense and random probes as controls in a subsequent experiment found the nonspecific probe binding to be about 0.3 silver grain/cell in both euthyroid and hypothyroid pituitary tissue. Thus, when the background is properly allowed for, we detected about a doubling of the STase mRNA in hypothyroid thyrotrophs compared to euthyroid thyrotrophs in this preliminary experiment.

Kinetic experiment

The kinetic experiment was carried out to confirm the existence of this modulation of STase mRNA by performing several independent replications at different durations of hypothyroidism and to study the time course of alterations

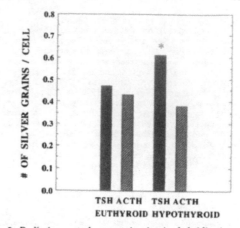

FIG. 5. Preliminary study comparing *in situ* hybridization of STase probe in thyrotrophs of euthyroid *vs.* hypothyroid mice treated with PTU for 6 weeks. TSH, Thyrotrophs; ACTH, corticotrophs. A total of 985 silver grains and 2033 cells were scored. Using χ^2 analysis, there was a significant ($P < 0.05$) increase in the number of silver grains per cell in hypothyroid compared to euthyroid thyrotrophs. The hybridization in corticotrophs from the same mice, an internal control, was not changed by hypothyroidism. Later use of control probes determined that nonspecific binding was 0.3 silver grain/cell; if this amount is subtracted from each of the four bars, the observed difference becomes more striking.

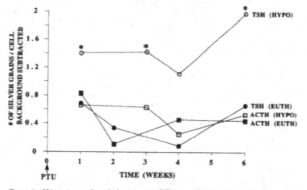

FIG. 6. Kinetic study of the rise in STase mRNA. Mice were treated for 1, 2, 3, 4, or 6 weeks with PTU. PTU was added to the drinking water at time zero, and the first mice were killed at 1 week. There was a significant ($P < 0.05$) increase in the number of silver grains per thyrotroph in the hypothyroid group (HYPO) compared to the euthyroid thyrotrophs (EUTH) at 1 week. The increase in the hybridization of the STase probe in hypothyroid thyrotrophs remained at 6 weeks.

in STase mRNA. Pituitary tissue from euthyroid mice and from mice treated with PTU for 1, 2, 3, 4, and 6 weeks was studied. A total of 4031 cells and 5588 silver grains were recorded for the kinetic study. Sense and random probes were used to determine nonspecific binding (0.3 silver grain/cell), and that amount was subtracted from the results reported below (Fig. 6). There was a significant increase in the number of silver grains per cell representing STase mRNA in hypothyroid thyrotrophs compared to euthyroid thyrotrophs (1.41 *vs.* 0.69 silver grains/cell) as early as 1 week after PTU treatment was started (Fig. 6). This increased hybridization of the STase probe in hypothyroid thyrotrophs compared to euthyroid thyrotrophs persisted at weeks 3 and 6. A caveat is that tissue slices from some animals at weeks 2 and 3 could not be analyzed due to tissue fragmentation caused by a defective microtome knife. In spite of the fact that Fig. 6 lacks data points from specific groups of animals at certain time points, the mean increase in probe hybridization in hypothyroid thyrotrophs compared to euthyroid thyrotrophs over the course of the 6-week experiment was obvious, highly significant by analysis of variance, and calculated to be approximately 170%.

Blood samples were taken from each mouse at the time of death, and serum T_4 levels were measured. T_4 levels fell from 72.3 ng/ml in euthyroid mice to 17.9 ng/ml in hypothyroid mice treated with PTU for 1 week. T_4 levels remained suppressed for the entire 6 weeks in the PTU-treated mice.

The cut surface areas of the immunostained thyrotrophs were measured to determine whether there was a change in the size of the thyrotrophs during hypothyroidism (Fig. 7). Very small immunostained areas represented tangential cuts of thyrotrophs. In euthyroid pituitaries there appeared to be two populations of thyrotrophs, medium (<160 μm^2) and large (>160 μm^2). The thyrotrophs became larger in hypothyroid mice after 1 week of PTU treatment, but did not become progressively larger in direct proportion to the duration of hypothyroidism after 3 weeks. Even in hypothyroid pituitaries there were two populations of thyrotrophs, medium and large in size. Silver grains were present in thyrotrophs of all cell sizes.

A potentially confounding issue was that a change in the cell size alone theoretically could account for an increase in the number of silver grains per cell. The size of the thyro-

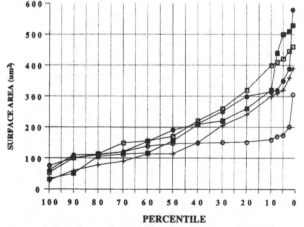

FIG. 7. Sizes of thyrotrophs. Immunostained thyrotrophs in the photomicrographs were traced. The paper tracings were weighed to determine the mean thyrotroph size in euthyroid mice and the groups of hypothyroid mice. The paper tracings of individual thyrotrophs also were sorted by hand and ranked according to size in each group of animals, so that the median size and percentile distribution were determined. The abrupt changes in the slopes of these lines, shown at the *right*, indicated that at least two populations of thyrotrophs existed. Although few large thyrotrophs were present in euthyroid mice, thyrotrophs grew larger in hypothyroid mice. O, Euthyroid; □, week 1; ●, week 3; ■, week 4; +, week 6 of PTU treatment.

trophs, as determined by the more accurate of the two methods used (weighing groups of cell tracing cut-outs), increased from a mean of 97 μm^2 in euthyroid thyrotrophs to a mean of 140 μm^2 in hypothyroid thyrotrophs, for a mean increase of about 40%. Therefore, only 40% of the increased number of silver grains per thyrotroph could have been due to an increase in the sizes of the cells alone, whereas the remaining increase was due to a specific increase in hybridization of the STase probe, indicating the presence of truly higher amounts of STase mRNA.

Discussion

These represent the first studies to look at the underlying cellular mechanisms responsible for the increase in sialic acid residues on TSH during hypothyroidism. No previous study of glycosyltransferase mRNA abundance has been performed in any glycoprotein hormone-synthesizing tissue. We hypothesized that more STase mRNA might be detectable in hypothyroid vs. euthyroid thyrotrophs.

The technique of in situ hybridization was employed because thyrotrophs were present among other cell types in pituitary tissue. An alternative technique, employing Northern analyses to quantitate STase mRNA, was thought to be unsuitable because hypothyroidism might cause STase mRNA to increase in thyrotrophs but decrease in other cell types, so that no net effect would be detectable. Purification of thyrotrophs for subsequent analyses of mRNA also was viewed as unsatisfactory because there might be variable contamination with other cell types, variable yields, and poor quantifiability. Ideally, we would have performed in situ hybridization and immunocytochemistry on the same tissue slices, but a variety of technical problems prevented this. We settled for performing immunocytochemistry for thyrotrophs and corticotrophs on the two adjacent tissue slices to that slice used for in situ hybridization. We then worked from photomicrographs to score silver grains in either thyrotrophs or corticotrophs, and this scoring was performed without knowledge at the time as to whether thyrotrophs or corticotrophs were being scored, to eliminate observer bias.

In a preliminary study we detected a significant increase in the hybridization of the STase probe in thyrotrophs of hypothyroid mice after 6 weeks of PTU treatment compared to that in euthyroid thyrotrophs. This finding was confirmed by a later kinetic study that found significant increases in the hybridization of the STase probe in hypothyroid thyrotrophs as early as 1 week after PTU treatment was started as well as in replicate experiments performed at other durations of hypothyroidism. The levels of STase mRNA in hypothyroid thyrotrophs remained elevated for the 6-week duration of the study. By measuring serum T_4 levels, the mice were confirmed to be hypothyroid by week 1 of the study and for the remaining weeks. At the same time, there was no change in the level of STase mRNA in corticotrophs from the same mice evaluated in the same tissue. Additionally, the size of the thyrotrophs increased during hypothyroidism, as had been previously reported (40, 41), but by carefully sizing thyrotrophs we were able to calculate that the change in size of the thyrotrophs could have been responsible for only a

40% increase in silver grains per cell. The observed specific increase in hybridization of the STase probe may represent an increase in transcription of the mRNA, a stabilization of newly transcribed mRNA, or a combination of both.

It should be emphasized that the experimental design allowed use of a valuable internal control. Immunostaining allowed identification of corticotrophs as well as thyrotrophs on each pituitary slice subjected to *in situ* hybridization. Thus, we demonstrated that specific hybridization increased in thyrotrophs, but not corticotrophs, in the same tissue slice, eliminating confounding factors, such as potential differences in washing of the tissue.

Terminal oligosaccharide residues are determined by the presence of specific glycosyltransferases in the Golgi of cells. A glycosyltransferase, α-2,6-STase, adds sialic acid to maturing glycoproteins with exposed galactose residues. This STase protein consists of a short N-terminal cytoplasmic domain, a transmembrane-spanning domain, and an intralumenal catalytic domain (42). The up-stream regulatory region of this STase gene has several putative thyroid hormone-responsive elements and, therefore, could be regulated by changes in the levels of T_3. Hypothyroidism may lead to an increased production of STase mRNA and a subsequent increase in the level of STase in the Golgi. The physical presence of more STase in the Golgi would lead to an increased sialylation of glycoproteins being synthesized by thyrotrophs, such as TSH.

In fact, two different sialyltransferase enzymes may be active in pituitary tissue (46, 47). Our 48-basepair probe was probably specific for the α-2,6-STase, because the analogous sequence in that region of the α-2,3-STase had only 33% homology. In future studies a series of carefully chosen probes might allow relative modulation of these two STases to be studied.

Analogous regulation of glycosyltransferases may occur during the synthesis of other glycoprotein hormones. Recently, Dharmesh and Baenziger (44) measured glycosyltransferase enzyme activity in rat pituitary tissue and found that estrogen modulated the activity of GalNAc transferase and sulfotransferase, thereby affecting the sulfation of the oligosaccharides of lutropin. One may speculate that in some pathological conditions the improper modulation of glycosyltransferases may cause the release of glycoprotein hormones with inappropriate properties. For example, heterogeneity of TSH secreted by rare patients with TSH-producing pituitary tumors has been documented (45). Perhaps, pituitary tumor tissue may express particular glycosyltransferases in a fixed unregulated manner, thereby secreting a particular subset of TSH isoforms that have more or less bioactivity than called for by a patient's thyroid status. Thus, further studies of the modulation of glycosyltransferases in glycoprotein hormone-secreting tissues may elucidate normal physiological processes and provide insight into pathological conditions.

Acknowledgments

The efforts of two students, Carla Gaskins and Jörg Trojan, are appreciated.

References

1. **Pierce JG, Parsons TF** 1981 Glycoprotein hormones: structure and function. Annu Rev Biochem 50:465–495
2. **Magner JA** 1990 Thyroid-stimulating hormone: biosynthesis, cell biology, and bioactivity. Endocr Rev 11:354–385
3. **Magner JA, Weintraub BD** 1982 Thyroid-stimulating hormone subunit processing and combination in microsomal subfractions of mouse pituitary tumor. J Biol Chem 257:6709–6715
4. **Chin WW, Habener JF, Kieffer JD, Maloof F** 1978 Cell-free translation of the messenger RNA coding for the α-subunit of thyroid-stimulating hormone. J Biol Chem 253:7985–7988
5. **Shupnik MA, Ridgway EC, Chin WW** 1989 Molecular biology of thyrotropin. Endocr Rev 10:459–475
6. **Constant RB, Weintraub BD** 1986 Differences in the metabolic clearance of pituitary and serum thyrotropin (TSH) derived from euthyroid and hypothyroid rats: effects of chemical deglycosylation of pituitary TSH. Endocrinology 119:2720–2727
7. **Keel BA** 1989 Thyroid-stimulating hormone microheterogeneity. In: Keel BA, Grotjan HE (eds) Microheterogeneity of Glycoprotein Hormones. CRC Press, Boca Raton, pp 203–215
8. **Thotakura NR, Desai RK, Bates LG, Cole ES, Pratt BM, Weintraub BD** 1991 Biological activity and metabolic clearance rate of a recombinant human thyrotropin produced in Chinese hamster ovary cells. Endocrinology 128:341–348
9. **Drickamer K** 1991 Clearing up glycoprotein hormones. Cell 67:1029–1032
10. **Morell AG, Gregoriadis G, Scheinberg IH, Hickman J, Ashwell G** 1971 The role of sialic acid in determining the survival of glycoproteins in the circulation. J Biol Chem 246:1461–1467
11. **Webster BR, Hummel BCW, McKenzie JM, Brown GM, Paice JC** 1972 Isoelectric focusing of human thyrotropin: identification of multiple components with dissociation of biological and immunological activities. In: Margoulies M, Greenwood FC (eds) Structure-Activity Relationships of Protein and Polypeptide Hormones. Int Congr Ser 241, Excerpta Medica, Amsterdam, pp 369–378
12. **Pekonen F, Carayon P, Amr S, Weintraub BD** 1981 Heterogenous forms of thyroid-stimulating hormone in mouse thyrotropic tumor and serum: differences in receptor-binding and adenylate cyclase-stimulating activity. Horm Metab Res 13:617–620
13. **Joshi LR, Weintraub BD** 1983 Naturally occuring forms of thyrotropin with low bioactivity and altered carbohydrate content act as competitive antagonists to more bioactive forms. Endocrinology 113:2145–2154
14. **Berman MI, Thomas CG, Manjunath P, Sairam MR, Nayfeh SN** 1985 The role of the carbohydrate moiety in thyrotropin action. Biochem Biophys Res Commun 133:680–687
15. **Amr S, Menezez-Ferreira M, Shimohigashi Y, Chen HC, Nisula B, Weintraub BD** 1985 Activities of deglycosylated thyrotropin at the thyroid membrane receptor-adenylate cyclase system. J Endocrinol Invest 8:537–541
16. **Amir SM, Kubota K, Tramontano D, Ingbar SH, Keutmann HT** 1987 The carbohydrate moiety of bovine thyrotropin is essential for full bioactivity but not for receptor recognition. Endocrinology 120:345–352
17. **Nissim M, Lee KO, Petrick PA, Dahlberg PA, Weintraub BD** 1987 A sensitive thyrotropin (TSH) bioassay based on iodide uptake in rat FRTL-5 thyroid cells: comparison with the adenosine 3',5'-monophosphate response to human serum TSH and enzymatically deglycosylated bovine and human TSH. Endocrinology 121:1278–1287
18. **Thotakura NR, LiCalzi L, Weintraub BD** 1990 The role of carbohydrate in thyrotropin action assessed by a novel approach using enzymatic deglycosylation. J Biol Chem 265:11527–11534
19. **Ryan RJ, Charlesworth MC, McCormick DJ, Keutmann HT** 1988 The glycoprotein hormones: recent studies of structure-function relationships. FASEB J 2:2661–2669
20. **Pickles AJ, Peers N, Robertson WR, Lambert A** 1992 Different isoforms of human pituitary thyroid-stimulating hormone have different relative biological activities. J Mol Endocrinol 9:251–256
21. **Sairam MR, Bhargavi GN** 1985 A role for glycosylation of the a subunit in transduction of biological signal in glycoprotein hor-

mones. Science 229:65–67

22. **Endo Y, Tetsumoto T, Nagasaki H, Kashiwai T, Tamaki Amino N, Miyai** 1990 The distinct roles of α- and β-subunits of human thyrotropin in the receptor binding and post-receptor events. Endocrinology 127:149–154

23. **Papandreou MJ, Sergi I, Medri G, Labbe-Jullie C, Braun J, Canonne C, Ronin C** 1991 Differential effect of glycosylation on the expression of antigenic and bioactive domains in human thyrotropin. Mol Cell Endocrinol 78:137–150

24. **Sergi I, Papandreou MJ, Medri G, Canonne C, Verrier B, Ronin C** 1991 Immunoreactive and bioactive isoforms of human thyrotropin. Endocrinology 128:3259–3268

25. **Yora T, Matsuzaki S, Kondo Y, Ui N** 1979 Changes in the contents of multiple components of rat pituitary thyrotropin in altered thyroid states. Endocrinology 104:1682–1685

26. **Mori M, Murakami M, Iriuchijima T, Ishihara H, Kobayashi I, Kobayashi S, Wakabayashi K** 1984 Alteration by thyrotropin-releasing hormone of heterogenous components associated with thyrotropin biosynthesis in the rat anterior pituitary gland. J Endocrinol 103:165–171

27. **Faglia G, Bitensky L, Pinchera A, Ferrari C, Paracchi A, Beck-Peccoz P, Ambrosi B, Spada A** 1979 Thyrotropin secretion in patients with central hypothyroidism: evidence for reduced biological activity of immunoreactive thyrotropin. J Clin Endocrinol Metab 48:989–998

28. **Taylor T, Weintraub BD** 1985 Differential regulation of thyrotropin subunit apoprotein and carbohydrate biosynthesis by thyroid hormone. Endocrinology 116:1535–1542

29. **Taylor T, Weintraub BD** 1985 Thyrotropin (TSH)-releasing hormone regulation of TSH subunit biosynthesis and glycosylation in normal and hypothyroid rat pituitaries. Endocrinology 116:1968–1976

30. **Taylor T, Scouten CW, Jacobowitz DM, Weintraub BD** 1986 The effects of anterior hypothalamic deafferentiation on thyrotropin (TSH) biosynthesis and response to TSH-releasing hormone. Endocrinology 118:2417–2424

31. **DeCherney GS, Gesundheit N, Gyves PW, Showalter CR, Weintraub BD** 1989 Alterations in the sialylation of secreted mouse thyrotropin in primary hypothyroidism. Biochem Biophys Res Commun 159:755–763

32. **Gyves PW, Gesundheit N, Stannard BS, DeCherney GS, Weintraub BD** 1989 Alterations in the glycosylation of secreted thyrotropin during ontogenesis: analysis of sialylated and sulfated oligosaccharides. J Biol Chem 264:6104–6110

33. **Gyves PW, Gesundheit N, Thotakura NR, Stannard BS, DeCherney GS, Weintraub BD** 1990 Change in the sialylation and sulfation of secreted thyrotropin in congenital hypothyroidism. Proc Natl Acad Sci USA 87:3792–3796

34. **Miura Y, Perkel VS, Papenberg KA, Johnson MJ, Magner JA** 1989 Concanvalin-A, lentil and ricin affinity binding characteristics of human thyrotropin: differences in the sialylation of thyrotropin in

sera of euthyroid, primary and central hypothyroid patients. J Clin Endocrinol Metab 69:985–995

35. **Papandreou MJ, Persani L, Asteria C, Ronin C, Beck-Pecoz P** 1993 Variable carbohydrate structures of circulating thyrotropin as studied by lectin affinity chromatography in different clinical conditions. J Clin Endocrinol Metab 77:393–398

36. **Amano J, Kobata A** 1993 Direct interaction of the sialic acid residue of human lutropin and chorionic gonadotropin with target cell is necessary for the full expression of their hormonal action. Arch Biochem Biophys 305:618–621

37. **Szkudlinski MW, Thotakora NR, Bucci I, Joshi LR, Tsai A, East-Palmer J, Shiloach J, Weintraub BD** 1993 Purification and characterization of recombinant human thyrotropin isoforms produced by Chinese hamster ovary cells: the role of sialylation and sulfation in thyrotropin bioactivity. Endocrinology 133:1490–1503

38. **Weinstein J, Lee EU, McEntee K, Lai P-H, Paulson JC** 1987 Primary structure of β-galactoside α2,6-sialyltransferase. J Biol Chem 262:17735–17743

39. **Helton T, McGinty J** 1993 Intrahippocampal NMDA administration alters Fos, Fos-related antigens, and opioid peptide immunoreactivity and mRNA in rats. Mol Cell Neurosci 4:319–334

40. **Farquhar MG, Rinehart JF** 1954 Cytologic alterations in the anterior pituitary gland following thyroidectomy: an electron microscope study. Endocrinology 55:857–876

41. **Farquhar MG** 1971 Processing of secretory product by cells of the anterior pituitary gland. In: Heller H, Lederis K (eds) Subcellular Organization and Function in Endocrine Tissues. Cambridge University Press, London, vol 1:79–124

42. **Svensson EC, Soreghan B, Paulson JC** 1990 Organization of the β-galactoside α2,6-sialyltransferase gene. J Biol Chem 265:20863–2086843

43. **Magner JA, Novak W, Papagiannes E** 1986 Subcellular localization of fucose incorporation into mouse thyrotropin and free α-subunits: studies employing subcellular fractionation and inhibitors of the intracellular translocation of proteins. Endocrinology 119:1315–1328

44. **Dharmesh SM, Baenziger JU** 1993 Estrogen modulates expression of the glycosyltransferases that synthesize sulfated oligosaccharides on lutropin. Proc Natl Acad Sci USA 90:11127–11131

45. **Magner J, Klibanski A, Fein H, Smallridge R, Blackard W, Young, Jr W, Ferriss JB, Murphy D, Kane J, Rubin D** 1992 Ricin and lentil lectin-affinity chromatography reveals oligosaccharide heterogeneity of thyrotropin secreted by 12 human pituitary tumors. Metabolism 41:1009–1015

46. **Gillespie W, Kelm S, Paulson JC** 1992 Cloning and expression of the Galβ1,3GalNAcα2,3-sialyltransferase. J Biol Chem 267:21004–21010

47. **Wen DX, Livingston BD, Medzihradszky KF, Kelm S, Burlingame AL, Paulson JC** 1992 Primary structure of Galβ1,3(4)GlcNAcα2,3-sialyltransferase determined by mass spectrometry sequence analysis and molecular cloning. J Biol Chem 267:21011–21019

TRH Alters the Types of TSH Released From the Pituitary in Man

Endocrinologists are interested in regulation – what are the controls that cause certain processes to speed up or slow down appropriately in light of changing situations encountered by animals? In multicellular organisms some messages to increase or decrease an activity are sent by nerves, but other signals are sent by hormones that circulate in the blood. TSH is such a hormone, and it causes the thyroid gland to speed up. TSH can act as a signal by increasing in quantity in the blood, but some of us in the 1980s came to believe that the qualitative structure of the TSH molecule might also be changed in different physiologic situations to add to the message. The pituitary gland, where TSH is made, receives a signal itself from a higher center in a brain region known as the hypothalamus. This signal from above is a small peptide called TRH. I wanted to test in humans in a clinical experiment whether exposure to TRH caused not only an increase in the amount of TSH in the blood, but also caused a qualitative change in the sugars on the TSH molecules, as compared to the TSH molecules present in blood before the TRH is given (the basal condition).

Proposing to inject a chemical into humans is serious business, and the exact written protocol, with provisions for obtaining informed consent, must be approved by a committee at a hospital. I chose my experiment wisely, however, because injectable TRH was a drug on the market that then was used from time to time for stimulatory testing in some endocrine patients. So the procedure was known to be safe and was not too exotic. The amount of blood to be drawn during the experiment was reasonable and not dangerous. The experiment would serve a credible scientific purpose, since I had the scientific techniques in my research laboratory to purify the TSH from the blood samples and definitively analyze whether qualitative changes became evident in TSH molecules after TRH exposure. Changes would not likely happen in the amino acid sequence of the protein, of course, but might happen in the sugars bound to the TSH.

As shown in Table 1, I found eleven normal subjects who were willing to receive the injection and have blood drawn. There is a secret not shown in the table. I was subject A! You can see that I was aged 40 and weighed 71.2 kg. And there is another secret. My wife, Glenda, was subject I, and she was aged 40 and weighed 58.8 kg. So now it can be told. There is a long history in science of self-experimentation – but I would never attempt anything foolishly dangerous. I recall reading that Isaac Newton while studying light with prisms once tried to push a metal probe behind one of his eyes to test the effect – that, frankly, is a bit over the top.

The study showed that the isoforms of TSH in blood changed after TRH injection as compared to the basal state, and it was the first such demonstration in man.

Free to Decide

0021-972X/92/7406-1306$03.00/0
Journal of Clinical Endocrinology and Metabolism
Copyright © 1992 by The Endocrine Society

Vol. 74, No. 6
Printed in U.S.A.

Intravenous Thyrotropin (TSH)-Releasing Hormone Releases Human TSH That Is Structurally Different from Basal TSH*

JAMES A. MAGNER, JOHN KANE, AND ERIC T. CHOU

Division of Endocrinology, Humana Hospital-Michael Reese, University of Illinois, Chicago, Illinois 60616

ABSTRACT. To determine whether basal TSH differed structurally from TRH-released TSH, the TSH obtained from 11 normal subjects before and after the iv administration of TRH was characterized using lectin-affinity chromatography. TSH was applied to the following lectins: lentil, ricin (both before and after TSH treatment with neuraminidase), Concanavalin-A, wheat germ, *Glycine max, Helix pomatia, Dolichos biflorus, Arachis hypogaea,* and *Vicia villosa* (isolectin B₄). After each column was washed to elute unbound TSH, the bound TSH was eluted using the appropriate specific sugar, and TSH in the column fractions was measured by immunoradiometric assay. Basal TSH was found to have a different oligosaccharide composition than TSH in serum 30 min after TRH administration. The basal TSH had fewer core fucose residues and more exposed galactose residues than the TSH released after TRH treatment. The amounts of oligosaccharide branching and the amounts of N-acetylglucosamine were similar, and the degrees of sialylation for both basal TSH and TRH-released TSH were highly variable. No exposed N-acetylgalactosamine residues were detected in either type of TSH; if present, these residues may have been uniformly sulfated. The biochemical differences detected in basal TSH *vs.* TRH-released TSH may reflect different posttranslational processing and storage of these molecules in thyrotrophs. These data provide an example of the release of particular isoforms of human TSH depending on a hypothalamic factor, a general principle that may be important in the physiological control of thyroid function by the pituitary. (*J Clin Endocrinol Metab* **74:** 1306–1311, 1992)

TSH FROM several species, including man, has three N-linked oligosaccharide chains that are very heterogeneous in composition and structure (reviewed in Refs. 1 and 2). Thus, although clinicians order serum TSH measurements to evaluate thyroid function in their patients, in fact, many isoforms of TSH exist. Different isoforms have different rates of metabolic clearance (3), and there is some evidence that different isoforms of TSH may have different biopotencies (4–16). The types of TSH isoforms released in particular physiological states may be controlled, to a greater or lesser degree, by endocrine factors, so that hormone with advantageous biological properties might circulate when conditions demand.

Although several animal studies found that different isoforms of TSH were present in different physiological states (17–23), our experiments showing that TSH in the serum of hypothyroid patients was more sialylated than TSH from euthyroid patients was one of the first such reports in man (24); altered isoforms of human TSH also have been reported in a different condition, nonthyroidal illness (25). We implicated hypothalamic factors, such as TRH, as potential modulators of human TSH isoforms since we demonstrated that TSH with euthyroid-type oligosaccharide chains circulated in a patient with hypothalamic disease in spite of the hypothyroid clinical state (24). The notion that TSH had altered bioactivity in central hypothyroidism was previously proposed (26–29), but other than the determination that the TSH was of normal molecular size, no biochemical characteristics of the TSH in central hypothyroidism were known.

We now extend these observations by reporting structural characteristics of human TSH present in serum before and after the administration of TRH. We found that the isoforms of TSH present in the basal state in normal subjects differ from the isoforms present after the administration of TRH.

Subjects and Methods

Normal subjects

The clinical characteristics of the 11 normal subjects are summarized in Table 1. None had serious medical illnesses, a history of thyroid disease, or symptoms or signs of thyroid disease. All signed informed consent for this Institutional Review Board-approved study. Serum was obtained at 10 min

Received September 26, 1991.
Address all correspondence and requests for reprints to: James A. Magner, M.D., Division of Endocrinology, Humana Hospital-Michael Reese, 2929 South Ellis Avenue, Chicago, Illinois 60616.
* This work was supported by USPHS Grant DK-38835 and Biomedical Research Support Grant 233–4706.

1306

TABLE 1. Clinical parameters of the 11 normal subjects

Subject	Age (yr)	Sex	Wt (kg)	T$_4$ (51–141 nmol/L)	T$_3$RU (25–35%)	Basal TSH (0.2–6 mU/L)	Peak TSH post-TRH (6–35 mU/L)	TSH 60 min post-TRH (mU/L)	Antimicro antibody	Anti-Tg antibody
A	40	M	71.2	107	29.9	5.0	19.4	15.5	Neg	Neg
B	41	M	89.5	81	33.9	2.4	13.7	10.0	Neg	Neg
C	25	M	76.4	86	33.7	2.7	17.8	13.8	Neg	Neg
D	59	F	59.0	103	31.5	0.7	7.7	5.7	Neg	Neg
E	31	F	47.3	172	23.8	0.6	6.2	4.9	Neg	Neg
F	34	M	69.5	69	31.5	3.1	16.3	3.3	1:1600	Neg
G	29	M	68.7	85	31.1	0.8	6.0	5.8	Neg	Neg
H	46	M	66.3	76	31.3	3.8	29.3	25.6	Neg	Neg
I	40	F	58.8	105	30.6	1.4	13.2	11.2	Neg	Neg
J	23	M	82.2	118	31.8	0.9	8.9	6.7	Neg	Neg
K	24	F	66.0	83	26.4	1.7	13.0	9.7	Neg	Neg

T$_3$RU, T$_3$ resin uptake; Anti-micro, antimicrosomal; Anti-Tg, antithyroglobulin.

before and 0, 20, 30, and 60 min after the iv administration of 300 μg TRH (Relefact, Hoechst-Roussel Pharmaceuticals, Summerville, NJ). All subjects had basal TSH values in the normal range. After TRH treatment, serum TSH levels peaked at 20–30 min and returned toward normal levels at 60 min.

Lectins

Lectins, insolubilized on beaded agarose or Sepharose, were obtained from commercial sources. Concanavalin-A (ConA), lentil, and wheat germ were purchased from Pharmacia Fine Chemicals (Piscataway, NJ). *Ricin communis* (RCA$_{120}$), *Helix pomatia*, *Dolichos biflorus*, *Vicia villosa* (isolectin B$_4$), and *Arachis hypogaea* were purchased from Sigma (St. Louis, MO). All sugars and other chemicals used for the chromatography were obtained from Gibco (Grand Island, NY) and Sigma.

Lectin affinity chromatography

Columns of 1–3 mL of each lectin were constructed using glass Pasteur pipettes or glass 5-mL pipettes. For all lectins except ricin, small volumes (0.5–1.5 mL) of serum were loaded directly onto each column. For ricin, TSH was first immunoconcentrated (24) using antihuman TSH monoclonal antibody-coated polystyrene tubes (Diagnostic Product Corp., Los Angeles, CA) and then incubated without or with neuraminidase (24) before application to the column. No detectable TSH remained in serum from which TSH was immunoconcentrated.

Each specimen was allowed to interact with the column for 60 min at room temperature, followed by a wash with 8 mL column buffer (1-mL fractions collected), a wash with 10 mL column buffer (found to contain <5% of the applied TSH and so discarded), then elution of bound TSH using 8 mL column buffer containing the appropriate sugar (1-mL fractions collected).

The details of the column chromatography for ConA, lentil, and ricin have been previously reported (24). In brief, the column buffer for ConA and lentil lectins contained 10 mM Tris-HCl, 150 mM sodium chloride, and 1 mM each of magnesium chloride, manganese chloride, calcium chloride, 0.1% sodium azide, and 0.1% BSA, pH 8.0. TSH weakly bound to ConA was eluted with 10 mM α-methylglucopyranoside, and TSH

tightly bound to ConA was eluted with 500 mM α-methylmannopyranoside. TSH bound to lentil was eluted with 500 mM α-methylmannopyranoside. For the remaining lectins, the column buffer was 18 mM phosphate, 138 mM sodium chloride, 2.7 mM potassium chloride, 0.1% sodium azide, and 0.1% BSA, pH 7.4. To elute bound TSH from ricin lectin, the column buffer was supplemented with 200 mM galactose. To elute bound TSH from wheat germ lectin, the column buffer was supplemented with 0.5 M N-acetylglucosamine. To elute bound TSH from the N-acetylgalactosamine-specific lectins, the column buffer was supplemented with 0.2 M N-acetylgalactosamine. The recoveries from the columns were 80–120%, in most cases near 100%. In view of its extreme toxicity, ricin was used following the directions suggested by the manufacturer and was destroyed using alkali.

Immunoradiometric assay (IRMA) of TSH

TSH in each serum specimen and column fraction was measured in duplicate using a commercial TSH IRMA kit (Bio-Rad, Hercules, CA). The minimum detectable dose was 0.02 mU/L. Individual column fractions generally contained TSH in the 0.1–2.0 mU/L range. Different TSH isoforms were detected similarly in this assay, as judged by measurements made before and after neuraminidase treatment. The presence or absence of sugars in specimens, as occurred in some lectin column fractions, did not affect the TSH assay (24).

Calculation and statistical analyses

For each column run, two well defined peaks (three for ConA) of TSH were seen, designated the unbound TSH and bound TSH (unbound TSH, weakly bound TSH, and tightly bound TSH for ConA). Each serum sample was subjected to two or three independent column runs for each lectin, and the percentages of TSH bound generally agreed closely. The mean ± SD percentage of TSH bound was calculated. Significant differences were determined using Student's t test.

Results

Lentil lectin chromatography

For each of the 11 normal subjects tested (Fig. 1), TSH present in serum 30 min after the iv administration of

1308   MAGNER, KANE, AND CHOU   JCE & M • 1992
                                                                                         Vol 74 • No 6

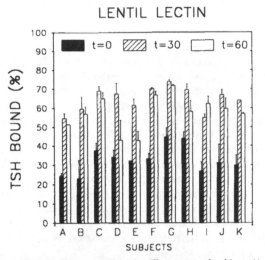

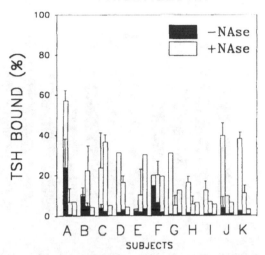

FIG. 1. TSH binding to lentil lectin. Eleven normal subjects (A-K) each received an iv injection of 300 μg TRH. Serum was obtained at 0 min (■), 30 min (▨), and 60 min (□) after the TRH injection. Each serum specimen was applied to a lentil lectin column; unbound TSH was washed off the column, then bound TSH was eluted from the column using 500 mM α-methylmannopyranoside. Values shown are the percentages of TSH (mean ± SD; n = 2–4) that bound to the lentil column. For every subject tested, a higher percentage of TRH-released TSH bound to the lentil column than that of basal TSH; the binding was greater at 30 min than at 60 min in all but one of the subjects.

TRH exhibited greater binding to lentil than did basal TSH (mean ± SD, 64.4 ± 6.8% vs. 32.5 ± 8.0%; P < 0.001). TSH present in serum 60 min after TRH treatment had less lentil binding than TSH at 30 min (57.8 ± 9.5% vs. 64.4 ± 6.8%; P < 0.01), but the binding had not yet returned to the basal amounts (57.8 ± 9.5% vs. 32.5 ± 8.0%; P < 0.001).

Ricin lectin chromatography

The ricin-binding characteristics of TSH are shown in Fig. 2. For subject H, for example, about 2% of his basal TSH bound to ricin, and after neuraminidase treatment to remove sialic acid residues to expose more galactose residues, the ricin binding of this basal TSH increased to 15%. TSH from this subject obtained 30 min after TRH administration exhibited only 1% binding to ricin, and binding increased to 6% after treatment with neuraminidase. For the group of 11 subjects, in every case TSH binding to ricin increased after neuraminidase treatment regardless of whether the TSH was from serum obtained before or after TRH treatment. The degree of ricin binding showed considerable heterogeneity from individual to individual. Before neuraminidase treatment, more basal TSH bound to ricin than did TSH obtained 30 min after TRH (6.9 ± 8.8% vs. 2.1 ± 2.0%; P < 0.05). There was only 1 sample (subject D) that was

FIG. 2. TSH binding to ricin lectin. Aliquots of the 0, 30, and 60 min serum specimens described in Fig. 1 were studied. For each specimen, TSH was immunoaffinity concentrated, divided equally, and incubated without or with neuraminidase. TSH was loaded onto a ricin lectin column; unbound TSH was washed off the column, then bound TSH was eluted from the column with 0.2 M galactose. Values shown are the percentages of TSH (mean ± SD; n = 1–3) that bound to the ricin column (in some cases, the SD was too small to be represented). For each of the 11 subjects (A-K), the *left bar* shows results for 0 min, the *middle bar* for 30 min, and the *right bar* for 60 min. For example, for subject A, about 24% of the basal TSH bound to ricin, and this increased to 57% after neuraminidase digestion; at 30 and 60 min, only 1% of the TSH bound to ricin, and this increased only to 6% after neuraminidase digestion.

an exception to this trend. After neuraminidase treatment, the basal TSH again had higher binding with ricin than did TSH obtained 30 min after TRH treatment (25.5 ± 17.8% vs. 14.6 ± 11.2%; P < 0.05), but there was substantial variability in this result, with 3 samples behaving in the opposite direction. The change in ricin binding caused by neuraminidase was 18.7 ± 15.5% for basal TSH and 12.5 ± 10.5% for TSH obtained 30 min after TRH administration, and these were not significantly different (P = 0.11).

ConA lectin chromatography

As shown in Fig. 3, there was substantial heterogeneity in the TSH-ConA binding among the 11 subjects. The percentages of TSH that failed to bind to ConA were similar for the basal TSH and the TSH 30 min after TRH treatment (5.3 ± 3.4% vs. 2.8 ± 5.8%; P = 0.0882); the percentages of TSH that bound weakly to ConA also were similar (81.1 ± 12.0% vs. 76.7 ± 7.6%; P = 0.1632). There was slightly less tight binding to ConA by the basal TSH than the 30 min post-TRH TSH (13.7 ± 9.4%

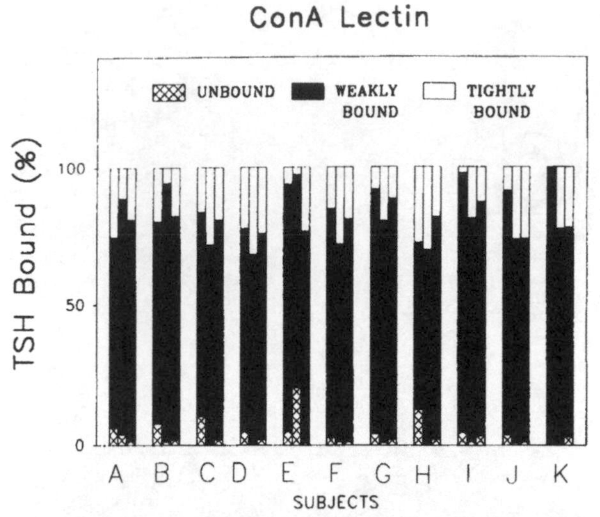

ConA Lectin

FIG. 3. TSH binding to ConA lectin. Aliquots of the 0, 30, and 60 min serum specimens described in Fig. 1 were studied. Each serum specimen was applied to a ConA column; unbound TSH was washed off the column, then weakly bound TSH was eluted using 10 mM α-methylglucopyranoside, and tightly bound TSH was eluted using 500 mM α-methylmannopyranoide. The *hatched, solid,* and *open areas* of each bar each represent the mean percentage of TSH that was unbound, weakly bound, or tightly bound, respectively (mean of 1–4 closely agreeing replicates). For each of the 11 subjects (A-K), the *left bar* shows results for 0 min, the *middle bar* for 30 min, and the *right bar* for 60 min. For example, for subject A, at 0 min, about 6% of the TSH was unbound, 69% was weakly bound, and 25% was tightly bound; at 30 min, about 4% of the TSH was unbound, 85% was weakly bound, and 11% was tightly bound.

vs. 20.5 ± 9.9%; $P = 0.0256$); 3 of the subjects (A, B, and E) clearly demonstrated the opposite.

Wheat germ lectin chromatography

Unlike the other lectins tested, wheat germ lectin was particularly susceptible to overloading. In only a few instances was enough TSH present before TRH treatment to allow chromatography of sufficiently small volumes of serum and still permit an accurate calculation of the percentage of TSH bound to wheat germ. In these instances, there was no significant difference between basal TSH and post-TRH TSH binding to wheat germ lectin.

N-Acetylgalactosamine-specific lectin chromatography

Small volumes of serum (0.1–0.5 mL) from euthyroid subject H and from three patients with primary hypothyroidism were loaded onto columns containing 1 mL *Glycine max, Helix pomatia, Dolichos biflorus, Vicia villosa,* and *Arachis hypogaea.* For every patient and for each lectin there was no detectable binding of TSH observed.

Discussion

TSH obtained from 11 normal subjects before and after the iv administration of TRH has been characterized using lectin affinity chromatography. TRH-released TSH was found to be structurally different from basal TSH. Direct structural characterization of TSH in the serum of these euthyroid patients was not possible because of the very small amounts present. Nevertheless, the use of lectins and a sensitive and specific IRMA allowed inferences to be made about the biochemical compositions of basal TSH and TRH-released TSH. Specific lectins were selected because of their availability and because their sugar binding specificities had been well characterized in the biochemical literature. Additional biochemical differences between basal TSH and TRH-released TSH might be disclosed by use of other lectins or other techniques.

Lentil lectin has affinity for oligosaccharides that bear a fucose residue on the inner *N*-acetylglucosamine residue, in the so-called core region of the oligosaccharide (30). The lentil data suggested that basal TSH had fewer core fucose residues, on the average, than TSH released after TRH. In most subjects, by 60 min after TRH treatment the character of the population of circulating TSH isoforms was returning toward that of basal TSH. In contrast, our prior analyses (24) of circulating human TSH from 10 euthyroid subjects and 40 patients with primary hypothyroidism detected no significant increase in the core fucosylation of TSH in primary hypothyroidism, a condition believed to be associated with increased secretion of TRH. The discrepancy between the present report and our prior study appears to be explained by the fact that TRH was given acutely in the present study, probably causing the acute degranulation of thyrotrophs and the release of TSH molecules that had been stored for some time; this differs from the presumed chronic increase in TRH tone in primary hypothyroidism. In that condition, thyrotrophs enlarge, develop large cisternae, and have few secretory granules (31). Thus, core fucosylation might be a marker for TSH molecules that had been stored in secretory granules. To our knowledge, no subcellular fractionation study has been performed to analyze structural differences in TSH present in secretory granules *vs.* other cellular compartments, although our prior studies have addressed the fucosylation of mouse TSH in the rough endoplasmic reticulum and Golgi (32) and determined that most of the fucose present in TSH heterodimers is bound to the β-subunit (33).

Ricin lectin (RCA$_{120}$) has affinity for oligosaccharides with exposed galactose residues (34). The ricin data suggested that both basal TSH and TRH-released TSH were sialylated, but there was substantial variation in the degree of sialylation from subject to subject. The

Free to Decide

basal TSH had significantly more galactose residues exposed, both initially and after neuraminidase treatment, than did the TRH-released TSH.

The oligosaccharide structures that interact with ConA have the following characteristics: triantennary, tetraantennary, and bisecting oligosaccharides do not bind to ConA; biantennary and truncated hybrid oligosaccharides bind weakly to ConA; high mannose and hybrid oligosaccharides bind firmly to ConA (35). Wheat germ lectin binds oligosaccharides with N-acetylglucosamine (35). ConA and wheat germ lectins were not very informative in this study. Compared to basal TSH, the TRH-released TSH may have had somewhat more tightly ConA-binding isoforms, species that may contain high mannose, or hybrid oligosaccharides.

No TSH binding to N-acetylgalactosamine-specific lectins was detected, suggesting that either these residues were not abundant or not exposed. Perhaps nearly uniform sulfation of N-acetylgalactosamine residues prevented binding to these lectins; the appropriate sulfatase to test this hypothesis is not yet available.

Further studies will be necessary to discover the cellular mechanisms by which basal TSH and TRH-released TSH come to differ structurally. Perhaps, for example, different isoforms of TSH are targeted for direct secretion vs. storage in granules. Alternatively, identical TSH molecules might be randomly sorted to immediate secretion vs. storage, but then TSH molecules are exposed to different posttranslational processing environments during late biosynthesis and/or storage.

The clinical significance of our findings remains to be determined. Because different isoforms of TSH appear to have different biological properties, the biosynthesis, storage, and release of different isoforms of TSH may be a normal part of the physiological control of thyroid function. Although not physiological, the present study provides a clear example of the release of different isoforms of TSH under two different conditions, euthyroidism vs. postpharmacological TRH. It may well be, for example, that as thyroid hormone suppression therapy is being monitored in certain patients (i.e. thyroid nodules or thyroid cancer) by using TRH testing and third or fourth generation TSH assays, the qualitative nature of the TSH as well as the amount of TSH might be of significance.

NOTE ADDED IN PROOF

Recently Flete et al (36) found that lutropin is rapidly cleared from the circulation by a hepatic receptor specific for sulfate-GalNAc, GlcNAc, Man. Perhaps we detected no TSH having GalNAc because it also is subject to rapid clearance by this receptor.

Acknowledgments

The dedication of the Clinical Metabolic Unit nurses, Edna McIntyre and Rosemary Dawkins, is acknowledged. Clinical laboratory data were obtained with the help of Leonida Sinio, Dr. Farhat Quadri, Kathy Lueth, and Robin Kane. Expert secretarial assistance was provided by Mrs. Margaret Nickless.

References

1. Magner JA. Thyroid-stimulating hormone: biosynthesis, cell biology, and bioactivity. Endocr Rev. 1990;11:354–85.
2. Wondisford FE, Magner JA, Weintraub BD. Chemistry and biosynthesis of thyrotropin. In: Braverman LE, Utiger RD, eds. The Thyroid, 6th ed. Philadelphia: Lippincott; 1992;257.
3. Constant RB, Weintraub BD. Differences in the metabolic clearance of pituitary and serum thyrotropin (TSH) derived from euthyroid and hypothyroid rats: effects of chemical deglycosylation of pituitary TSH. Endocrinology. 1986;119:2720–7.
4. Webster BR, Hummel BCW, McKenzie JM, Brown GM, Paice JC. Isoelectric focusing of human thyrotropin: identification of multiple components with dissociation of biological and immunological activities. In: Margoulies M, Greenwood FC, eds. Structure-activity relationships of protein and polypeptide hormones. Excerpt Med Int Congr Ser. 1972;241:369–78.
5. Takai NA, Filetti S, Rapoport B. Studies on the bioactivity of radioiodinated highly purified bovine thyrotropin: analytical polyacrylamide gel electrophoresis. Endocrinology. 1981;109:1144–9.
6. Pekonen F, Carayan P, Amr S, Weintraub BD. Heterogeneous forms of thyroid-stimulating hormone in mouse thyrotropic tumor and serum: differences in receptor binding and adenylate cyclase-stimulating activity. Horm Metab Res. 1981;13:617–20.
7. Joshi LR, Weintraub BD. Naturally occurring forms of thyrotropin with low bioactivity and altered carbohydrate content act as competitive antagonists to more bioactive forms. Endocrinology. 1983;113:2145–54.
8. Dahlberg PA, Petrick PA, Nissim M, Menezes-Ferreira MM, Weintraub BD. Intrinsic bioactivity of thyrotropin in human serum is inversely correlated with thyroid hormone concentrations: application of a new bioassay using the FRTL-5 rat thyroid cell strain. J Clin Invest. 1987;79:1388–94.
9. Sairam MR, Bhargavi GN. A role for glycosylation of the α-subunit in transduction of biological signal in glycoprotein hormones. Science. 1985;229:65–7.
10. Berman MI, Thomas CG, Manjunath P, Sairam MR, Nayfeh SN. The role of the carbohydrate moiety in thyrotropin action. Biochem Biophys Res Commun. 1985;133:680–7.
11. Amr S, Kubota K, Tramontano D, Ingbar SH, Keutmann HT. The carbohydrate moiety of bovine thyrotropin is essential for full bioactivity but not for receptor recognition. Endocrinology. 1987;120:345–52.
12. Amr S, Menezes-Ferreira MM, Shimohigashi Y, Chen HC, Nisula B, Weintraub BD. Activities of deglycosylated thyrotropin at the thyroid membrane receptor-adenylate cyclase system. J Endocrinol Invest. 1986;8:537–41.
13. Nissim M, Lee KO, Petrick PA, Dahlberg PA, Weintraub BD. A sensitive thyrotropin (TSH) bioassay based on iodide uptake in rat FRTL-5 thyroid cells: comparison with the adenosine 3',5'-monophosphate response to human serum TSH and enzymatically deglycosylated bovine and human TSH. Endocrinology. 1987;121:1278–87.
14. Thotakura NR, LiCalzi L, Weintraub BD. The role of carbohydrate in thyrotropin action assessed by a novel approach using enzymatic deglycosylation. J Biol Chem. 1990;265:11527–34.
15. Thotakura NR, Desai RK, Bates LG, Cole ES, Pratt BM, Weintraub BD. Biological activity and metabolic clearance of a recombinant human thyrotropin produced in Chinese hamster ovary cells. Endocrinology. 1991;128:341–8.
16. Sergi I, Papandreou M-J, Medri G, Canonne C, Verrier B, Ronin C. Immunoreactive and bioactive isoforms of human thyrotropin.

Endocrinology. 1991;128:3259–68.

17. Yora T, Matsuzaki S, Kondo Y, Ui N. Changes in the contents of multiple components of rat pituitary thyrotropin in altered thyroid states. Endocrinology. 1979;104:1682–5.

18. Mori M, Murakami M, Iriuchijima T, et al. Alteration by thyrotropin-releasing hormone of heterogeneous components associated with thyrotropin biosynthesis in the rat anterior pituitary gland. J Endocrinol. 1984;103:165–71.

19. Gesundheit N, Magner JA, Chen T, Weintraub BD. Differential sulfation and sialylation of secreted mouse thyrotropin (TSH) subunits: regulation by TSH-releasing hormone. Endocrinology. 1986;119:455–63.

20. Gesundheit N, Fink DL, Silverman LA, Weintraub BD. Effect of thyrotropin-releasing hormone on the carbohydrate structure of secreted mouse thyrotropin: analysis by lectin affinity chromatography. J Biol Chem. 1987;262:5197–203.

21. Gyves PW, Gesundheit N, Taylor T, Butler J, Weintraub BD. Changes in thyrotropin (TSH) carbohydrate structure and response to TSH-releasing hormone during postnatal ontogeny: analysis by Concanavalin-A chromatography. Endocrinology. 1987;121:133–40.

22. Taylor T, Weintraub BD. Altered thyrotropin (TSH) carbohydrate structures in hypothalamic hypothyroidism created by paraventricular nuclear lesions are corrected by in vivo TSH-releasing hormone. Endocrinology. 1989;125:2198–203.

23. Gyves PW, Gesundheit N, Thotakura NR, Stannard BS, DeCherney GS, Weintraub BD. Changes in the sialylation and sulfation of secreted thyrotropin in congenital hypothyroidism. Proc Natl Acad Sci USA. 1990;87:3792–6.

24. Miura Y, Perkel VS, Papenberg KA, Johnson MJ, Magner JA. Concanavalin-A lentil and ricin lectin affinity binding characteristics of human thyrotropin: differences in the sialylation of thyrotropin in sera of euthyroid, primary, and central hypothyroid patients. J Clin Endocrinol Metab. 1989;69:985–95.

25. Lee H-Y, Suhl J, Pekary AE, Hershman JM. Secretion of thyrotropin with reduced Concanavalin-A-binding in patients with severe nonthyroid illness. J Clin Endocrinol Metab. 1987;65:942–5.

26. Peterson VB, McGregor AM, Belchetz PE, Elkeles RS, Hall R. The secretion of thyrotropin with impaired biological activity in patients with hypothalamic-pituitary disease. Clin Endocrinol (Oxf). 1978;8:397–402.

27. Faglia G, Bitensky L, Pinchera A, et al. Thyrotropin secretion in patients with central hypothyroidism: evidence for reduced biological activity of immunoreactive thyrotropin. J Clin Endocrinol Metab. 1979;48:989–98.

28. Faglia G, Beck-Peccoz P, Ballabio M, Nava C. Excess of β-subunit of thyrotropin (TSH) in patients with idiopathic central hypothyroidism due to the secretion of TSH with reduced biological activity. J Clin Endocrinol Metab. 1983;56:908–14.

29. Beck-Peccoz P, Amr S, Menezes-Ferreira MM, Falia G, Weintraub BD. Decreased receptor binding of biologically inactive thyrotropin in central hypothyroidism. N Engl J Med. 1985;312:1085–90.

30. Kornfeld K, Reitman HL, Kornfeld R. The carbohydrate-binding specificity of pea and lentil lectins: fucose is an important determinant. J Biol Chem. 1981;256:6633–40.

31. Farquhar MG. Processing of secretory products by cells of the anterior pituitary gland. In: Heller H, Lederis K, eds. Subcellular organization and function in endocrine tissues. Cambridge: Cambridge University Press; 1971;1:79–124.

32. Magner JA, Novak W, Papagiannes E. Subcellular localization of fucose incorporation into mouse thyrotropin and free α-subunits: studies employing subcellular fractionation and inhibitors of the intracellular translocation of proteins. Endocrinology. 1986;119:1315–28.

33. Magner J, Papagiannes E. Studies of double-labeled mouse thyrotropin and free alpha-subunits to estimate relative fucose content. Proc Soc Exp Biol Med. 1986;183:237–40.

34. Baenziger JU, Fiete D. Structural determinations of Ricinus communis agglutinin and toxin specificity for oligosaccharides. J Biol Chem. 1979;254:9795–9.

35. Cummings RD, Kornfeld S. Fractionation of asparagine-linked oligosaccharides by serial lectin-agarose affinity chromatography: a rapid, sensitive, and specific technique. J Biol Chem. 1982;257:11235–40.

36. Flete D, Srivastava V, Hindsgaul O, Baenziger JU. A hepatic reticuloendothelial cell receptor specific for SO_4-4GalNAcβ1, 4GlcNAcβ1,2Manα that mediates rapid clearance of lutropin. Cell. 1991;67:1103–10.

The Inherent Uncertainty of Nature Essay, and Krauss Book Review

I won a scholarship to spend time on the campus of the University of Illinois in Urbana during the summer of 1968. These were the months between my Junior and Senior years of high school. I had free room and board in a college dormitory (Barton Hall) since Urbana was about 200 miles east of my hometown. I worked on a small research project related to human lipoprotein biochemistry in the laboratory of Dr. Nishida at Burnsides Research Laboratory. At first most of my time was spent shadowing an experienced laboratory technician, who assigned me to do small tasks – weigh out ingredients using a balance to make buffers, wash glassware, check pH of samples, etc. Eventually I graduated to more sophisticated tasks, such as using a stopwatch to collect data about solutions containing macromolecules using a large water bath at a carefully maintained temperature that contained a glass capillary viscometer. I also learned how to use an ultracentrifuge, which was a bit frightening in view of the complexity and power of the machine.

No abstract or co-authorship resulted from this summer experience, but I gained invaluable hands-on training using scientific equipment that was far more sophisticated than the simple tools I had used in my high school lab sessions. Another benefit was my exposure to the campus of the University, so a few months later I felt very comfortable applying there for college. And a third benefit was free time to read several books, including a new 1967 edition of a 1947 classic: *One Two Three...Infinity*, by George Gamow. Because I had gotten an excellent refractor telescope the prior summer, I had already read several books about astronomy, so I was well prepared for Gamow's book. This book provided a foundation for my reading during the next decade about cosmology, special and general relativity, and quantum mechanics.

As a budding scientist, I was troubled a bit in high school and college by the tension between religion and science. In those years, as now, I was both a devout Catholic and also a firm believer in Darwinian evolution. I intuitively firmly believed in the unity of truth, however, so I knew that somehow the religious and scientific arenas could not be fundamentally contradictory. So my heart and mind were basically at peace. During college I happened to read a collection of scientific essays that by chance contained the amazing book chapter, The Decline of Determinism, by Arthur Stanley Eddington. I was riding on a bus as I first read that chapter, and it was as though I had been struck by lightning, so I will never forget

that hour. Eddington argued persuasively that many truths of quantum mechanics meant that there was plenty of intellectual space to believe in free will. A few years later I was influenced by the philosopher Mortimer Adler, especially his book, *How To Think About God*. As an adult I remain an active scientist and an active participant in my religious community, and there are many such professionals, including Francis Collins, who has written of his religious and scientific experience.

Back in 1988 I was stunned when I read a December issue of *The Scientist*. An essay by Dr. William Provine, an atheist, claimed that religion was bunk and science had all the answers. I wrote a short essay in response to Dr. Provine that was printed in *The Scientist* a couple of weeks later. A number of letters subsequently appeared with various comments – several were very critical of my essay. But no matter; I wanted to present a few ideas that might make scientists think more broadly.

Years later I read a book by cosmologist Dr. Lawrence Krauss, *A Universe From Nothing*. It seemed scientifically superb but philosophically shallow, so in 2013 I posted on Amazon.com a book review so entitled. It was not just his book, but also a YouTube posting by Krauss that surprised me by its shallowness, so readers may judge for themselves.

Then I made a new valuable discovery. Martin Gardner, the mathematician who wrote a column for *Scientific American* for many years, died in May, 2010 at the age of 95. In subsequent years several essays about his life and work appeared, and I read one that mentioned one of his books that sounded interesting, so I ordered a copy. It was *The Whys of a Philosophical Scrivener*, originally published in 1983, but then republished with updates in 1999. It is a treasure! It is both scientifically and philosophically profound, and includes a bit of humor here and there so typical of Gardner. Unbeknownst to me, Gardner in 1983 was exploring some of the same ideas that I was thinking about by the mid-1980s. But his training in philosophy and breadth of reading were much more extensive than mine, and I take my hat off to him in praise of this entertaining and thoughtful book that covers such questions as the existence of free will, and whether atheism makes sense. I was gratified to see on the Amazon web site that most reviews of Gardner's book were highly positive, although some were highly critical – just as several letters in *The Scientist* had been very critical of my short essay in 1988.

Free to Decide

The Inherent Uncertainty Of Nature Is A Basis For Religion

by James A. Magner

In his eloquent article, "Scientists, Face It! Science And Religion Are Incompatible," William Provine raised points that have troubled many thoughtful scientists who find themselves unable to reconcile their views about science and religion in an intellectually honest way. He could have raised other compelling arguments against the meaningfulness of our lives, such as the prevalence of horrible human ills and suffering, shared even by innocent infants.

In spite of these observations, however, I believe that scientists can rationally justify a belief in God and in the meaningfulness of human life.

The use of the word "rational" in this context is exceedingly important. I have had long and generally unsatisfactory discussions with many religious persons; on occasion these led to painful or embarrassing incidents when my questions were perceived as threats or insults. When asked to explain why they believe in God, many such persons exhibit a profound lack of critical thinking, and appear to hold their beliefs on the basis of intuition. Many describe an unanticipated turn of events in their lives, or an emotional experience of special significance, and I have regarded these, in general, as wholly unconvincing.

Ultimate Meaning

I believe that Dr. Provine, however, too hastily excludes the God hypothesis. If a biologist is willing to work for a year to sequence a single gene, certainly it is worth years of thought and effort to explore whether or not human existence is ultimately meaningless, as Dr. Provine insists it is.

Science Permits A Belief In Free Will

Because "random genetic drift, natural selection ... and many other purposeless mechanisms" were responsible for the origin of life and the course of evolution, Dr. Provine suggests that life is meaningless and that we have no free will. But here he is wrong. It is the very randomness and unpredictability of these processes that allow for the possibility of free will. This argument was lucidly outlined by Arthur Stanley Eddington in his much debated essay, "The Decline of Determinism" (*New Pathways In Science*, Macmillan, 1935, Chapter IV). Nineteenth-century physicists envisioned a "billiard ball" universe in which, if the position and motion of every atom could be known

at a point in time, it necessarily followed that the position and motion of every atom could be known for all times in the past, and predicted for all times in the future. Although the feat of actually charting every atom was far beyond technical capabilities, the intellectually honest physicist of that era would have been unable to believe in free will --- or indeed in any creative force, such as a god, outside of natural processes.

But with the discovery of radioactivity and the rise of quantum physics, randomness and unpredictability entered the scene. Although Einstein and a number of scientists disliked the new indeterminism ("You believe in God playing dice," Einstein wrote to Max Born in 1944), other physicists accepted quantum mechanics with a sense of liberation. "The old classical determinism of Hobbes and Laplace need not oppress us any longer," wrote Hermann Weyl in *The Open World* (Yale University Press, 1932).

Because of these new discoveries in physics, Dr. Provine is incorrect when he argues that our choices "are determined by the interaction of heredity and environment." By demonstrating a fundamental uncertainty in the basic processes of nature, science allows for the existence of free will --- and for a belief in God.

Thus, I claim that Dr. Provine's "common sense" views about the nature of life and the world are flawed because they are based on an insufficiently representative sample of reality; he has sampled the universe only within a very limited range of temperatures pressures, velocities and times. As he well knows, we live in a relativistic and not a Newtonian universe, and this must be taken into account in the pursuit of intellectually honest religious views. Therefore, scientists can believe in God while still acknowledging that the world they study offers no empirical evidence for such an entity.

I also believe that there is a reasonable argument for the existence of God. In his book *How To Think About God* (Bantam Books, 1980), philosopher Mortimer Adler reasoned that God may be presumed to exist only if it can be shown that the universe is created continuously, rather than having been created only once in the distant past. Many phenomena in quantum physics suggest to me that, in fact, the universe is being caused continuously. To cite but one example, an electron and a positron may suddenly appear out of nothingness due to a quantum fluctuation, whirl about, and then totally annihilate each other, all within a fraction of a second. Such quantum phenomena fulfill Adler's critical condition for the existence of God: the "dice" that Einstein had complained about actually are being cast continuously.

Reasonable Alternative

Of course, it still takes an intuitive leap to say that the existence of free will and a belief in God imply that human life is meaningful. That intuitive leap is one that I am willing to make because it seems more reasonable than the alternative --- that God exists, but that in a universe that must be continuously willed into existence, a self-aware, rational creature is of no consequence to God.

The age-old riddle of human suffering, as well as other obstacles to faith, must then be viewed in the context of a vast complex universe which is itself impersonal and cares nothing for man, but in which conditions permit life and cognition to arise through natural and random processes. The same nerves that allow an organism to delight in the warmth of spring sunshine unfortunately also confer the ability to sense the pain of seared flesh. To wax theological, God is behind it all and provides the possibilities. He lets us find our own way through the maze of existence, laughing when we laugh and hurting when we hurt. The latter may be dismissed as wishful thinking, but it is one important concept in my own personal struggle to make sense of the world.

James A. Magner, M.D., is a clinician at Michael Reese Hospital in Chicago and an assistant professor of medicine at the University of Chicago.

Reprinted with permission of *The Scientist*. The original essay appeared in *The Scientist* on December 26, 1988.

Scientifically Superb, Philosophically Shallow

Book Review by James Magner

I greatly enjoyed reading *A Universe From Nothing* by Lawrence Krauss, and I found it to be scientifically clear and very well written -- but in my view the book glossed over too quickly the profound philosophical implications of modern cosmology. The afterward by Richard Dawkins suffered the same shortcoming.

The book prompted me to watch Krauss' Sept. 11, 2011 talk posted on YouTube that briefly summarized the key ideas. Krauss' side-comments during the talk, as well as the introduction by Richard Dawkins, again declared in which philosophical camp they wished to pitch their tent. But I worry that the elegant scientific concepts summarized do not so clearly lead to that depressing existential position. Krauss jokingly shared his view of the human situation near the start of his talk when he remarked that he had considered using the title, *We Are All Fu..ed!* Humorous, but is it true?

The eminent philosopher Bertrand Russell (1872-1970) was a bit more poetic in his choice of language as he wrote in 1903 of humanity's desperate situation (I quote from a rendition published by Augros and Stanciu in *The New Story of Science* (1984), an interesting book but one with major flaws of its own):

"That man is the product of causes which had no provision of the end they were achieving; that his origins, his growth, his hopes and fears, his loves and beliefs are but the outcome of accidental collocations of atoms; that no fire, no heroism, no intensity of thought and feeling, can preserve an individual life beyond the grave; that all the labors of the ages, all the devotion ... all the noonday brightness of human genius are destined to extinction ... all these things, if not quite beyond dispute, are yet so nearly certain, that no philosophy which rejects them can hope to stand. Only within the scaffolding of these truths, only on the firm foundation of unyielding despair, can the soul's habitation henceforth be safely built."

In sum, in his book Krauss wonderfully recounts in an approachable style the key concepts of modern cosmology, but falls with rather startling self-certainty into the depressing philosophical notions voiced by Russell more than a century ago. Krauss was a bit more flexible in his YouTube talk when for one brief moment he showed one slide and remarked about the element of mystery in all this. But he radically undervalues this element. As I will explain, mystery is fundamental in view of a necessary first logical but unprovable step required in all complex arguments.

In spite of the keen desire by Krauss and Dawkins to be, I presume, purely rational scientists untainted by wishful thinking, these sorts of truly strong scientific intellectuals must recognize that any argument must begin with one or a few key unproven assumptions -- this is unavoidable. As has been elegantly proven by Kurt Gödel (1906-1978), no complex system of thought, even formal mathematics, can be built up from scratch and be internally fully consistent without resort to at least one external assumption or definition that cannot be definitively proven within that complex system. This is Gödel's water-tight "incompleteness theorem" (1931), and its surprising truth has to do with the contradictions necessarily encountered regarding self-referential sets. Descartes (1596-1650), for example, in his *Discourse on the Methods* (1637) began with the fundamental proposition, "I think, therefore I am." When considering the modern "Theory of Mind," to cite another example, one could propose that a human person is in reality just an isolated brain floating in an oxygenated physiologic solution in a vast alien experiment, and all mental experiences, sensations, interactions with other persons, etc. result from a gigantic simulation --- other persons actually have no minds at all. Alternatively, even though we cannot prove that other persons exist and have independent minds, we can reasonably assume that is truly the case, and move ahead from there as we try to grasp "reality."

Coming to unavoidable unprovable assumptions related to cosmology, which sorts of assumptions make most sense? In science we often resort to Occam's razor -- the principle of parsimony: an explanation should be as simple as possible until a somewhat more complex explanation is actually required to fit with the facts. Krauss along with modern cosmologists seem to find that all the mass and energy in the universe apparently sum to zero, and the argument is convincing and, I think, probably true. And he also invokes a sort of anthropic principle: that humans exist because in this present universe, as opposed to many other unfavorable universes, the natural laws crystalized in forms that made human beings physically possible. But is this parsimonious? There certainly is a heavy burden of "specialness" if one believes that there has been only a single universe, this is it, and it is exactly perfect so that intelligent beings can exist and evolve. But there may be arguably an even more heavy burden to the alternative view favored by Krauss; that there are billions of parallel universes -- the "multi-verse" --- or perhaps billions of sequential universes. Krauss thinks that in nearly all of these many universes the conditions were not right for sentient beings, but in at least one very rare case, a universe came into existence that made life possible. So has there been only one universe that is unique and special, or have there been billions of random universes? My belief is that, at the present time, reasonable persons have no basis by which to settle definitively which of these assumptions is the closest to the truth. Moreover, my intuition is that it is precisely this question that is the crux of the fundamental unprovable assumption that we must make when thinking about the ultimate meaning of life -- or lack thereof. In view of Gödel, it is fully scientific and allowed for each person to consider and to make this choice of a key starting assumption, and then thereafter one must logically develop a consistent world view based on observed facts. Perhaps I am wrong, but I believe that Krauss and Dawkins should carefully think about this. Gödel is the key.

A particular aspect of Krauss' argument bothers me, however. The billions of universes are supposedly arising from nothing, and actually are nothing since in each universe the total mass and energy sums to zero. But Krauss invokes that this is possible because within quantum nothingness there are virtual particles that are rapidly entering and exiting existence. But if there is truly nothing, then how do the newly formed virtual particles "know" what characteristics to briefly assume? Must there not be "laws" to guide them? In other words, it appears that there may be "several types of nothing" -- one type is seething with virtual particles of certain types that are rapidly appearing and disappearing, but I am interested really in another type of nothing -- absolutely nothing, lacking even in the virtual particles. Can there be different types of nothing? This calls to mind the work of the German mathematician Georg Cantor (1845-1918), the expert in set theory, who proved that there were different types of infinity. He showed, for example, that the real numbers are "more numerous" than the natural numbers, even though both are infinite.

Thus, my view, in agreement with Arthur Stanley Eddington's (1882-1944) famous essay *The Decline of Determinism* (1935), is that we do not live in a "billiard ball" deterministic universe. Quantum mechanics allows for indeterminism, and also, in my view, free will. I tried to make such a case in my brief essay *The Inherent Uncertainty of Nature Is a Basis for Religion* published in *The Scientist* in December, 1988. Various influences that shaped my thinking have been described in a book, *Chess Juggler* (2011). I'll admit to being influenced over the years also by the profound insights of the philosopher Mortimer Adler (1902-2001) -- one of his many books was *How to Think About God* (1980). Even Isaac Newton (1642-1727) reflected philosophically in his *Opticks* (1704) that he wanted to learn "Whence it is that Nature doth nothing in vain; and whence arises all that Order and Beauty which we see in the World." Let me close with what the naturalist and anthropologist Loren Eiseley (1907-1977) wrote in *The Immense Journey*, "Rather, I would say that if 'dead' matter has reared up this curious landscape of fiddling crickets, song sparrows, and wondering men, it must be plain to even the most devoted materialist that the matter of which he speaks contains amazing, if not dreadful powers, and may not impossibly be, as Hardy has suggested, 'But one mask of many worn by the Great Face behind.'"

Book review posted on Amazon.com in 2013 by James Magner.

Historical Essays

I loved history classes in elementary and high school. During every summer in the 1950s and 1960s, when I was a youngster at home, my father loaded up his young family for a two week vacation drive around the USA in our non-air conditioned sedan. We usually slept in a tent at campgrounds, which was great fun for me and my young brother, although it is only as an adult that I now realize what a great sport my mother was – and I can tell you that she was genuinely perfectly happy to rough it that way. I always had a vote on destinations and I insisted that we plan routes so as to make lots of stops to see museums, battlefields, national parks and famous places.

During high school and college I read extensively about the history of science, and I have done so ever since as pure entertainment. My global travels with Bayer and also Genzyme allowed many opportunities for historical side trips, including to rather obscure places such as the preserved homes of Christian Huygens, Isaac Newton, Charles Darwin, William Herschel and others.

My first serious essay on a topic in the history of science was "Emil Fischer (1852–1919): The stereochemical nature of sugars" published in The Endocrinologist 2004; 14(4):239-244. My second such essay was "Seymour D. Van Meter, MD (1865–1934): The Texan who wielded a scalpel in Denver and left a lasting legacy" published in The Endocrinologist 2007; 17(2):71-77. When the latter appeared I was contacted immediately by the American Thyroid Association, which has a named annual award in honor of Van Meter, and I was asked if that organization could republish my essay. After minor tweaking, the essay was republished in Thyroid 2007; 17(8):779-785. Both of these essays are reproduced here with permission of the publisher, and no further reproduction in all or part may be used without written permission.

I have served for several years on the History and Archives Committee of the American Thyroid Association, and in late-2012 the several members were asked if anyone might be interested in writing a short historical essay related to research or discoveries in thyroid disease. I volunteered to write something because over the years I had photocopied many old publications about discoveries related to thyroid stimulating hormone (TSH), the pituitary hormone that was my main academic research interest. I stored these old publications in a box in my garage, and I actually intended someday to write something using them. The essay took shape during odd hours during 2013, and was published in 2014. The original citation is Magner J, Historical note: Many steps led to the discovery of thyroid-stimulating hormone. Eur Thyroid Journal 2014; 3 (no. 2): 95-100 (DOI:10.1159/000360534), and it is reproduced in this collection with permission of the publisher.

HISTORICAL NOTE

Emil Fischer (1852–1919)
The Stereochemical Nature of Sugars

James A. Magner, MD

Emil Fischer (1852–1919) made pioneering insights into the stereochemistry of the simple sugars, used the analogy of a lock-and-key fit between an enzyme and its substrate, and discovered that proteins are polypeptides. He published about organic dyes, characterized and synthesized caffeine and theobromine, and made landmark contributions regarding purines. He was awarded the Nobel Prize in Chemistry in 1902, and his work influences every endocrinologist to this day.

A RITE OF PASSAGE

Memorizing structures of organic molecules remains a rite of passage for premedical college students studying organic chemistry. This is often a class that separates those who choose to remain premedical versus students who fall back to another college major. The situation was no different for me at the University of Illinois, Urbana, in the early 1970s. It was striking even to a novice that several simple sugars (including glucose) had the identical chemical formula, $C_6H_{12}O_6$, yet had different properties and biochemical roles in living tissues. The explanation rests on the nature of the asymmetric carbon atom.

From the Genzyme Corporation, Cambridge, Massachusetts.

Reprints: James Magner, MD, Genzyme Corporation, 500 Kendall Street, 6th Floor, Cambridge, MA 02142. E-mail: James.magner@genzyme.com.

The orientation of a hydroxyl (-OH) group pointing to one side or the other of these molecules makes a difference in the way enzymes interact with that sugar. Late one night, while memorizing sugar structures based on so-called "Fischer diagrams," I read a historical note in my textbook about Emil Fischer. (My class used *Organic Chemistry*, 2nd Edition, edited by Robert Morrison and Robert Boyd, a wonderful book with a dark green cover.[1] Many readers may have used that squat text during that era.) I was impressed by the ingenuity, clarity, and importance of Fischer's contribution, and I vowed someday to find out a little more about who Emil Fischer was and how he came to these wonderful insights.

As I reviewed materials to prepare this article, I was struck once again by the excellence of German science in the late 19th and early 20th centuries. This was probably in part the result of the enlightened reform of the German educational system in the 19th century, far ahead of other European countries or the United States, and the cultural emphasis on academic achievement and scientific knowledge. My reading brought to mind the apocryphal Cold War story about a U.S. official and a Soviet official arguing about which social system was better. After a few minutes, it became clear that the American official was much better informed and had extensive details about industrial production, agricultural efficiency, and so on, to back his case. Growing more and more frustrated, the exasperated Soviet official, red-faced and eyes bulging, suddenly

leaped from his chair, pounded his fist on the table, and blurted, "Our German scientists are better than your German scientists!"

THE YOUNG EMIL FISCHER AND THE PATH TO BERLIN

Hermann Emil Fischer (Fig. 1) was born near Cologne, Germany, at Euskirchen on October 9, 1852.[2,3] His father ran a prosperous lumber business, and it was Emil's good fortune throughout his life to have substantial financial resources as a result of the family enterprise. Business did not interest him, however, and his fledgling mistakes were more a signal to his father that he wanted to do something else with his life. He loved physics, but a mentor at the University of Bonn, Adolf von Baeyer (1835–1917), who had worked with August Kekulé (1829–1896; of benzene ring fame), advised Fischer in 1871 to study chemistry (von Baeyer was destined to win the Nobel Prize in Chemistry in 1905, 3 years after his student).[4]

After receiving his PhD in 1874, Fischer became an assistant instructor at Strasbourg University, where he discovered phenylhydrazine, the first hydrazine base. This discovery would influence his later work, for the chemical would become a useful tool for analyzing sugars. After the death of the prominent chemist Justus von Liebig in 1873, von Baeyer was invited to move to the University of Munich in 1875, and Fischer followed him there. Fischer rose to the rank of Associate Professor of Analytical Chemistry in 1879, and then

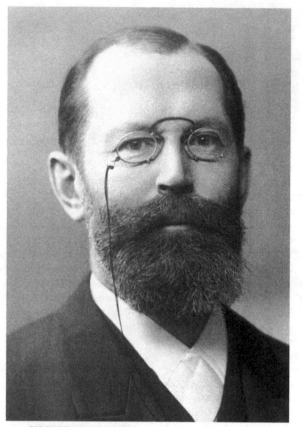

FISCHER, Hermann Emil
Nobel Laureate CHEMISTRY 1902
© Nobelstiftelsen

FIGURE 1. Emil Fischer in 1902 near the time that he was awarded the Nobel Prize in Chemistry. Copyright, The Nobel Foundation.

was appointed Professor of Chemistry in 1881 at the University of Erlangen.

He was approached in 1883 to take the position of scientific director at a private firm, Badische Anilin- und Soda-Fabrik, which we in the United States today would better recognize as BASF (founded in 1865).[5] This was a major opportunity for Fischer. Graebe and Lieberman at BASF had synthesized alizarin, a red dye for clothing, to compete with the natural product, "madder," in 1869. The company then lavished funding over the next 2 decades in a focused but high-risk effort to discover a synthetic indigo. This triumph was accomplished in 1880, and as the blue

dye was commercialized, a disaster was perpetrated on the British in India as the demand for natural indigo declined precipitously (down to 641,000 hectacres in 1896 and to 114,000 hectacres by 1909). Although Fischer was tempted, he loved academic research, and the family money gave him the freedom to turn down the offer.

In 1887, Fischer experienced a bout of severe gastritis and took a 1-year leave of absence before moving to the University of Wurzburg. After 4 highly productive years as Professor of Chemistry there (more about glucose, see subsequently), in 1892 he made his final academic move to the University of Ber-

lin, where he succeeded A. W. Hoffman as the Chair of Chemistry. Fischer (Fig. 2) retained the Chair until his death in 1919.

OPTICAL ACTIVITY

Jean-Baptiste Biot (1774–1862)[6] experimented with light, magnetism, and electricity in Paris, and discovered in 1815 that some chemicals in solution rotated the plane of polarized light, although he had no insight into the cause. The young Louis Pasteur (1822–1895),[7] while pursuing his first important experiments in the late 1840s, noted that the tiny crystals of tartaric acid (a key chemical present in French wine) seemed to come in 2 varieties. Using a magnifying glass, Pasteur observed that the shapes of the 2 crystal types appeared to be mirror images of each other. He tediously used tweezers to separate the 2 types of crystals and found that when dissolved, a solution of 1 type of crystal rotated polarized light in 1 direction, whereas a solution of the other type of crystal rotated polarized light in the opposite direction. Pasteur's insight was that the molecule of tartaric acid must come in 2 forms that were mirror images of each other, like right and left gloves. However, structural chemistry was not yet advanced enough to allow Pasteur to associate this finding with bonds to carbon. (Years later, Fischer mentioned Pasteur's experiments in his Nobel Prize lecture.)[8]

During the early 1870s, Jacobus H. van't Hoff (1852–1911) and J. A. Le Bel independently came on the concept of the asymmetric carbon atom.[9] Although his doctoral thesis in 1874 dealt with cyanoacetic acids and malonic acid, van't Hoff's early fame actually derived from a small pamphlet that he published a few months before entitled "Voorstel tot Uitbreiding der Tegenwoordige in de Scheikunde gebruikte Structuurformules in de Ruimte" and so on. ("Proposal for the Development of 3-Dimensional Chemical Structural Formulae"). Consisting of 12 pages of text and 1 page of diagrams, the paper

240

The Endocrinologist • Volume 14, Number 5, October 2004

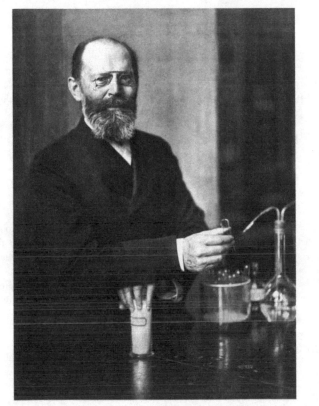

FIGURE 2. Emil Fischer a few years after receiving the Nobel Prize in Chemistry. Copyright, Science Museum/Science & Society Picture Library.

showed that the asymmetric carbon atom could explain the occurrence of isomers of compounds despite their identical chemical formulae. van't Hoff also explained how such stereochemistry could be related to optical activity. These revolutionary ideas began to find acceptance the next year after publication of "Chimie dans l'Espace" ("Chemistry in Space"), although the German translation did not appear until 1877 and the English in 1891. He later acknowledged in "Dix Années dans l'Histoire d'une Théorie" ("Ten Years in the History of a Theory") that J. A. Le Bel had independently arrived at the identical concepts, although without pragmatic detail. The first publication about the asymmetric carbon atom occurred just as Fischer was finishing his doctorate. (van't Hoff later was awarded the Nobel Prize in Chemistry in 1901.) The assignment as a D- or L-sugar began based on whether the plane of polarized light was rotated to the right or left (dextrorotary or levorotary). Today, optical isomers of monosaccharides are assigned as either D- or L- based on their absolute configurations as relative to D-glyceraldehyde, as proposed by Rosanoff, an American chemist, in 1906.[1]

A FAMILY OF ALDOHEXOSES

As shown in Figure 3, the structural formula for an aldohexose (such as glucose) contains 4 asymmetric carbon atoms, each marked by an asterisk.[1] Thus, there are 2^4 or 16 possible stereoisomers having this general formula, 8 pairs of enantiomers, as we would say today. This is the family of aldohexoses.

All 16 compounds have been created by synthesis or isolated from nature, and include the very common compounds glucose, mannose, and galactose (each with a D- and an L-form). The generic structural formula as drawn in Figure 3 could represent any of the aldohexoses. Only when one has specified the configuration about each of the asymmetric carbon atoms will the formula refer to a unique aldohexose. The carbon atoms are numbered in Figure 3 from the "top" downward in the usual convention. A specific natural 5-carbon sugar, L-arabinose, which will play an important part in this story, is depicted to the right in Figure 3. Note that the 5 carbon atoms in L-arabinose correspond to carbons 2 through 6 of the generic aldohexose formula. Another caveat is that in these types of diagrams, the bonds on a given carbon atom depicted horizontally by convention are meant to be projecting out from the page, whereas the vertical bonds are projecting into the page.[1]

The way that Fischer worked out the correct configurations of the aldohexoses demanded years of trial and error, ingenuity, and logic. We return now to the reagent phenylhydrazine, which Fischer discovered early in his career. Aldoses react with this compound to form phenylhydrazones, and when both the first and second carbon have reacted, the product is called an osazone[1] (Fig. 4). Note the loss of asymmetry about carbon 2 after this reaction, because there are now only 3 atoms bound to that carbon instead of 4. Moreover, 1 of the difficulties of studying monosaccharides was their tendency to form syrups rather than solids that could be dissolved and crystallized easily. While working at the University of Munich in the early 1880s, Fischer found that his reagent, phenylhydrazine, converted sugars into osazones that could be isolated easily, and their crystals had characteristic forms that could be identified. Fischer found that 2 distinct monosaccharides, D-glucose and D-mannose, yielded the same osazone. Because osazone formation destroyed

241

1	CHO	
2	*CHOH	
3	*CHOH	CHO
4	*CHOH	HO – C – H
5	*CHOH	H – C – OH
6	CH₂OH	H – C – OH
		CH₂OH

Generic Aldohexose **L-Arabinose**

FIGURE 3. Generic structure of an aldohexose (left) such as glucose or mannose. The conventional numbering of the carbon atoms is shown, and the 4 asymmetric carbons are marked with asterisks. Correct structure of L-arabinose (right). Fischer determined this structure as a stepping stone on the way to learning the structure of glucose. Fischer discovered and then built on the fact that the 5 carbons in L-arabinose correspond to carbons 2 through 6 in glucose.

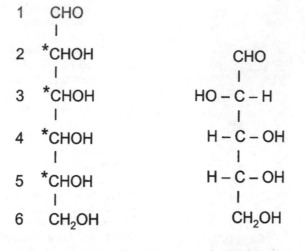

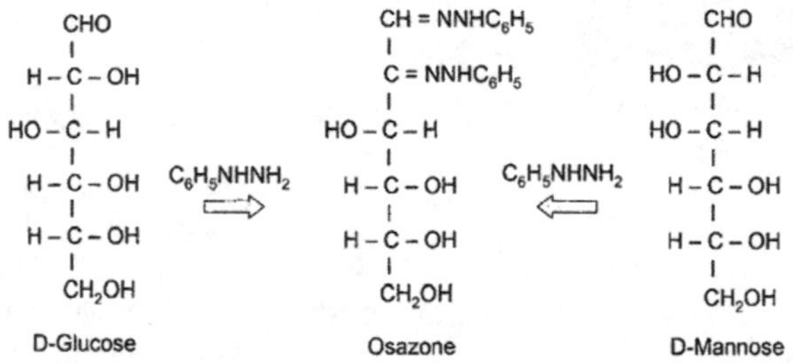

FIGURE 4. Structures of D-glucose, D-mannose, and their common osazone. Fischer discovered that after reacting D-glucose or D-mannose with phenylhydrazine, the asymmetry of carbon 2 was destroyed, and these 2 sugars formed the identical osazone. Although at first Fischer did not know the configurations at carbons 3, 4, and 5, he knew at that stage that these configurations would turn out to be identical in D-glucose and D-mannose. The configuration at carbon 5 was assumed to have the -OH to the right (this arbitrary assumption was found to have been correct only years later when absolute configurations could be established). Then Fischer deduced the relative configurations about carbons 3 and 4 by studies of L-arabinose. Finally, the correct configuration at carbon 2 was assigned after complex studies of D-gulose.

asymmetry about carbon 2 without changing the configuration of the rest of the molecule, it followed logically that D-glucose and D-mannose were identical (but still with unknown structures at this point) except that they had configurations about carbon 2 that were mirror images (Fig. 4). Today we call D-glucose and D-mannose epimers.[1]

A CHAIN OF LOGIC TO THE STRUCTURE OF D-GLUCOSE

In 1886, Heinrich Kiliani at the Technische Hochschule in Munich dis-

covered a method for lengthening the carbon chain of sugars (the added carbon was at the "top" of the chain, as oriented in the figures—an important detail).[1] Fischer extended that method with a reduction step to be able to study the reaction products as aldoses, the so-called Kiliani-Fischer synthesis.[1] Fischer knew that D-glucose, the most important monosaccharide, was an aldohexose, and in 1888 he set out to learn which of the 16 possible configurations of $C_6H_{12}O_6$ was the correct formula for naturally occurring glucose. Fischer took as a necessary arbitrary starting assumption that the -OH group of D-glucose at carbon 5 was on the right side, and he then worked out the relative configurations about the other carbon atoms. Thus, he was determining (by internal consistency of all of the classic chemical reactions) which of 8 possible structures represented D-glucose. We know today, now that absolute configurations can be established, that the -OH group at carbon 5 of D-glucose actually is on the right side, so Fischer happens to have guessed correctly in terms of the absolute configuration.

The path that Fischer took to learn the structure of D-glucose remains a complicated one to explain, so I will only mention the highlights here, and the interested reader wanting additional details will need to peruse Chapter 33 in Morrison and Boyd.[1] Fischer started by deciphering the correct configuration of the 5-carbon sugar, L-arabinose (Fig. 3). He found that oxidation of L-arabinose yielded a product that was optically active, implying that if the -OH group on the last asymmetric carbon was assumed to be on the right side, then the -OH group 2 carbons away was on the left side (or else there would have been no optical activity). Thus, these L-arabinose data provided the detail that in D-glucose, carbon 3 had a -OH group on the left.

Fischer next found that L-arabinose was converted in the Kiliani-Fischer synthesis (by adding a carbon to the "top") into both D-glucose and

242

The Endocrinologist • Volume 14, Number 5, October 2004

D-mannose. These 2 sugars, therefore, must have the same configurations about carbons 3, 4, and 5 as did the analogous carbons in L-arabinose. Fischer then discovered that, when oxidized by acid, both D-glucose and D-mannose yielded dicarboxylic acids that were optically active, implying that the -OH group on carbon 4 is on the right side (because if it had been on the left side, one of the resulting compounds would not have been optically active). This established that the analogous carbon in L-arabinose must have had the -OH group on the right side, which established the correct formula for L-arabinose.

Finally, Fischer determined that the oxidation of another hexose, D-gulose (which he was required to synthesize), yielded the same dicarboxylic acid as did oxidation of D-glucose. A somewhat complex chain of logic based on this observation established that the -OH on carbon 2 in D-glucose must be on the right side. It followed that the correct structure of D-glucose must be as shown in Figure 4, with D-mannose having the opposite configuration about carbon 2.

Fischer published[10] this result in 1891 while at the University of Wurzburg, and this triumph of determination and logic was primarily responsible for his being awarded the Nobel Prize in Chemistry in 1902, although he was also well known by that time for his landmark work on purines. During his Nobel Lecture,[8] delivered on December 12, 1902, he proudly showed the structures of a family of purines and made several jokes about wonderful compounds that had come from foul-smelling substances such as guanine from guano. He also showed the 16 formulae of the aldohexoses (Fig. 5), of which only 12 substances had actually been synthesized or isolated from nature at that time.

PROTEINS ARE POLYPEPTIDES

During the early 20th century, Fischer turned his attention to identifying the individual amino acids and was the discoverer of proline. He coined

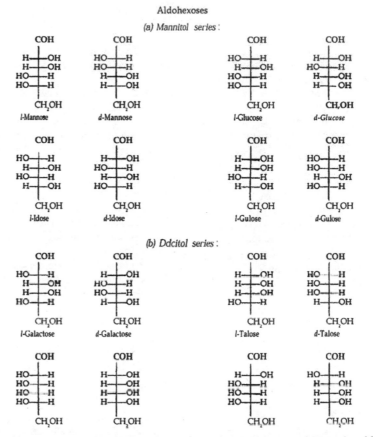

FIGURE 5. Figure used by Emil Fischer in his Nobel Prize lecture of December 12, 1902, to illustrate the 16 structures of the family of aldohexoses. Copyright, The Nobel Foundation.

the term "peptide bond." Fischer then started with individual purified amino acids and synthesized short peptides. He also studied enzymes and fats, and even analyzed lichen brought back from Black Forest holidays. In 1902, at the meeting of the Society of German Scientists and Physicians in Karlsbad, Fischer followed the eminent chemist Franz Hofmeister (1850–1922) on the program. Hofmeister presented a plenary lecture about the possible structure of proteins; then Fischer spoke about the isolation of amino acids from protein hydrolysates and suggested that proteins were made from amino acids linked together. Thus was born the Fischer-Hofmeister theory of protein structure.

PERSONAL LIFE

A brilliant and patient man, Fischer is said to have had a keen memory, and he made up for his poor speaking ability by being able to memorize many pages of lecture notes. In 1888, Fischer married Agnes Gerlach, who was the daughter of the anatomy professor at Erlangen. Although she died in the seventh year of their marriage, they had 3 sons. Unhappily, 1 was killed in the First World War, and another took his own life at age 25 while distraught over compulsory military service. A third son, Hermann Otto Laurenz Fischer (died 1960), eventually became a Professor of Biochemistry at the University of California

243

Free to Decide

at Berkeley. In the early years of World War I, Emil Fischer is said to have been a patriot, but later became disenchanted with Germanic folly. Shortly after the war, his health failed, possibly as a result of chronic exposure to multiple chemical solvents, and it is believed that he developed a type of cancer. Amid the shambles of postwar Germany, these problems overwhelmed him and it is believed that he took his own life[11] in 1919.

THE LEGACY

Shortly after Fischer's death, the German Chemical Society established the Emil Fischer Memorial Medal, viewed as a prestigious scientific award. The field of carbohydrate chemistry moved onward. In the 1890s, Fischer himself had provided evidence that glucose actually was a cyclic structure, and Tollens, Tanret, and many others contributed to this concept.[1] In 1909, C. S. Hudson of the U.S. Public Health Service made proposals about nomenclature that were widely accepted (and the enantiomer of alpha-D-[+]-glucose became alpha-L-[−]-glucose), although in 1926 the ring size was corrected.[1] The -OH groups pointing to the right in Fischer diagrams were agreed to be pointing downward in the cyclic structures. Although some of these conven-

tions were initially based on questionable relationships postulated to exist between configuration and optical rotation, subsequent enzymatic and x-ray evidence have bolstered the choices made.

Emil Fischer was an inspiration to students and colleagues. He made many fundamental contributions to modern biochemistry that we take for granted today. He had a special influence on me, apparently, after I read about his diagrams in college. That lesson may have predisposed me, perhaps, to have a bit of extra interest in carbohydrate biochemistry. When chance factors years later provided certain opportunities for me, I chose to study the oligosaccharides of the glycoprotein hormones. A few months ago my office moved to a new building in which the conference rooms were being named for famous scientists, and Fischer was selected to be so honored. This coincidence prompted me to keep my promise from decades before—to find a few minutes to learn more about this remarkable man's life.

REFERENCES

1. Morrison RT, Boyd RN, eds. *Organic Chemistry*. 2nd ed. Boston: Allyn and Bacon; 1969.
2. Emil Fischer—Biography (official web site of the Nobel Foundation). January 30, 2004. Available at: http://www.nobel.se/chemistry/laureates/1902/fischer-bio.html. Accessed April 19, 2004.
3. Hermann Emil Fischer 1852–1919 (web site of Peptides International). Available at: http://www.pepnet.com/fischerbio.html. Accessed April 19, 2004.
4. Adolf von Baeyer—Biography (official web site of the Nobel Foundation). June 23, 2003. Available at: http://www.nobel.se/chemistry/laureates/1905/baeyer-bio.html. Accessed April 19, 2004.
5. Lecture 5: Organic Chemistry & International Politics (web site of University of Toronto). Available at: http://www.chass.utoronto.ca/~bhall/hps282f/LECTURE%205%20Organic%Chemistry.html. Accessed May 7, 2004.
6. Jean-Baptiste Biot (web site of School of Mathematics and Statistics, University of St. Andrews, Scotland). January 1997. Available at: http://www.history.mcs.st-andrews.ac.uk/Mathematicians/Biot.html. Accessed May 5, 2004.
7. Geison GL. *The Private Science of Louis Pasteur*. Princeton, NJ: Princeton University Press; 1995.
8. Emil Fischer-Nobel Lecture (official web site of the Nobel Foundation). April 7, 2004. Available at: http://www.se/chemistry/lauretes/1902/fischer-lecture.html. Accessed April 19, 2004.
9. Jacobus H. van't Hoff—Biography (official web site of the Nobel Foundation). April 15, 2004. Available at: http://www.nobel.se/chemistry/laureates/1901/hoff-bio.html. Accessed April 19, 2004.
10. McBride JM. Emil Fischer: On the configuration of grape sugar and its isomers. I. Classic paper as first published in Berichte d d chem Gesellsch 24:1836 (1891) (web site of J. M. McBride, Yale). Available at: http://classes.yale.edu/chem125a/125/history99/6Stereochemistry/Fischer/FischerGlucosePrf.pdf. Accessed May 6, 2004.
11. Reynolds R, Tanford C. Enzyme action. Emil Hermann Fischer 1852–1919. In: Tallack P, ed. *The Science Book*. London: Weidenfeld & Nicolson; 2003:218–219.

THYROID
Volume 17, Number 8, 2007
© Mary Ann Liebert, Inc.
DOI: 10.1089/thy.2007.0141

Thyroid History

Seymour D. Van Meter, M.D. (1865–1934):
The Texan Who Wielded a Scalpel in Denver and
Left a Lasting Legacy

James A. Magner

SEYMOUR DOSS VAN METER (1865–1934) (Figs. 1 and 2) was a skilled general and abdominal surgeon who had a successful practice in Denver, in partnership with his daughter, Virginia. He had a reputation for particular skill with goiter operations and was known as a kind man who provided care to patients of all financial means. He served as president of the American Association for the Study of Goiter in 1929, an organization that later became the American Thyroid Association. Although he published little, his keen belief that the scientific method was the true hope of humankind led him to donate funds to establish a prestigious annual award given to a person who has made outstanding contributions to research on the thyroid gland or related subjects and who is not older than the age of 45 in the year of the award. (Funds have been supplemented over the years by industry.) The winner customarily delivers a 60-minute talk at the annual meeting of the American Thyroid Association, and since 1930 the list of awardees has included many young stars of the thyroid world. Many of the awardees, however, probably know little about the life of Dr. Van Meter.*

A Confederate Soldier Has a Son

The hot south Texas sun blazed down on the scrawny cattle grazing between the clumps of prickly pear, mesquite, blackbrush, and a few small live oak trees. Irish immigrants had settled near Sulfur Creek, and the little town of Oakville was made the county seat in 1856 and was granted a post office in 1857 (1). A small stone courthouse was built, and the hanging tree nearby had plenty of use. Several stores, two hotels, a livery stable, a school, and two churches were established. In 1861, of 150 voters in Live Oak County, only 9 had opposed secession (2). Men raised cattle and drove the herds to coastal towns or broke wild mustangs, which could be sold a few miles north in San Antonio or in east Texas. Families captured and slaughtered as many as a hundred wild hogs in a year, and their hides, meat, and tallow provided supplementary income. During the war, the demand

for cattle increased and the business became more profitable. Although the war ended badly for the Confederacy, by 1867 Rep. Samuel T. Foster boasted that Live Oak County was one of the finest stock-raising areas in the state. There was little

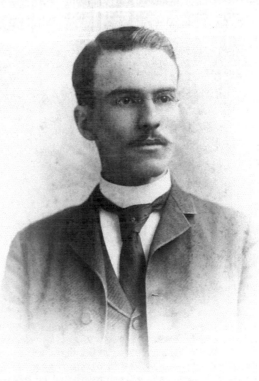

FIG. 1. Dr. Seymour Doss Van Meter at about the time of his graduation from medical school, 1889. Reprinted with permission from the Archives of the University of Pennsylvania, Philadelphia. All rights reserved.

Genzyme Corporation, Cambridge, Massachusetts.
*This historical article was first published in *The Endocrinologist* 17(2): 71–77, 2007, and has been republished with permission.

779

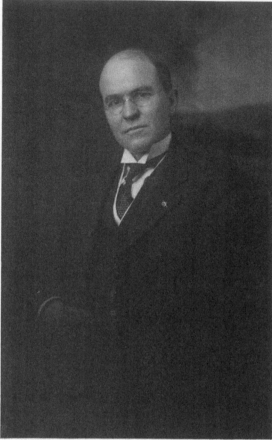

FIG. 2. Dr. Seymour D. Van Meter near the height of his career, approximately 1910. Undated photograph. Reprinted with permission, Denver Public Library, Western History Collection, all rights reserved.

agriculture in the area in the 1860s, but in 20 years there would be growing tension between the farmers who fenced the land and the cattlemen who cut the fences.

William Cunningham Van Meter was a farmer who had attended Hampden-Sydney College in Virginia between 1849 and 1851 (3). This all-male, Presbyterian, liberal arts school is the 10th oldest college in the United States (founded 1775). He expressed an interest in engineering, but he did not obtain a degree. No record remains of his hometown. After serving in the Confederate Army, he brought his wife, formerly Elfrida Victoria Wright, to Oakville, Texas. Their son, Seymour, was born there on October 18, 1865 (4). The boy attended the public school, and he must have been a bright student. Due to scant information available at present, it is hard to imagine now what prompted his choice at age 20 to

attend the University of Pennsylvania in Philadelphia, but he matriculated there in medical courses in September 1886. He was awarded the MD degree in May 1889 and was honored as sixth in his class (5). After completing an internship at Presbyterian Hospital in Philadelphia, he married Annie Virginia Cunningham, the daughter of a farmer, on May 1, 1893, in Moorefield, West Virginia, and their first daughter, Elfrida Victoria, was born the next year.

Denver Becomes a Booming City

Gold was discovered in Colorado on Cherry Creek in 1858, and within 25 years the tiny settlement there, Denver, became a populous city, second only to San Francisco in the West. Railroads further contributed to the success of the economy there, but the lack of medical facilities was only addressed in 1883 when the Union Pacific Railroad built a 66-bed hospital at 40th and York Street (6). But nurses were needed. Colorado's first bishop, Joseph Machebeuf, wrote to the sisters in Lafayette, Indiana, for assistance. Seven German-speaking nuns, members of the Poor Sisters of St. Francis Seraph of Perpetual Adoration, arrived in Denver in 1884. But after 6 years, Sister Mary Huberta believed that the order needed its own, larger hospital. The bishop urged caution, but Sister Huberta believed that St. Anthony, who traditionally aids the despairing, would help. The sisters sought donations at the mining camps and stood with their tin cups outside saloons, barbershops, and especially at the paymasters as railroad workers collected their wages. In May 1892, the new hospital, named for the saint who had helped it come into being, opened on West 16th Avenue and Raleigh Street, with 120 ward beds and 60 private beds. By then, other small hospitals also were opening.

Booming Denver seemed an opportune place for a young surgeon, and Dr. Van Meter first established an office there in the early 1890s. A photo (Fig. 3) from about 1895, taken from the Central Presbyterian Church tower on Sherman Street, shows the state capitol building under construction,

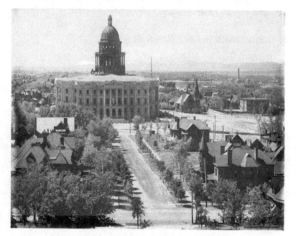

FIG. 3. Panorama of Denver, circa 1895, with the capitol building under construction. Reprinted with permission, Colorado Historical Society, creator William Henry Jackson (1843–1942), No. CHS.J2616, all rights reserved.

fine homes, and tree-lined streets (7). The buildings and smokestack of Denver General Hospital can be seen in the distance. Dr. Van Meter's home, at 1723 Tremont Place, located about six blocks northwest of the capitol building, was not far from where this photo was taken. (The photos in this article have not been previously published,* to my knowledge, except for the photo of Virginia Van Meter, which appeared in her medical school yearbook.)

Dr. Van Meter first served as a staff surgeon at St. Francis Hospital from 1894 to 1897. He practiced at the City and County Hospital, starting in 1902, and also served at Mercy Hospital from 1905 until 1908. His offices were located at Suite 619 of the Majestic Building, and another address given was 1326 Columbine Street (5). He took two postgraduate trips to European surgical clinics, but details of these trips have been lost. Starting in 1901, he was a member of the Colorado State Board of Medical Examiners, and he eventually served as secretary-treasurer and executive officer of that organization. He belonged to the county and state medical associations and the American Medical Association, and he later served as president of the Denver City and County Medical Society. By 1910, he published short articles on topics such as "Medical Licensure" and "Medical Laws and the Influences Which Mould Them," demonstrating his interest in how the young scientific practice of medicine was being organized in the United States. His early articles also dealt with surgical topics, such as "A New Operation for the Ingrown Toenail" and "Spontaneous Rupture of the Uterus."

A second daughter, Virginia Cunningham, was born in 1896, and his third daughter, Jane, was born in 1907.

In 1914, a book was prepared for distribution at a dinner at the University Club of the University of Pennsylvania to celebrate the 25th anniversary of Van Meter's class of '89. He had listed as his hobbies, "Team work in operating and up-stream superiority in trout fly fishing" (5). In Denver, he was a member of the Wigwam Club, named after the American Indian dwelling, which celebrated fishing and other outdoor activities. He was also a member of the Cherry Hills Country Club.

He served in the Medical Reserve Corps, United States Army. After World War I, he took on additional surgical patients at Children's Hospital, Beth Israel Hospital, and St. Luke's Hospital, although most of his work was performed

at Denver General Hospital, where he served on staff for 25 years (4).

A photo (Fig. 4) from about 1891 to 1900 shows St. Luke's Hospital to consist of two substantial three-story brick buildings, each with a high roof with more than a dozen gables (7). Two stone crosses are prominent, and the tall brick chimney from the heating plant emerges from behind one of the buildings. A horse-drawn buggy waits in front of the main entrance, with its white stone arch. The first x-ray department there, depicted in a photo (Fig. 5) dated 1896, shows eight large lead batteries on the floor, with cables stretched over chairs to electrical equipment on small tables, with a stout wooden table also available (7). An apparatus with a dozen large light bulbs is mounted prominently on the wall. The human skeleton hanging in the back corner likely was a handy reference when viewing a dim image of a bloody and bruised patient. Another photo (not shown) of the same hospital from about 1910 reveals that by then a third large adjoining brick building had been built.

Several old photos survive that capture scenes of Denver General Hospital, which was located at West 6th Avenue and Cherokee Street (7). One photo (Fig. 6) shows that the hospital was a two-and-a-half–story brick building with dormers and projecting bays. Best shown is the west wing, where the surgical ward, operating rooms, tuberculosis ward, and administrative offices were located. The east wing, where the women's, children's, and typhoid wards were located, is in the distance. A sign near the curb reads, "Keep Space Open for Ambulance." A photo (Fig. 7) from about 1905 captures the linen-covered tables of the doctors' and nurses' dining room (7). It seems that coat and tie for doctors and white uniforms with high hats for nurses were standard. One can imagine a leisurely discussion ensuing about a difficult case. A view (Fig. 8) of the men's chronic ward from 1907 shows metal beds, white starched sheets, dedicated nurses and orderlies, and a few patients; it appears that all of the window shades are drawn during the daytime (7). Years later, in 1927, a photo (Fig. 9) captures nurses and technicians

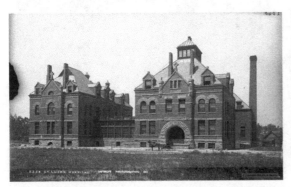

FIG. 4. St. Luke's Hospital, Denver, circa 1891–1900. Reprinted with permission, Colorado Historical Society, creator William Henry Jackson (1843–1942), No. CHS.J71, all rights reserved.

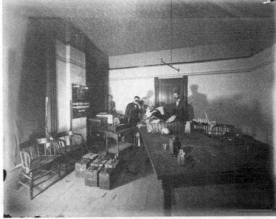

FIG. 5. The first x-ray department in St. Luke's Hospital, Denver, circa 1896. Harry Buckwalter and Dr. C. E. Tennant prepare to x-ray Central City Marshal Mike Kehler. Reprinted with permission, Colorado Historical Society, creator Harry H. Buckwalter, No. CHS-B1470, all rights reserved.

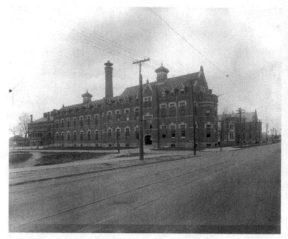

FIG. 6. Denver General Hospital, circa 1910–1920. Reprinted with permission, Denver Public Library, Western History Collection, No. X-28546, all rights reserved.

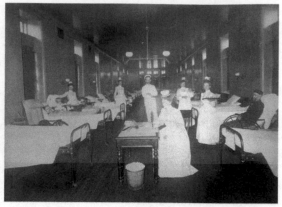

FIG. 8. Men's chronic ward, Denver General Hospital, circa 1907. Reprinted with permission, Denver Public Library, Western History Collection, No. X-28572, all rights reserved.

at work in the laboratory at Denver General Hospital, which has a wall of windows, sinks, glass bottles, and an icebox (7). To the modern eye, it looks like the space into which the laboratory has yet to be moved. A photo (Fig. 10) taken in 1931 captured a nurse standing at the large porcelain sinks in the wash-up room at the Denver General Hospital, and a photo (Fig. 11) of an operating room taken that same year reveals a modern design (7). The Romanesque-style surgical wing of General Hospital, built in 1892, has been captured in another photo (Fig. 12) taken between 1930 and 1940 (7).

Thyroid Surgery in the Early Twentieth Century

No records remain to tell of Dr. Van Meter's surgical practice. But contemporary texts have many surprises for modern readers. One must remember that in the era before widespread iodine supplementation, many otherwise healthy

persons had substantial goiters that were both a cosmetic and medical problem. Moreover, surgery was the remedy not only for simple and multinodular goiters and for thyroid tumors but also for hyperthyroidism. One wanted to avoid the necessity of operating on a severely hyperthyroid patient, but diagnosing mild or early hyperthyroidism was tricky. A text from 1922 describes the usual medical and surgical methods at Western Reserve University in Cleveland. Dr. Robert S. Dinsmore, the Third Resident Surgeon at Lakeside Hospital in Cleveland, elaborates on the "Goetsch test," which was used to differentiate between hyperthyroidism and early tuberculosis in a patient with weight loss, weakness, fatigue, and slight elevation of temperature but in whom the physical signs and x-ray findings of tuberculosis were negative (8). To perform this test, the patient was admitted to the hospital and allowed to have a quiet and calm environment. On the second day, the patient was injected subcutaneously with

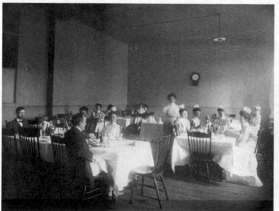

FIG. 7. Doctors' and nurses' dining room, Denver General Hospital, circa 1905. Reprinted with permission, Denver Public Library, Western History Collection, No. X-28565, all rights reserved.

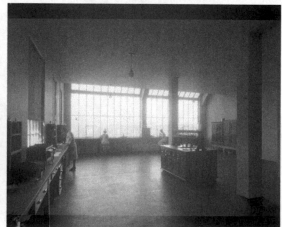

FIG. 9. Nurses and technicians at work in the laboratory, Denver General Hospital, circa 1927. Reprinted with permission, Denver Public Library, Western History Collection, No. X-28585, all rights reserved.

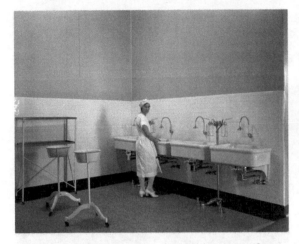

FIG. 10. The large porcelain sinks in the wash-up room, Denver General Hospital, 1931. Reprinted with permission, Denver Public Library, Western History Collection, No. X-28594, all rights reserved.

six minims of adrenalin chlorid [sic] 1:1000 (although this should be avoided if the blood pressure was above 160). At 5-minute intervals for 40 to 60 minutes, the observer was to score the blood pressure, pulse rate, respiration rate, nervousness, tremor of the fingers, hyperhidrosis, size of pupils,

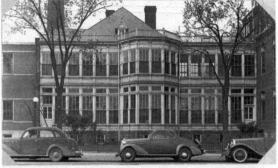

FIG. 12. The surgical wing of Denver General Hospital on 6th Avenue, circa 1930–1940. Reprinted with permission, Denver Public Library, Western History Collection, No. X-20559, all rights reserved.

and pallor or flushing of the skin, as well as record verbal symptoms from the patient, and thereby achieve the differentiation of hyperthyroidism from tuberculosis. Patients with hyperthyroidism had more effects during the test, although Dr. Dinsmore reports that he has tested 251 patients, and 89% had positive reactions of varying degrees.

A big controversy during this era was whether the glands of hyperthyroid patients should be treated with exposure to strong x-rays, usually a "maximum dose every 3 weeks" or, alternatively, whether the thyroid should be surgically removed. Dr. George Crile, in his 1922 chapter, noted that 239 drugs had been credited with the cure of hyperthyroidism and that several hundred articles had reported use of x-ray therapy to treat this condition (9). Dr. Crile put emphasis on the 1916 report in the St. Paul Medical Journal by Dr. D. M. Berkman at the Mayo Clinic that "Although in their experience the results of x-ray treatment were good, they were temporary; that the results were delayed and required many repetitions of treatment; that practically no dependable beneficial results were obtained in less than a month; and that in the more serious cases 'the excitement and mobilization incident to x-ray treatment usually offset whatever early benefits may be received.'" Thus, by about 1920, many experts were concluding that surgery was the better treatment. A commonly reported mortality rate for such operations, which likely were partial thyroidectomies, was about 1%. Infection postoperatively was a problem, but for more serious cases, the wounds commonly would be left wide open and dressed with 1:5000 flavine gauze (10). The opinion was that it was important to allow the aseptic wound secretions to drain away from the patient to prevent fever. Delayed closure of the wound then was performed a day or two after the primary surgery. Drs. Crile and W. E. Lower report that of 485 wounds left open in this manner, the mortality rate was 3.9%. Most patients were not severely hypothyroid after surgery, which was just as well since Dr. Chester D. Christie at Western Reserve University found that thyroid extract did not reliably improve his patients with myxedema (11). Tetany due to hypoparathyroidism occurred on occasion, and Dr. Crile by 1922 preferred to attempt to visualize the parathyroid glands during the operation, although he feared that doing so might damage their blood supply.

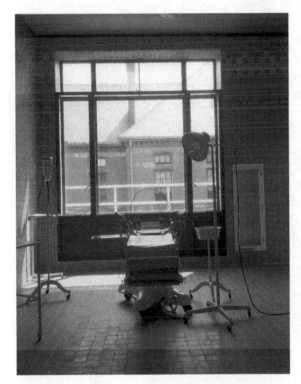

FIG. 11. Operating room, Denver General Hospital, 1931. Reprinted with permission, Denver Public Library, Western History Collection, No. X-28583, all rights reserved.

More shocking to the modern reader is the fact that some degree of deception routinely was practiced on hyperthyroid patients who were being admitted for thyroid surgery, although it was felt that this was for their own good. A frightened and excited hyperthyroid patient was felt to be at greatly increased risk for surgical mortality. Dr. Crile describes this method briefly as follows: "The patient is protected from worry, anxiety and fear by tactful management" (10). A more detailed description is provided by Drs. W. R. Goff and E. O. Rushing, both physicians at Lakeside Hospital.

"Because of the nervousness of these patients and their poor tolerance for suspense they are usually not told when the operation is to be performed; in fact, if possible, the subject of operation is altogether avoided, and stress is laid upon treatment. To prevent the patient from knowing exactly when the operation is to take place the following routine is carried out daily for several days beforehand.

"The operating-room clothes are put on usually the day after admission. Some kind of explanation has to be given for each move to satisfy the curiosity of the patient. He is told the pneumonia jacket and leggings are kept on to insure an even temperature of the body, etc.

"A hypodermic injection of sterile water is given every morning about 8 and breakfast is deferred.

"At 9 each morning, before the patient's breakfast is served, the anesthetist takes a nitrous oxid-oxygen [sic] machine to the bedside and, after explaining to the patient that she is going to give him some oxygen for his heart, the mask is held lightly over the face, and a small amount of nitrous oxid and oxygen is given, never allowing the patient to become unconscious. This procedure is usually explained by the ward physician the night before during his social call. In some cases several mornings are required to get the inhalations started, because if the patient becomes at all disturbed, the maneuver is suspended, to be tried again the next morning.

"On the morning of the operation a hypodermic injection of morphin, gr. 1/6, and atropin, gr. 1/150, is substituted for the sterile water. The patient is not disturbed by nurses or visitors after the hypodermic injection has been given, and at the usual time the anesthetist gives the inhalation. This time the patient is allowed to pass into the analgesic or anesthetic stage, and in this condition is operated upon in his bed, if the sensitivity of the case demands it, or is transferred to the operating room" (12).

A Daughter as a Partner

Dr. Van Meter's oldest daughter, Elfrida, married a man named Packard, and his youngest daughter, Jane, studied at the Sorbonne in Paris (4). It was his middle daughter, Virginia, who followed most closely in her father's footsteps. After attending Manual Training High School, the University of Colorado (1913–1915), and the University of Pennsylvania premedical (1915–1917), she was awarded the MD degree by that institution in 1922 (13). Her photo (Fig. 13) in *The Scope*, the yearbook in 1921, reveals her at age 25 to have attractive features and an intelligent expression. After additional training at Robert Packer Hospital in Sayre, PA, she returned to Denver in 1925 to practice with her father, becoming the first female surgeon in Colorado. In 1927, she surprised friends by completing an operation, then walking from the

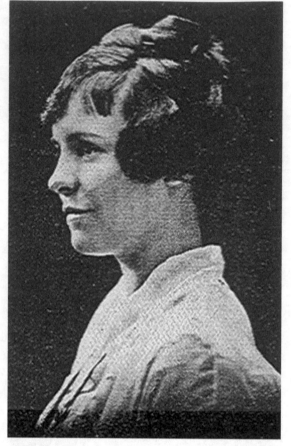

FIG. 13. Virginia Van Meter, 1921. Reproduced with permission, Archives of the University of Pennsylvania, all rights reserved.

hospital to a church where she married the prominent surgeon Dr. William C. Finnoff. In 1929, her husband developed appendicitis, and the *Denver Post* on March 29 made much of the fact that Virginia and her father, Dr. S. D. Van Meter, together operated on William to save his life (13). Not only did she practice medicine with her father, her home at 1621 Court Place was only a block from her father's former house. Tragically, her husband preceded her in death, and their only son, Seymour, was killed in a plane crash on December 1, 1946. After practicing medicine in Denver for 25 years, during which time she witnessed countless medical innovations, she moved to Tucson. She suffered a heart attack and died at the Medical Center on August 31, 1962, at age 66.

The Legacy

Dr. Seymour Van Meter served in 1929 as president of the organization that later would be known as the American Thyroid Association. In that day, most of the members were surgeons. Only later, after the introduction of radioiodine and various medical treatments for thyroid diseases, did the membership shift largely to internists and endocrinologists.

Dr. Van Meter donated a sum of money to support the annual award that bears his name, and he knew the first awardee, another surgeon, Dr. William F. Rienhoff, Jr., who went on to a long career at Johns Hopkins (14).

In January 1934, at age 68, Dr. Van Meter was stricken with cancer, and he died the next month at St. Luke's Hospital. The obituary, which appeared on page 1 of the *Denver Post* on that same day, Tuesday, February 27, stressed that he had devoted his lifetime to the advancement of medical science (4). The newspaper did not mention his wife, so she may have preceded him in death. The obituary stated that, "During his last conscious hour he requested his daughter, Dr. Virginia C. Finnoff, to arrange for an autopsy that will enable his colleagues to discover the cause of his malady and asked that immediately thereafter his body should be cremated, without funeral services" (4). This was done at Riverside cemetery crematory that same afternoon.

Every life can teach a lesson, and the life of Dr. Van Meter teaches many. We all can try to emulate his roles as head of a family and skillful and hardworking medical practitioner. We can admire his rise from small town obscurity and wonder if we would have had such courage in the 19th century to study far from home and begin new ventures in unfamiliar cities. We can envy his good fortune of being blessed with children, including one who was a bright child who understood and shared his art. But perhaps we especially should take note of the service he provided to many organizations and to his faith in the importance of science to humanity. I suspect that his autopsy failed to advance medical knowledge very much, in spite of his brave wish. But his generous donation, which established the Van Meter Award, definitely has played an important role over many years to encourage and reward young scientific investigators in the thyroid field.

Acknowledgments

Deserving of special thanks for helping me obtain materials are Nancy R. Miller of the University of Pennsylvania Archives, Judy Brown and Coi Drummond-Gehrig of the Western History/Genealogy Department of the Denver Public Library, Bobbi Smith of the American Thyroid Association, and John Brinkley of the Hampden-Sydney College Archives.

References

1. Oakville Texas! Available at: www.geocities.com/oakvilletx/?200612. Accessed November 12, 2006.
2. Handbook of Texas online, Live Oak County. Available at: www.tsha.utexas.edu/handbook/online/articles/OO/hlo4.html. Accessed November 10, 2006.
3. Archives of Hampden-Sydney College, Hampden-Sydney, Virginia.
4. Dr. Van Meter dies and leaves body to science. *Denver Post.* February 27, 1934.
5. University of Pennsylvania Archives, Philadelphia, PA. Alumni records collection. Folder title: Van Meter, Seymour Doss, MD, 1889.
6. St. Anthony Hospitals, our history, 2005. Available at: www.stanthonyhosp.org/index.php?shistory. Accessed November 13, 2006.
7. Denver Public Library western history photos. Available at: http://photowest.org/cgibin. Accessed November 17, 2006.
8. Dinsmore RS 1922 Adrenalin sensitization test for hyperthyroidism. In: Rowland AF (ed) The Thyroid Gland Clinics of George W. Crile and Associates. W. B. Saunders, Philadelphia, pp 99–104.
9. Crile GW 1922 Surgery vs. x-ray in the treatment of hyperthyroidism. In: Rowland AF (ed) The Thyroid Gland Clinics of George W. Crile and Associates. W. B. Saunders, Philadelphia, pp 185–194.
10. Crile GW, Lower WE 1922 The technic of operations on the thyroid gland. In: Rowland AF (ed) The Thyroid Gland Clinics of George W. Crile and Associates. W. B. Saunders, Philadelphia, pp 223–252.
11. Christie CD 1922 The value of basal metabolism studies in exophthalmic goiter. In: Rowland AF (ed) The Thyroid Gland Clinics of George W. Crile and Associates. W. B. Saunders, Philadelphia, pp 141–158.
12. Goff WR, Rushing EO 1922 Preoperative management of exophthalmic goiter. In: Rowland AF (ed) The Thyroid Gland Clinics of George W. Crile and Associates. W. B. Saunders, Philadelphia, pp 195–199.
13. University of Pennsylvania Archives, Philadelphia, PA. Alumni records collection. Folder title: Van Meter, Virginia Cunningham, MD, 1921.
14. Longmire WP, Rienhoff WF Jr. 2001 A not-to-be-forgotten mentor. Surgery **129:**110–113.

Address reprint requests to:
James A. Magner, M.D.
500 Kendall Street
Genzyme Corporation
Cambridge, MA 02142

E-mail: james.magner@genzyme.com

Basic Thyroidology / Review

European Thyroid Journal

Eur Thyroid J
DOI: 10.1159/000360534

Received: January 9, 2014
Accepted after revision: February 11, 2014
Published online: March 13, 2014

Historical Note: Many Steps Led to the 'Discovery' of Thyroid-Stimulating Hormone

James Magner

Genzyme, a Sanofi company, Cambridge, Mass., USA

Key Words

Thyroid-stimulating hormone · Discovery · History of science

Abstract

Finding thyroid-stimulating hormone was a process rather than a circumscribed event, and many talented persons participated over many years. Key early participants were Bennet M. Allen and Philip E. Smith who had the misfortune just prior to World War I of independently and simultaneously starting very similar experiments with tadpoles. This led to a series of back and forth publications attempting to establish priority for finding evidence of a thyrotropic factor in the anterior pituitary. Decades of work by others would be required before sophisticated biochemical techniques would bring us to our modern understanding.

© 2014 European Thyroid Association
Published by S. Karger AG, Basel

Introduction

Who discovered insulin? Penicillin? These questions have answers although they involve caveats and stories rather than one-word responses. So, who discovered thyroid-stimulating hormone (TSH)? In fact, the answer includes many stories and many names. This short paper is intended simply to present some little-known facts about the early discernment that there existed a thyrotropic factor in the pituitary, with emphasis on the activities of two biologists in the early 20th century. This is not intended as a comprehensive review but instead highlights that our thyroid field has stories of human interest and illustrates that finding TSH was a process rather than a circumscribed event.

Development of Knowledge of TSH: Period 1

Table 1 lists some key events that gradually led to a fuller understanding that there existed a pituitary factor that stimulated thyroid tissue, followed by the isolation and characterization of that factor. The development of knowledge of TSH occurred in three periods. First, there was general recognition that the pituitary contained a thyrotropic substance. Two young biologists (Bennett M. Allen of the University of Kansas, and Philip E. Smith of Cornell University and the University of California, Berkeley) independently used tadpoles as inexpensive model systems since it was known (in large part due to Allen) that the thyroid was necessary for the tadpole to go

James Magner
Genzyme, a Sanofi company
500 Kendall St., 7th Floor
Cambridge, MA 02142 (USA)
E-Mail james.magner@genzyme.com

Table 1. Some names and events in TSH history

Niépce [21] (1851): observed at autopsy that the pituitary of a cretin was grossly enlarged.

Cushing's group [22] (1910): noted thyroid atrophy after some pituitary surgeries.

Adler [23] (1914): preliminary studies of hypophysectomy of mammals and tadpoles causing thyroid atrophy.

Allen [1] (1916) and Smith [2] (1916): careful experiments using tadpoles proved that a thyrotropic substance existed and was present in the anterior portion of the pituitary.

Aron [24] (1929) and Loeb and Bassett [25] (1929): developed bioassay of pituitary gland extracts in guinea pigs.

Jansen and Loesser [26] (1931): first partially purified a preparation of TSH (still with critical contaminants, such as LH).

Greep [27] (1935), White and Ciereszko [28] (1941), and Bates et al. [29] (1959): many methods used to purify TSH activity by 50–300 fold.

Hoskins [30] (1949): concept of 'feedback' in the 'thyroid-pituitary axis'.

Heideman [31] (1953) and Crigler and Waugh [32] (1955): improved purification of TSH by ion-exchange chromatography. In the 1950s and 1960s, attempts to sequence the peptide of TSH provided confusing data.

Condliffe and Bates [33, 34] (1957): much improved ion exchange chromatography. TSH was found to be retained on diethylaminoethyl cellulose (DEAE cellulose) only at high pH and low ionic strength, while LH was not absorbed.

Papkoff and Samy [35] (1967): recognized that ovine LH had two nonidentical subunits.

Liao and Pierce [36] (1970): recognized the subunit nature of TSH and described a common subunit in bTSH and bLH.

Liao and Pierce [37] (1971): determined the peptide sequences of bTSH α- and β-subunits.

Fiddes and Goodman [38] (1981): cloned the common α-subunit of the human glycoprotein hormones, while Wondisford et al. [11] (1988) and (independently) Guidon et al. [12] (1988) and Tatsumi et al. [13] (1988) cloned the β-subunit of hTSH.

Chin et al. [39], Ridgway, Shupnick (1980s), and others studied the transcriptional regulation of the subunits.

Weintraub, Magner [40] and Szkudlinski and others [41] (1980s and 1990s) studied the oligosaccharides of TSH and structure-function correlates.

through metamorphosis into a frog. Larval amphibians survived 'small cut and needle scoop surgeries' (my term) better than did young mammals. In addition, using a microscope, anterior pituitaries of larval amphibians could be removed relatively precisely during a certain anatomically favorable stage of larval development; then one could watch for a subsequent biological effect on the thyroid follicle structure. Both Allen and Smith were doing such experiments. In July 1916, Allen was traveling through Berkeley on his way to a scientific meeting to be held in San Diego, and he met Smith. To their mutual consternation, they were both scheduled to present similar data at the Western Society of Naturalists on August 9–12, 1916! They both wrote summaries of their presentations at that August meeting which only appeared in print several months later in the *Anatomical Record* [1, 2]. Both had noted that many of the hypophysectomized tadpoles developed thyroid follicular changes with less colloid, the tadpoles grew slowly, the legs did not enlarge,

and the dark pigment granules in the skin shrank so that the tadpoles took on a creamy silver color that was quite striking (fig. 1) – we now know that the color change was probably due to the absence of MSH. While the creative and insightful Bennet Allen was taking the long, slow train ride back to Lawrence, Kansas, the ambitious and talented young Smith [3], not wanting to be scooped, was able to return rapidly to Berkeley and wrote a 3-page article that was quickly published in the August 25, 1916, issue of *Science*, only 13 days after the close of the San Diego conference. In that paper, Smith inserted a sentence stating that he had first attempted such experiments in 1914. Allen [4] was necessarily later in submitting his results to *Science*, and his article appeared in the November 24, 1916, issue.

Both Smith and Allen were smart, skilled, and ambitious, and this collision of careers was unfortunate. It is painful today to read a paragraph inserted by Allen into his November 1916 article, as follows:

Eur Thyroid J
DOI: 10.1159/000360534

Magner

This phase of my work was duplicated by Dr. P.E. Smith, who published a preliminary account of his work in the August 25, 1916, number of *Science*. During the month of July prior to this time I had the pleasure of discussing my work with Dr. Smith at Berkeley. Previous to this time I had no knowledge of his work nor of his plans and he assures me that he was equally ignorant of my work. We both presented papers upon our experiments at the meeting of the Western Society of Naturalists at San Diego, August 9 to 12. On June 7, before starting west, I demonstrated specimens and explained my results to a number of scientists, including Dr. Frank R. Lillie, Dr. Emil Goetsch, Dr. Chas H. Swift and a number of others whom I met in Chicago at that time. It is thus clear that these experiments were independently conceived by Dr. Smith and myself and that we worked contemporaneously upon them each without knowledge of the other's work until July, 1916, two months after the experiments had been performed. [4]

Although Smith had published first in *Science* with amazing rapidity, and Smith also included interesting photographs of specimens in his 1916 *Anatomical Record* report, one can tell by the tone of Allen's 1916 *Science* publication that he was not about to fade into the night. Allen [5, 6] published a detailed 14-page summary of his data in the *Biological Bulletin* in 1917, followed by another paper in *Science* in 1920, this time describing how pituitaries from adult *Rana pipiens* could be transplanted under the skin of hypophysectomized tadpoles to partially restore their thyroid follicles. These papers were impressive counterpunches. Smith responded in a 1922 paper that showed that administration of bovine anterior pituitary to hypophysectomized tadpoles could repair and activate their thyroids, and Smith published other papers in the mid-1920s extending the work to mammals. Allen then responded by publishing a book chapter in January 1927 summarizing data about the influence of the hypophysis upon the thyroid gland in amphibian larvae. The passing of years would eventually prove both gentlemen to be superb biologists, keen intellects, and skilled researchers who accidentally started simultaneously on the same path.

Smith was invited to participate in the Harvey Lectures Series of 1930. In the 1931 publication of his lecture, Smith [7] illustrated how extracts from ox pituitaries partially restored the thyroid follicular structure in hypophysectomized tadpoles and how rat pituitaries when administered daily to hypophysectomized rats could partially restore their thyroid follicular structure.

Smith (1884–1970) (fig. 2) was born in De Smet, South Dakota, and earned a BS from Pomona College and a PhD from Cornell. He worked briefly at Berkeley and Stanford before moving to the Department of Anatomy at Columbia University in 1927, where he remained until his retirement in 1952 [8]. He became an expert at performing hypophysectomy in the rat and played a role in the elucida-

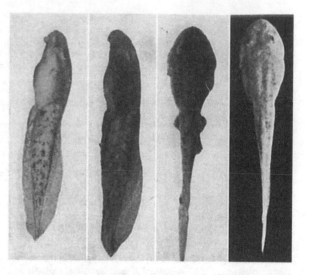

Fig. 1. Tadpoles as published in the *Anatomical Record* by Smith [2] in 1916.

tion of several important pituitary hormones. Smith served as president of the Endocrine Society in 1939–1940.

Bennet Allen (1877–1963) (fig. 3) was born in Indiana, attended college at DePauw University, and received a doctorate in zoology from the University of Chicago in 1903. After teaching at the University of Wisconsin, he became professor of zoology at the University of Kansas in 1913 and headed the department. He moved to the nascent Southern Branch of the University of California at Los Angeles in 1922. During his long career there he served as chairman of the Department of Zoology and as a dean. He served as officer in several scientific societies and was a respected research investigator. Even before good research facilities were available, he mentored many students in research projects and developed a loyal following of trainees. Over the years, he pushed for funding better facilities, with huge influence. He 'retired' at age 70 in 1947 but then began a new career in the Atomic Energy Project at UCLA, and he published 26 additional scientific papers, many about amphibians, reptiles, and aspects of radiation exposure (details courtesy of UCLA).

Development of Knowledge of TSH: Periods 2 and 3

The second period of increased understanding about TSH began in 1953 when ion exchange chromatography was applied to prepare much more pure preparations of

Many Steps Led to the 'Discovery' of TSH

Eur Thyroid J
DOI: 10.1159/000360534

3

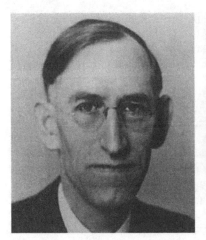

Fig. 2. Philip E. Smith, undated.

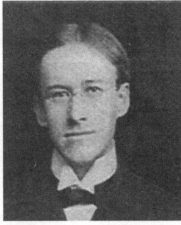

Fig. 3. Bennet M. Allen, 1899.

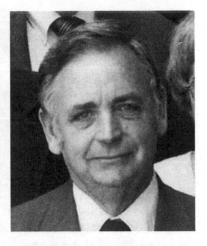

Fig. 4. John G. Pierce, undated.

TSH, although LH was still a confounding contaminant [9]. Attempts to perform peptide sequencing were unsuccessful. In the late 1950s the third period of understanding was entered when a much improved ion exchange chromatography technique led to purer preparations of TSH along with recognition that TSH consisted of 2 peptide chains (that were heavily glycosylated).

Dr. John Pierce (fig. 4) and his team at UCLA separated the α- from the β-subunits of bovine TSH, which allowed proper amino acid sequencing. Pierce was known as a brilliant and kind man who shared reagents generously. He was born in 1920 and received his BA, masters, and PhD (1944) degrees from Stanford University in California [10]. He served in the navy during World War II, was a postdoctoral fellow at Stanford and Cornell, served as a faculty member at Cornell for 4 years, and then moved to UCLA in 1952. Pierce served as chairman of biological chemistry from 1979–1984, and at the end of his career he served as associate dean of the School of Medicine. Pierce died in 2006 and is fondly remembered. It was my privilege to have met him in the 1980s.

The work by Pierce and his colleagues led others to find the subunit genes in several species. Analogous to the contemporaneous work of Dr. Smith and Dr. Allen, the sequence of the human TSH β-subunit gene was reported by three groups working independently, all published in 1988 [11–13]. The human TSH subunit gene sequences were essential for the preparation of recombinant human TSH, which is made in large bioreactors using Chinese hamster ovary cells, since the posttranslational glycosylation achieved by eukaryotic cells is important in human TSH.

The Phenomenon of Simultaneous Discovery

I was struck by the example of simultaneous discovery illustrated by Smith and Allen. For context, it is interesting to reflect on other instances. Science is conducted by curious humans who can also be ambitious and competitive. Oftentimes great advances in science have been spurred by this competition, although there can be a darker side. Scientists have long known this, but the general public was not as aware until the publication of the remarkable book *The Double Helix*, by James Watson [14], in 1968. Watson [14] and Crick were substantially aided by helpful colleagues who pointed out the correct molecular configurations (under physiological conditions) of the purine and pyrimidine bases – a lack of this precise chemical knowledge would have severely impaired their model building. Watson [14] and Crick also had a helpful sneak peek at Rosalind Franklin's unpublished X-ray crystallography films, and they were also aware via a draft manuscript that Linus Pauling was about to publish an incorrect 3-chain model of DNA structure, yet they did not contact Pauling to stop him from making this error. Competition probably also spurred progress in the Human Genome Project after Craig Venter decided to attempt to outcompete the huge government program. After the two groups essentially ended in a tie, it took efforts by the president of the USA and scheduling of a White House ceremony in June 2000 to bring the situation to a reasonably peaceful resolution. The president of the USA and the prime minister of France also had to become involved to settle an acrimonious dispute between

Eur Thyroid J
DOI: 10.1159/000360534

Magner

Robert Gallo and Luc Montagnier regarding priority of the discovery of the human immunodeficiency virus (HIV). The Nobel Prize in Physiology or Medicine then was awarded to Montagnier and Francoise Barré-Sinoussi in 2008 for the discovery of that virus (and also to Harald zur Hausen for work on the papilloma viruses and cervical cancer). As has been widely discussed by historians interested in these events, Gallo was not recognized by the Nobel committee.

Numerous entertaining and fascinating examples of simultaneous work as well as competitive (mis)adventures abound in the history of science, and some are succinctly summarized in *Great Feuds in Science,* by Hal Hellman [15], and *Prize Fight: the Race and the Rivalry to be the First in Science,* by Morton A. Meyers [16], which has a good discussion of the Gallo-Montagnier controversy as well as other examples.

Within endocrinology there have been several other notable examples of intense rivalry between investigators. Roger Guillemin (born in 1924) of the Salk Institute, La Jolla, California, competed for more than 20 years against Andrzeg 'Andrew' Schally (born in 1926) of Tulane University, New Orleans, Louisiana, as both teams worked intensely on hypothalamic hormones. In 1977 both men were awarded the Nobel Prize, shared with Rosalind Yalow, for their work on neurohormones, most importantly TRH and GnRH. A New York Times science writer, Nicholas Wade, subsequently prepared a somewhat controversial book about this competition, *The Nobel Duel* [17]. Persons who worked in one of the laboratories report that the book captures well the intense activity required 7 days per week as the groups competed, and is basically factually true and is recommended, although some errors in fact are claimed. In another instance of rivalry, teams of researchers in Belgium and California competed to report the sequence of the TSH receptor. Gilbert Vassart and his colleagues at the Free University of Brussels competed with Basil Rapoport and others in

California, and both groups published key data in 1989 [18–20].

In this article I elaborated on the Allen versus Smith situation. As things turned out, subsequent advances made by many people produced a detailed molecular and physiological understanding of a very important hormone, TSH. One application of that knowledge was the production of recombinant human TSH, to the great benefit of our patients.

In sum, important advances in the knowledge of TSH, as is true in nearly all scientific fields, were the work both of a few talented, insightful individuals and a large number of hard-working, dedicated, and skilled people who over time compiled key information that contributed to the whole. We should all keep in mind these aspects of discovery as we seek to make our contributions. We must be stimulated by healthy competition, but avoid overly competitive or rancorous activities. We must enjoy the human stories as well as the science, and appreciate the privilege of participating in the enterprise of science.

Acknowledgements

Carol Balsamo of the Endocrine Society kindly removed a photo of P.E. Smith from the office wall and scanned it for inclusion into this article. Mike Reid, Director of the Kansas University History Project, provided information. Sarah Myers of the DePauw University Archives kindly provided the photo of Bennet Allen. Nae Saeteurn and Penny Jennings of UCLA briefly borrowed photos of John Pierce from walls at that institution, which enabled me to prepare the photo of John Pierce.

Disclosure Statement

James Magner is an employee of Genzyme, a Sanofi company, the manufacturer of recombinant human TSH. He is also a shareholder of Sanofi.

References

1 Allen BM: Extirpation of the hypophysis and thyroid glands of *Rana pipiens.* Anat Rec 1916;11:486.
2 Smith PE: The effect of hypophysectomy in the early embryo upon the growth and development of the frog. Anat Rec 1916;11:57–64.
3 Smith PE: Experimental ablation of the hypophysis in the frog embryo. Science 1916;44:280–282.
4 Allen BM: The results of extirpation of the anterior lobe of the hypophysis and of the thyroid in *Rana pipiens* larvae. Science 1916;44:755–758.
5 Allen BM: Effects of the extirpation of the anterior lobe of the hypophysis of *Rana pipiens.* Biol Bull 1917;32:117–130.
6 Allen BM: Experiments in the transplantation of the hypophysis of adult *Rana pipiens* to tadpoles. Science 1920;52:274–276.
7 Smith PE: Relations of the activity of the pituitary and thyroid glands. Harvey Lect Ser 1931;25:129–143.

8 Medvei VC: The Americans; in Medvei VC (ed): The History of Clinical Endocrinology. Carnforth, Parthenon, 1993, pp 275–305.

9 Pierce JG: Chemistry of thyroid-stimulating hormone; in Handbook of Physiology. Washington, American Physiological Society, 1974, section 7, vol 4, Knobil E, Sawyer WH (eds): The Pituitary Gland and Its Neuroendocrine Control, part 2. Bethesda, pp 79–101.

10 Puett D, Iles R, Huhtaniemi I: Tribute to a pioneer in the glycoprotein hormone field, Dr. John G. Pierce. Mol Cell Endocrinol 2010; 329:3.

11 Wondisford FE, Radovick S, Moates JM, Usala SJ, Weintraub BD: Isolation and characterization of the human thyrotropin β-subunit gene. J Biol Chem 1988;263:12538–12542.

12 Guidon PT, Whitfield GK, Porti D, Kourides IA: The human thyrotropin β-subunit gene differs in 5′ structure from murine TSH β genes. DNA 1988;7:691–699.

13 Tatsumi K, Hayashizaki Y, Hiraoka Y, Miyai K, Matsubara K: The structure of the human thyrotropin β-subunit gene. Gene 1988;73: 489–497.

14 Watson J: The Double Helix. New York, Atheneum, 1968.

15 Hellman H: Great Feuds in Science. New York, Wiley, 1998.

16 Meyers MA: Prize Fight: the Race and the Rivalry to be the First in Science. New York, Palgrave Macmillan, 2012.

17 Wade N: The Nobel Duel. New York, Anchor Press/Doubleday, 1981.

18 Parmentier M, Libert F, Maenhaut C, Lefort G, Perret J, Van Sande J, Dumont JE, Vassart G: Molecular cloning of the thyrotropin receptor. Science 1989;246:1620–1622.

19 Nagayama Y, Kaufman KD, Seto P, Rapoport B: Molecular cloning, sequence and functional expression of the cDNA of the human thyrotropin receptor. Biochem Biophys Res Commun 1989;165:1184–1190.

20 Libert F, Lefort A, Gerard C, Parmentier M, Perret J, Ludgate M, Dumont JE, Vassart G: Cloning, sequencing and expression of the human thyrotropin (TSH) receptor: evidence for binding of autoantibodies. Biochem Biophys Res Commun 1989;165:1250–1255.

21 Sawin CT: Defining thyroid hormone: its nature and control; in McCann SM (ed): Endocrinology, People and Ideas. Bethesda, American Physiological Society, 1988.

22 Crowe JS, Cushing HW, Homans J: Hypophysectomy. Bull Johns Hopkins Hosp 1910;21: 126–169.

23 Adler L: Metamorphosestudien an Batrachierlarven. 1. Extirpation endokriner Drüsen. 2. Extirpation der Hypophyse. Arch Entwickl Mech Org 1914;39:21–45.

24 Aron M: Action de la prehypophyse sur le thyroide chez le cobaye. O R Soc Biol (Paris) 1929;102:682.

25 Loeb L, Bassett RB: Effects of hormones of anterior pituitary on thyroid gland in the guinea pig. Proc Soc Exp Biol and Med 1929;26:860.

26 Jansen S, Loesser A: Die Wirkung des Hypophysenvorderlappens auf die Schilddrüse. Arch Exp Pathol Pharmakol 1939;163:517–529.

27 Greep RO: Separation of a thyrotropin from the gonadotrophic substances of the pituitary. Am J Physiol 1935;110:692.

28 White A, Ciereszko LS: Purification of the thyrotropic hormone of the anterior pituitary. J Biol Chem 1941;140:139.

29 Bates RW, Garrison MM, Howard TB: Extraction of thyrotrophin from pituitary glands, mouse pituitary tumors, and blood plasma by percolation. Endocrinology 1959; 65:7–17.

30 Hoskins RG: The thyroid-pituitary apparatus as a servo (feedback) mechanism. J Clin Endocrinol 1949;9:1429.

31 Heideman ML Jr: Purification of bovine thyrotropic hormone by ion exchange chromatography. Endocrinology 1953;53:640–652.

32 Crigler JF Jr, Waugh DF: Use of the carboxylic cation exchange resin IRC-50 in the purification of thyrotropic hormone (TSH). J Am Chem Soc 1955;77:4407–4408.

33 Condliffe PG, Bates RW: Chromatography of thyrotropin on diethylaminoethyl-cellulose. Arch Biochem Biophys 1957;68:229–230.

34 Condliffe PG, Bates RW, Fraps RM: Fractionation of bovine thyrotrophin and luteinizing hormone on cellulose ion exchange columns. Biochim Biophys Acta 1959;34:430–438.

35 Papkoff H, Samy TSA: Isolation and partial characterization of the polypeptide chains of ovine interstitial cell-stimulating hormone. Biochim Biophys Acta 1967;147:175–177.

36 Liao T-H, Pierce JG: The presence of a common type of subunit in bovine thyroid-stimulating hormone and luteinizing hormones. J Biol Chem 1970;245:3275–3281.

37 Liao T-H, Pierce JG: The primary structure of bovine thyrotropin. 2. The amino acid sequences of the reduced, S-carboxymethyl α and β chains. J Biol Chem 1971;246:850–865.

38 Fiddes JC, Goodman HM: The gene encoding the common alpha subunit of the four human glycoprotein hormones. J Mol Appl Genet 1981;1:3.

39 Chin WW, Carr FE, Burnside J, Darling DS: Thyroid hormone regulation of thyrotropin gene expression. Recent Prog Horm Res 1993; 48:393–414.

40 Magner JA: Thyroid-stimulating hormone: biosynthesis, cell biology, and bioactivity. Endocr Rev 1990;11:354–385.

41 Grossman M, Weintraub BD, Szkudlinski MW: Novel insights into the molecular mechanisms of human thyrotropin action: structural, physiological, and therapeutic implications for the glycoprotein hormone family. Endocr Rev 1997;18:476–501.

Genzyme Thyroid Remnant Ablation Follow-up Studies

Elisei et al. and Bartenstein et al.

I moved from academia to industry in February, 1997 when I started at Bayer Corporation in West Haven, CT. Although I loved being a university professor, the loss of my basic research funding required me to work in other roles as an endocrinologist to justify my faculty salary. The low reimbursement amounts for endocrinology clinic visits (as compared with cardiology, for example) would cause me to have essentially 100% of my time devoted to patient care at the university. I really enjoyed caring for patients, but I was certain that I was a scientist first and a physician second, so I wanted to spend only a maximum of about 50% of my working time seeing patients. That just was not feasible. I elected to change jobs and try instead to do clinical research in the pharmaceutical world.

Things went well at Bayer. In 1997 I wrote formal scientific company reports (Clinical Study Reports) for two large Phase 3 studies of type 2 diabetes patients. I then worked with the external investigators to publish those data: Rosenstock et al. Diabetes Care 1998; 21: 2050-2055 and Kelley et al. Diabetes Care 1998; 21:2056-2061. I also was involved in numerous early development programs, and assisted with clinical trials of Levitra. I then was recruited in 2003 to move to Cambridge, MA to work at Genzyme on clinical projects related to thyroid disease, which was more aligned with my research background, especially since Genzyme manufactured recombinant human TSH (rhTSH).

During 2003 and 2004 I evaluated clinical data related to use of rhTSH in certain patients with very advanced thyroid cancer, or other special clinical circumstances. With collaborators I published that data: Robbins R, Driedger A, Magner J, and the Thyrogen Compassionate Use Investigator Group. Recombinant human TSH-assisted radioiodine therapy for patients with metastatic thyroid cancer who could not elevate endogenous TSH or be withdrawn from thyroxine. Thyroid 2006; 16(11):1121-1130. I also worked on clinical studies about use of rhTSH in a benign thyroid disease, and published some of that work. Additional opportunities arose to assist publishing clinical data from an ongoing thyroid cancer clinical registry.

But my most important work in that era had to do with clinical studies testing use of rhTSH with oral radioactive iodine to achieve ablation of the thyroid remnant left behind in the neck after near-total thyroidectomy. I wrote the Clinical Study Report for a global study, and assisted getting data ready for publication that appeared in 2006. The Food and Drug Administration (FDA), however, was not yet quite convinced that Thyrogen should be approved for this new clinical indication. FDA instructed Genzyme that additional follow-up of patients treated in the prior study would be required before any new language could be added to Thyrogen's product label in the USA. So our team at Genzyme wrote a follow-up clinical protocol, and we engaged the investigators who had participated in the prior study to attempt to reexamine each of the treated patients to collect certain measurements. The clinical study data were limited but proved to be adequate. The data were submitted formally to the FDA, which then granted a new indication for use of Thyrogen in the USA for thyroid remnant ablation. This regulatory approval allowed many patients routinely to avoid severe hypothyroidism during clinical treatment for their cancer. I worked with the external investigators to write up these clinical data, which appeared as the Elisei et al. paper reproduced in this book.

During other later regulatory interactions with the European Medicines Agency (EMA) in London, I made the case on Genzyme's behalf to further update the Thyrogen European product label to allow for Thyrogen treatment of a broader range of thyroid cancer patients, including the unusual patients with large, locally invasive tumors – so-called T4 patients. As I stood before a committee known as the CHMP, I was told that Genzyme must do a prospective randomized study of scores of T4 patients in order to get this desired label language. After a few seconds of quick thinking, I responded from the podium that since T4 patients made up only about 5% of newly diagnosed thyroid cancer patients, it likely would take a decade for such a difficult study to achieve enrollment – but I wanted to offer the CHMP a counter-proposal. Could Genzyme do a retrospective data collection study at multiple European hospitals and thereby in only 2 years collect 10 years of past patient data? I assured the CHMP that creative attempts would be made to reduce bias regarding what patients were entered into the retrospective data base. After a few minutes further discussion, the CHMP agreed with my counter-proposal. But then I was on the hook to somehow make that happen. The Genzyme statistician and I designed a protocol that avoided need for patient informed consent (on the basis that patients that did poorly with the treatment would have died or become incapacitated, so would not be included in the data base, biasing the data). Our study design also had a novel way of sorting patient records in a structured manner to reduce the ability of investigators to pick and choose which past patients would be placed into the data base – this also helped to reduce bias. Finally, we applied a sophisticated statistical technique in the analysis making use of propensity scores, a tool that attempts to improve the quality of retrospectively collected data so as to more closely approach the gold standard of a prospective randomized clinical trial. The data were successfully collected and summarized for the EMA, which allowed the favorable language that had been granted in advance to remain in the European Thyrogen label. The investigators and I then published the clinical trial data as Bartenstein et al., reproduced in this book.

THYROID
Volume 24, Number 3, 2014
© Mary Ann Liebert, Inc.
DOI: 10.1089/thy.2013.0157

High-Risk Patients with Differentiated Thyroid Cancer T4 Primary Tumors Achieve Remnant Ablation Equally Well Using rhTSH or Thyroid Hormone Withdrawal

Peter Bartenstein,[1] Elisa Caballero Calabuig,[2] Carlo Ludovico Maini,[3] Renzo Mazzarotto,[4]
M. Angustias Muros de Fuentes,[5] Thorsten Petrich,[6] Fernando José Cravo Rodrigues,[7]
Juan Antonio Vallejo Casas,[8] Federica Vianello,[9] Michela Basso,[9] Marcelino Gómez Balaguer,[10]
Alexander Haug,[1] Fabio Monari,[4] Raquel Sánchez Vañó,[2] Rosa Sciuto,[3] and James Magner[11]

Background: Few data exist on using thyrotropin alfa (recombinant human thyroid-stimulating hormone [rhTSH]) with radioiodine for thyroid remnant ablation of patients who have T4 primary tumors (invasion beyond the thyroid capsule).

Methods: A retrospective chart review protocol at nine centers in Europe was set up with special waiver of need for informed consent, along with a careful procedure to avoid selection bias when enrolling patients into the database. Data on 144 eligible patients with T4 tumors were collected (T4, N0–1, M0–1; mean age 49.7 years; 65% female; 88% papillary cancer). All had received ^{131}I remnant ablation following TSH stimulation with rhTSH or thyroid hormone withdrawal (THW) since January 2000 (rhTSH $n=74$, THW $n=70$). The primary endpoint was based on evaluation of diagnostic radioiodine scan thyroid bed uptake more than six months after the ablation procedure, while stimulated serum Tg was a secondary endpoint. Safety was evaluated within 30 days after rhTSH or ^{131}I.

Results: Successful ablation judged by scan was achieved in 65/70 (92.9%) of rhTSH and in 61/67 (91.0%) of THW patients; the success rates were comparable, since noninferiority criteria were met. Although some patients in the initial cohort had tumor in cervical nodes and metastases, considering all evaluable patients regardless of various serum anti-Tg antibody assessments, the stimulated Tg was <2 ng/mL in 48/70 (68.6%) and 39/67 (58.2%) in rhTSH and THW groups respectively; if patients with anti-Tg antibody levels >30 IU/mL were excluded, the stimulated Tg was <2 ng/mL in 42/62 (67.7%) and 37/64 (57.8%) respectively. No serious adverse events occurred within the 30-day window after ablation.

Conclusions: Use of rhTSH as preparation for thyroid remnant ablation in patients with T4 primary tumors achieved a rate of ablation success that was high and noninferior to the rate seen after THW, and rhTSH was well tolerated.

Introduction

AN ELEVATED THYROTROPIN (TSH) level in the blood is essential for effective thyroid remnant ablation. Historically, TSH has been elevated in these patients to allow remnant ablation by using thyroid hormone withdrawal (THW).

Thyrotropin alfa (recombinant human thyroid-stimulating hormone [rhTSH], Thyrogen; Genzyme, Cambridge, MA) was developed to provide TSH elevation to stimulate ^{131}I uptake, thyroglobulin (Tg) secretion, or both while sparing patients the consequent hypothyroid morbidity and quality-of-life impairment from several weeks of THW (1–9). In the

The senior principal investigators are listed in alphabetical order, followed by secondary investigators.
[1]Department of Nuclear Medicine, University of Munich, Munich, Germany.
Departments of [2]Nuclear Medicine and [10]Endocrinology, University Hospital Dr. Peset, Valencia, Spain.
[3]Division of Nuclear Medicine, Regina Elena National Cancer Institute, Rome, Italy.
[4]Hematology-Oncology Department, Radiotherapy Section, S. Orsola-Malpighi Hospital, Bologna, Italy.
[5]Nuclear Medicine Department, Virgen de las Nieves University Hospital, Granada, Spain.
[6]Department of Nuclear Medicine, Hannover University School of Medicine, Hannover, Germany.
[7]Endocrinology Service, Portuguese Institute of Oncology of Coimbra Francisco Gentil, Coimbra, Portugal.
[8]Nuclear Medicine Service, University Hospital Reina Sofía de Córdoba, Córdoba, Andalucia, Spain.
[9]Department of Radiotherapy, Institute of Oncology Veneto-IRCCS, Padua, Italy.
[11]Global Medical Affairs, Endocrinology, Genzyme, Cambridge, Massachusetts.

United States, rhTSH was approved for diagnostic use in 1998, and for use for remnant ablation in 2007; these two indications were approved in Europe in 2000 and 2005 respectively. The remnant ablation indication was formally amended by regulators in Europe in 2009 to extend the indication from patients with "low-risk thyroid cancer," a term poorly defined at that time, to all patients with well-differentiated thyroid cancer without distant metastases (European Medicines Agency Web site: www.emea.europa.eu under Thyrogen decisions, November 2009). This same indication for use of rhTSH for remnant ablation in all types of patients with well-differentiated thyroid cancer who are not M1 has been adopted by the Food and Drug Administration in the rhTSH package insert. These regulatory steps were aided by data in published patient series showing that successful remnant ablation was achieved using rhTSH in patients with larger primary tumors, tumor-node-metastases (TNM) classed T3 and T4, with presence of cervical nodes, and even with distant metastases (10–12). Subsequently, more data about successful remnant ablation using rhTSH along with only 30 mCi ^{131}I in low-risk patients but also in patients having cervical node involvement (13,14), and primary tumors classed T3 (14) added useful information. But published data about ablation success using rhTSH in patients with T4 primary tumors were not extensive.

Such T4 patients are rare (approximately 5% of all thyroid cancers), and are the most locally advanced stage of well-differentiated thyroid cancer. T4 patients have tumor extension beyond the thyroid capsule with invasion into surrounding local structures. In addition, these patients may or may not have involved neck nodes and distant metastases, elements that could affect the interpretation of stimulated serum Tg levels, for example when using serum Tg to assess success of remnant ablation. The subset of T4 tumors comprises a heterogeneous population, which tends to result in individualized patient treatment based on the disease progression and medical situation.

The primary objective of this chart review protocol was to demonstrate noninferior thyroid remnant first ablation success (based on historical diagnostic whole body scan [WBS] records) using rhTSH plus ^{131}I compared to THW plus ^{131}I in patients with T4 tumors. Secondary objectives were to assess remnant ablation efficacy of the rhTSH versus THW methods in such patients based on historical stimulated Tg levels, and also based on other historical records beyond the scan and laboratory reports (such as comments in clinic progress notes), and to explore the safety profile of rhTSH in this setting.

Methods

The study was designed and funded by Genzyme. The investigators collected data from patient charts, the data were summarized, and statistical analyses were performed by Covance. Covance and Genzyme wrote the final study report and this manuscript with input from the investigators. This study was a retrospective, noninterventional study comparing the thyroid remnant ablation success of rhTSH (thyrotropin alfa; Genzyme) plus ^{131}I versus THW plus ^{131}I in patients with T4 tumors. The study consisted of reviewing and recording necessary efficacy and safety information from historical patient records. As this was a retrospective study, no investigational product was administered, and Good

Clinical Practice guidelines did not apply. Applicable local and national regulations were followed.

Eligible patients were thyroid cancer patients (living or deceased) who had undergone a near-total or total thyroidectomy of a well-differentiated T4 tumor on or after January 1, 2000. The chart reviews were conducted between May and August 2012. A T4 tumor was defined as a primary tumor of any size that extended beyond the thyroid capsule (referred to as TNM classification T4, N0–1, or M0–1). Eligible patients must have received their first remnant ablation attempt using THW or rhTSH (0.9 mg intramuscularly [IM] on two consecutive days) followed by high ablative activity of ^{131}I (≥ 28 mCi or ≥ 1.036 GBq).

Each site recorded study data into an electronic case report form (eCRF). There was no monitoring of data collected on the eCRF, although the site could be contacted (to seek clarification about missing, incomplete, or unclear data) by telephone or electronic communication to maintain patients' confidentiality.

Waiver of informed consent

This study was approved by the Institutional Ethics Committees of all involved sites. There was also approval of a waiver for the requirement of obtaining patient informed consent, a decision supported by the following rationale. First, there was no physical risk to the patients. This study consisted of retrospectively reviewing and recording necessary efficacy and safety information from historical patient records. Second, collection of the informed consent would make the study unfeasible due to unavailability of current addresses. Some eligible patients may have been seriously ill, very old, or have died. Not including these patients in the study would lead to a possible bias of only including patients who were not as ill. Third, not obtaining an informed consent would not adversely affect patients' rights and welfare. The information taken from patient charts did not include identifiable information.

Procedures to avoid enrollment bias

Historical records were reviewed by investigators in a systematic fashion to identify eligible patients. Each patient record reviewed but found not to be eligible was entered into the eCRF as a screen failure, and included selected limited demographic characteristics and listing of the inclusion/exclusion criteria not met. Each patient record reviewed and found to be eligible was entered into the eCRF, and included limited demographic characteristics, information about the patient's first thyroid remnant ablation treatment, and data related to ablation success or failure.

To avoid bias when looking at charts to select patients for inclusion into the study, investigators followed a systematic process, as follows:

1. Make a list of all T4-type patients fulfilling the study's inclusion and exclusion criteria.
2. Split the list into two lists, by treatment group (rhTSH vs. THW).
3. Order each list by date of ^{131}I ablation (most recent date on top).

Patient selection for enrollment and entry into the eCRF then occurred as follows:

1. Ensure patient source data are available for the first several patients at the top of each list to make it easier to

be able to select patients consecutively to complete the eCRFs.

2. Starting with one of the two lists, enter the first patient in the list into the eCRF.
3. Moving to the other list, enter the first patient on that list into the eCRF. At this point, the number of patients in the two treatment groups (rhTSH and THW) is balanced.
4. Descending down the first list, enter the next patient from the list into the eCRF.
5. Returning to the other list, enter the next patient into the eCRF.
6. Repeat the above steps until any one of the following conditions are met: (i) the rhTSH list is exhausted of eligible patients; (ii) the THW list is exhausted of eligible patients; (iii) 20 eligible patients have been entered onto the eCRF.

After written approval from Genzyme, recruitment could be continued beyond the initial number of patients to a new target number for enrollment. Because there was an enrollment cap due to budget limitations, this "stop at 20" rule gave each institution time to review charts and enter patients into the database, allowing for a broader multinational patient sample.

Number of patients planned and analyzed

Concerning enrollment at all centers, chart reviews to identify eligible patients were planned to continue until one of the following scenarios was achieved: (i) 63 or more eligible patients were enrolled who had undergone ablation by THW *and* 63 or more eligible patients were enrolled who had undergone ablation with appropriate use of rhTSH (0.9 mg IM on two consecutive days), *or* (ii) a maximum of 225 total eligible patients were enrolled altogether in the study.

Inclusion and exclusion criteria

Historical records from patients who met all of the following criteria were eligible for inclusion in this retrospective evaluation: male or female patients living or deceased, aged 18 years or older at the time of first ablation for thyroid cancer; diagnosed with a well-differentiated T4 tumor (a primary tumor of any size that extends beyond the thyroid capsule; TNM classification T4, N0-1, M0-1), excluding unusual histological types such as oncocytic (Hürthle cell carcinoma), tall cell, sclerosing, or cribriform thyroid cancers; undergone a near-total or total thyroidectomy on or after January 1, 2000; undergone first ablation of thyroid remnants with high activity ^{131}I (≥ 28 mCi or ≥ 1.036 GBq); undergone first ^{131}I remnant ablation using either rhTSH (0.9 mg IM on two consecutive days) or THW stimulation, excluding nonstandard rhTSH regimens; historical records available confirming ablation results by (i) diagnostic WBS (DxWBS) using a small (≥ 2 mCi or 74 MBq) activity of iodine ^{131}I (or ^{123}I) performed at least six months after administration of the first ablation activity of ^{131}I, and/or (ii) Tg measured at least six months after administration of the first ablation activity of ^{131}I.

Historical records from patients who met any of the following criteria were excluded from this retrospective evaluation: received propylthiouracil, methimazole, vitamins, or supplements containing kelp or iodine (taking a multivitamin that does not contain iodine or kelp is acceptable); received medications that significantly affect iodine handling such as high-dose corticosteroids, high-dose diuretics, or lithium in the 45 days before administration of first ablative activity of ^{131}I; received any iodine-containing contrast agents within three months prior to first ablative activity of ^{131}I administered; or used amiodarone within the two years prior to first ablative activity of ^{131}I administered.

Efficacy assessments

Primary endpoint. This was the first ablation success rate by DxWBS using a small activity (≥ 2 mCi or 74 MBq) of iodine ^{131}I (or ^{123}I) performed at least six months after administration of first ablation activity of ^{131}I. Success was defined as historical records with no visible uptake in the thyroid bed, an uptake in the thyroid bed of $< 0.1\%$ of the applied activity, or a trace amount. The word "trace" need not be present in the chart as long as the word used has the same meaning.

Secondary endpoints. These were (i) first ablation success based on stimulated Tg level of < 2 ng/mL performed at least six months after administration of first ablation activity of ^{131}I; and (ii) first ablation success based on other historical records (such as comments in clinic progress notes) performed at least six months after administration of first ablation activity of ^{131}I.

Safety evaluation

All serious adverse events (SAEs) within the safety review period were recorded on the eCRF. Events within the safety review period were defined as events that started within 30 days after rhTSH administration for rhTSH patients, or within 30 days after ablative ^{131}I activity for THW patients.

Statistical methods

Efficacy. The primary efficacy variable—ablation success rate—was analyzed by means of a generalized linear model (GLM) to compare the rhTSH and THW groups. The model was adjusted for the following covariates using a covariate selection process: center, N1 status (N1 vs. not N1), age, sex, and year of treatment. Covariate adjustment was performed by fitting each covariate separately to the model and retaining those covariates with $p \leq 0.2$. The retained covariates were included in the model together, and those with $p \leq 0.1$ were kept in the final model. The result used for inference was the confidence interval (CI) of the risk difference (rhTSH–THW), which was compared with the prespecified noninferiority margin of -0.2. If the lower bound of the confidence interval was > -0.2, noninferiority was concluded. The primary analysis was conducted on the full analysis set (FAS), which consists of all patients who were treated and who received a DxWBS to assess ablation success. Two supportive sensitivity analyses were conducted. The first utilized a simple GLM that did not adjust for covariates. The second utilized a GLM that adjusted for propensity score conducted on the propensity set (PS). The PS is defined as those patients in the FAS retained after the following propensity trimming criteria were applied. Propensity score was first estimated for each patient in the FAS using logistic regression. The logistic regression modeled the distribution of treatment (rhTSH, THW as the outcome variable) given the following covariates: center, N1 status (N1 vs. not N1), age, sex, and year of treatment. The propensity score was then ordered, ignoring treatment group. Subjects in the THW group with propensity scores higher than the maximum propensity score in the rhTSH group were removed from analysis. Similarly, subjects in the THW group with propensity scores lower than the minimum propensity score in the rhTSH group were removed. The patients remaining after this trimming process constitute the PS. The propensity score was used to balance the covariates in the two groups, and therefore reduce the bias in the comparison of two treatment groups in a nonrandomized study.

The secondary efficacy parameters were ablation success rate based on Tg level of $<2 \, \text{ng/mL}$ and ablation success rate based on other historical records, and were analyzed in the same way as for the primary efficacy parameter.

Sample size. Although this was a retrospective study, a sample size calculation was performed to provide an understanding of what power could be expected if a randomized study was conducted. This included the following assumptions:

- The success rate for THW under the null hypothesis. Success levels between 60% and 90% were modeled. Historically across a number of studies, the rate of ablation success has been around 80%. More recent studies comparing rhTSH to THW have seen ablation success rates around 90% or higher. These studies have generally not included T4 patients, and based on clinical experience, a value of 80% success was more realistic and assumed to be the rate for THW.
- Noninferiority margin. This was a heterogeneous population. A value of 20% was proposed.
- $\alpha = 0.05$.
- 80% power. It was determined that a sample size of 63 patients per treatment arm would provide 80% power, while 84 patients per treatment arm would provide 90% power.

Results

A total of 153 patients were entered into the study database. Nine of these patients did not meet all eligibility criteria and were therefore excluded from the study populations.

Of the 144 eligible patients in the treated/safety set, 74 received rhTSH plus ^{131}I administration (rhTSH group) and 70 received THW plus ^{131}I administration (THW group). Demographics are presented in Table 1. The mean age was 49.7 years, 65% female, with 88% papillary cancer and 12% follicular cancer. Demographics of patients in the two treatment groups were similar, although more patients in the THW group had involved cervical nodes, and the mean amount of radioiodine used for ablation was slightly lower in the rhTSH group (107.8 mCi) than in the THW group (128.6 mCi), $p = 0.0003$. Seven of these 144 patients did not receive a DxWBS for detecting ablation success, resulting in 137 (95.1%) eligible patients in the FAS. Of these patients, 70 received rhTSH and 67 received THW. One patient who was in the THW group had a calculated propensity score lower than the minimum propensity score in the rhTSH group and was therefore removed from the PS. This resulted in 136

(94.4%) of originally eligible patients in the PS, with 70 patients in the rhTSH group and 66 patients in the THW group.

Efficacy results

A summary of efficacy results is presented in Table 2. For the prespecified primary efficacy objective, 65/70 (92.9%) of rhTSH and 61/67 (91.0%) of THW patients had successful remnant ablation, defined as no uptake or only trace uptake in the thyroid bed on the DxWBS done more than six months later. The risk difference (rhTSH–THW) was 0.034 [CI−0.043, 0.112]. The covariate sex ($p = 0.054$) was retained in the final model following the covariate selection process. As the lower bound value of the CI for the risk difference was > -0.2, noninferiority was successfully met ($p = 0.386$), showing that thyroid remnant first ablation success of rhTSH plus ^{131}I was noninferior to THW plus ^{131}I in patients with T4 tumor based on historical DxWBS records.

The results from the first sensitivity analysis without adjusting for covariates were similar to the primary efficacy analysis. The risk difference (rhTSH–THW) was 0.018 [CI−0.073, 0.109] and $p = 0.697$. The results from the second sensitivity analysis adjusting for the covariate propensity score were also similar to the primary efficacy analysis. The risk difference was 0.017 with CI [−0.071, 0.105] and $p = 0.706$. The p-value for the covariate propensity score was 0.322. The results from the two sensitivity analyses demonstrated that any potential covariate imbalances between treatment groups were minimal and that the choice of covariates had minimal effect, supporting the primary efficacy endpoint result that rhTSH plus ^{131}I was noninferior to THW plus ^{131}I in patients with T4 tumor based on historical DxWBS records.

Because different types of anti-Tg antibody tests (or other such tests) were used at the different centers over the years, as a "first look" at ablation success based on the stimulated Tg result, no patient was excluded from the analysis because of anti-Tg antibody status. We suspected that tumor in neck nodes or in distant metastases also could confound this analysis of Tg values. Thyroid remnant first ablation success based on stimulated Tg level of $<2 \, \text{ng/mL}$ (done more than six months after the ablation procedure) was achieved in 48/70 (68.6%) and 39/67 (58.2%) patients in the rhTSH and THW groups respectively. The risk difference was 0.036, with CI [-0.117, 0.188] and $p = 0.645$.

A subgroup analysis was performed for the secondary endpoint of first ablation success based on historical stimulated Tg levels, excluding those with anti-Tg antibody level $>30 \, \text{U/mL}$, a cut-off value that had been adopted clinically at several centers, although the authors do not vouch for the validity of this approach. Removal of these patients' data resulted in 62 patients in the rhTSH group and 64 patients in the THW group for this subgroup analysis. Of these patients, 42/62 (67.7%) of rhTSH patients and 37/64 (57.8%) of THW patients had successful remnant ablation, defined as $<2 \, \text{ng/mL}$ serum Tg. The risk difference was 0.028, with CI (−0.130, 0.186] and $p = 0.730$. The covariates regional node status ($p = 0.002$) and year of treatment ($p = 0.020$) were retained in the model following the covariate selection process. Thus, among patients with anti-Tg antibody level $\leq 30 \, \text{U/mL}$, ablation success results were similar to those seen in the overall Tg analysis. Although these data clearly are confounded, for example by tumor in cervical nodes, had the ablation success

TABLE 1. DEMOGRAPHY AND BASELINE VARIABLES (ALL PATIENTS TREATED/SAFETY SET)

	rhTSH (n=74)	THW (n=70)	p-Value
Age (years)[a]			
n	74	70	
Mean±SD	50.6±17.3	48.7±13.7	0.4698
Median (min/max)	50.5 (20/86)	46.5 (20/78)	
Sex, n (%)			
n	74	70	
Female	50 (67.6)	44 (62.9)	0.6016
Male	24 (32.4)	26 (37.1)	
Histological tumor type, n (%)			
n	74	70	
Papillary thyroid cancer	64 (86.5)	63 (90.0)	0.6093
Follicular thyroid cancer	10 (13.5)	7 (10.0)	
Other thyroid cancer	0 (0.0)	0 (0.0)	
Tumor node classification, n (%)			
n	74	70	
N0	27 (36.5)	14 (20.0)	0.0444
N1	33 (44.6)	45 (64.3)	
Nx	14 (18.9)	11 (15.7)	
Tumor metastasis classification, n (%)			
n	74	70	
M0	30 (40.5)	28 (40.0)	0.9800
M1	5 (6.8)	5 (7.1)	
Mx	39 (52.7)	37 (52.9)	
Length of time between confirmed well-differentiated T4 tumor diagnosis and thyroidectomy (days)[b]			
n	74	70	
Mean±SD	5.8±8.5	5.8±8.1	0.9504
Median (min/max)	2.0 (0/37)	2.0 (0/40)	
Length of time between thyroidectomy and rhTSH use for ablation preparation (days)[c]			
n	74		
Mean±SD	90.1±70.7		
Median (min/max)	78.5 (6/508)		
Length of time between thyroidectomy and first remnant ablation with high activity ^{131}I (days)[d]			
n	74	70	
Mean±SD	92.1±70.7	87.7±59.6	0.6887
Median (min/max)	80.5 (8/510)	76.0 (14/245)	
Activity of ^{131}I used for first remnant ablation for each unit type (mCi)[e]			
n	74	70	
Mean±SD	107.8±22.5	128.6±40.3	0.0003
Median (min/max)	100.0 (56/205)	113.7 (50/300)	

The denominator for percentages is the number of patients in the treated/safety set for the relevant treatment group.
[a]Calculated as (date of confirmed well-differentiated T4 tumor diagnosis−date of birth+1)/365.25.
[b]Calculated as date of thyroidectomy−date of confirmed well-differentiated T4 tumor diagnosis.
[c]Calculated as date of first injection of rhTSH−date of thyroidectomy.
[d]Calculated as date of first remnant ablation with high activity ^{131}I−date of thyroidectomy.
[e]Units of Megabecquerels (MBq) were standardized into mCi by multiplying by 0.027; units of Gigabecquerels (GBq) were standardized into mCi by multiplying by 27.
rhTSH, recombinant human thyroid-stimulating hormone (rhTSH) and ^{131}I administration; THW, thyroid hormone withdrawal and ^{131}I administration.

rates (using stimulated Tg as the criterion) in the two treatment groups been very different, this would have been problematic.

Thyroid remnant first ablation success based on other (nonscan and non-Tg) historical records (such as comments in clinic progress notes) was achieved in 57/70 (81.4%) and 57/67 (85.1%) patients in the rhTSH and THW groups respectively. The risk difference was 0.040 with CI [−0.089, 0.168] and p=0.544. Thus, data collected for the prespecified secondary efficacy endpoints were consistent with the primary efficacy results. Other efficacy variables were summarized descriptively by treatment group for the FAS and showed similar trends between rhTSH and THW for: (i) frequency and percentage of patients with DxWBS showing similar amounts of regional or distant metastases, (ii) stimulated and nonstimulated Tg levels, and (iii) length of time between first remnant ablation with ^{131}I and DxWBS. However, an increased level of anti-Tg antibodies was observed in stimulated and nonstimulated samples in rhTSH patients compared to THW patients, and this remains without explanation.

TABLE 2. SUMMARY OF EFFICACY ENDPOINTS
(FULL ANALYSIS SET)

	rhTSH (n = 70)	THW (n = 67)	Total (n = 137)
DxWBS showing visible uptake in the thyroid bed,[a] n (%)			
n	70	67	137
No uptake seen	59 (84.3)	53 (79.1)	112 (81.8)
Significant uptake	5 (7.1)	6 (9.0)	11 (8.0)
Trace uptake	6 (8.6)	8 (11.9)	14 (10.2)
Clinicians' judgment of ablation success based on historical records,[b] n (%)			
n	70	67	137
Successful	57 (81.4)	57 (85.1)	114 (83.2)
Unsuccessful	13 (18.6)	10 (14.9)	23 (16.8)
Stimulated thyroglobulin levels,[c] n (%)			
n	70	65	135
<2 ng/mL	48 (68.6)	39 (58.2)	87 (63.5)
≥2 ng/mL	22 (31.4)	26 (38.8)	48 (35.0)

The denominator for percentages is the number of patients in the full analysis set for the relevant treatment group.

[a] Ablation success for the primary endpoint is defined as historical records of no visible uptake in the thyroid bed; an uptake in the thyroid bed (if measured quantitatively) of <0.1% of the applied activity; or a small amount of visible uptake seen in the thyroid bed but deemed to be a trace amount.

[b] Secondary efficacy variable: first ablation success based on historical records performed at least six months after administration of first ablation activity of [131]I.

[c] Secondary efficacy variable: first ablation success based on stimulated Tg level of <2 ng/mL performed at least six months after administration of first ablation activity of [131]I.

rhTSH, rhTSH and ^{131}I administration; THW, thyroid hormone withdrawal and ^{131}I administration.

Safety results

No treatment-related SAEs were identified, suggesting that both treatments are well tolerated and that rhTSH is not different from THW with regard to these safety endpoints.

Discussion

Limited data exist about use of rhTSH with ^{131}I for remnant ablation in patients with TNM T4 primary tumors because such differentiated thyroid cancers occur in less than 5% of newly diagnosed patients. This retrospective, noninterventional study was based on chart reviews at nine European centers to assess the efficacy and safety of rhTSH use in this setting. The study had some unusual features, including obtaining waivers so that informed consent was not required and use of a well-defined method to select which patients were entered into the study such that there would be minimal selection bias while at the same time keeping the two treatment arms numerically balanced.

The majority of the patients were middle-aged females with papillary cancers, and the treatment groups had similar distributions of sex, age, cancer type, and TNM classification. All rhTSH patients had consistent treatments, that is, two identical doses of rhTSH administered one day apart. There were more patients with involved cervical nodes in patients who received THW ($p = 0.0444$), and the activity of ^{131}I was greater in the THW treatment group ($p = 0.0003$). Slight differences in demographics and treatment history were not expected to impact the study results.

The primary efficacy analysis of first ablation success rate based on historical DxWBS in the FAS showed 92.9% of rhTSH patients and 91.0% of THW patients had successful remnant ablation, defined as "no uptake" or "trace uptake" in the thyroid bed on subsequent DxWBS (rhTSH was noninferior to THW). This major finding was also supported by the two sensitivity analyses, which showed that any potential covariate imbalances between treatment groups were minimal and that the choice of covariates in the primary model made no difference to the finding of noninferiority.

Thyroid remnant first ablation success based on stimulated Tg level of <2 ng/mL, or based on other historical records (e.g., comments in clinic progress notes), which were the prespecified secondary efficacy endpoints, also showed that the rhTSH treatment was noninferior to THW.

Although care was taken to avoid investigator bias regarding which patients were captured by the chart reviews, and a propensity analysis was performed, this retrospective study has limitations inherent in any nonrandomized series of patients who were not treated prospectively. The patients prescribed use of THW could have been viewed as more ill by their physicians and so were given a higher amount of ^{131}I for their ablation procedures, although we speculate that had the rhTSH patients received more ^{131}I, then there might have been criticism that the extra ^{131}I was favoring the ablation results seen after rhTSH. An additional weakness is that the study was very focused on testing just one hypothesis—assessing the ablation rates by nuclear medicine scanning after two methods of preparation for ablation. As the protocol was being designed, it became clear that over years, there was great variation in the types of Tg assays (and anti-Tg antibody assays and recovery tests) used at the institutions. Therefore, Tg data were collected but relegated to a secondary endpoint. Many other clinical care parameters (use of low-iodine diets, compliance with such diets, urine iodine measurements, etc.) were intentionally not collected in order to streamline the chart reviews and because a study of fewer than 150 patients was not expected to allow rigorous analyses of various treatment subgroups. For example, although 10 patients with M1 disease were enrolled and were equally divided between the two treatment groups, we did not collect data about the location of the metastases or their response to radioiodine treatment.

The first ablation success rates as assessed by scan in this study were high and similar to the rates seen in other published studies with thyroid tumors of a lower TNM status (4,13,14). In a randomized, controlled study ($n = 63$) by Pacini et al., designed to compare the efficacy and safety of rhTSH and THW in patients staged T0, T1, T2, and T4 with minor invasion of the thyroid capsule (with 90% of the patients staged T0–T2), N0–N1, and M0 or T0–T1, N1, and M0, it was found that successful ablation occurred in 100% of patients in both groups (4). In the HiLo study (14), 438 patients with differentiated thyroid cancer (tumor stage pT1–T3, Nx, N0 or N1, and M0) were randomized to one of four arms: 30 mCi or 100 mCi, each with either rhTSH or THW as preparation. Ablation success rates (as judged by both scan and stimulated Tg <2 ng/mL) were 85% in the group receiving 30 mCi versus 88.9% in the group receiving 100 mCi. The group that was prepared using rhTSH had a success rate of 87.1%, whereas patients prepared using THW had a success rate of 86.7%. The ESTIMABL study by Schlumberger *et al.* (13) compared the same four strategies for thyroid remnant ablation as evaluated in the HiLo study. Patients in ESTIMABL were, however, TNM stage pT1 <1 cm with N1, or pT1 >1–2 cm with either N0 or 1, or pT2 with N0, and for all these patient types, there could not be any distant metastases present. For the four groups, rhTSH+30 mCi, rhTSH+100 mCi, THW+30 mCi, and THW+100 mCi, the rates of ablation success (as judged by fulfilling both criteria of neck ultrasound and stimulated Tg<1 ng/mL by local assay) were 90%, 93%, 92%, and 94% respectively. No T4 patients had been included in the HiLo or ESTIMABL studies, but together with the present European chart review study of T4 patients, it appears that the success rates of remnant ablation using rhTSH or THW preparation are similar for patients with T0–4 primary tumor types of differentiated thyroid cancer.

No treatment-related SAEs were identified in patient records for either treatment, indicating that rhTSH plus ^{131}I and THW plus ^{131}I are not different from each other with regard to this safety endpoint.

In conclusion, this retrospective data collection indicates that preparation for thyroid remnant ablation using either rhTSH or THW is comparably effective and safe in such T4 type patients.

Acknowledgments

This study was a Genzyme-sponsored project, THYR04910, and was accomplished with the assistance of colleagues at Covance, including a skilled writer, Jeffrey Gardner. Funding for this study was provided entirely by Genzyme, a Sanofi company.

Author Disclosure Statement

J.A.V.C. received fees for speaking for Genzyme, Bayer, and Novartis Oncology, and participated in an advisory board for Covidien. J.M. is an employee of Genzyme. None of the remaining authors have anything to disclose.

References

1. Ladenson PW, Braverman LE, Mazzaferri EL, Brucker-Davis F, Cooper DS, Garber JR, Wondisford FE, Davies TF, DeGroot LJ, Daniels GH, Ross DS, Weintraub BD 1997 Comparison of administration of recombinant human thyrotropin with withdrawal of thyroid hormone for radioactive iodine scanning in patients with thyroid carcinoma. N Engl J Med **337:**888–896.

2. Haugen BR, Pacini F, Reiners C, Schlumberger M, Ladenson PW, Sherman SI, Cooper DS, Graham KE, Braverman LE, Skarulis MC, Davies TF, DeGroot LJ, Mazzaferri EL, Daniels GH, Ross DS, Luster M, Samuels MH, Becker DV, Maxon HR, Cavalieri RR, Spencer CA, McEllen K, Weintraub B, Ridgway EC 1999 A comparison of recombinant human thyrotropin and thyroid hormone withdrawal for the detection of thyroid remnant or cancer. J Clin Endocrinol Metab **84:**3877–3885.

3. Shroeder PR, Haugen BR, Pacini F, Reiners C, Schlumberger M, Sherman SI, Cooper DS, Schuff KG, Braverman LE, Skarulis MC, Davies TF, Mazzaferri EL, Daniels GH, Ross DS, Luster M, Samuels MH, Weintraub B, Ridgway EC, Ladenson PW 2006 A comparison of short-term changes in health-related quality of life in thyroid carcinoma patients undergoing diagnostic evaluation with recombinant human thyrotropin compared with thyroid hormone withdrawal. J Clin Endocrinol Metab **91:**878–884.

4. Pacini F, Ladenson PW, Schlumberger M, Driedger A, Luster M, Kloos RT, Sherman S, Haugen B, Corone C, molimaro E, Elisei R, Ceccarelli C, Pinchera A, Wahl RL, Leboulleux S, Ricard M, Yoo J, Busaidy NL, Delpassand E, Hänscheid H, Felbinger R, Lassmann M, Reiners C 2006 Radioiodine ablation of thyroid remnants after preparation with recombinant human thyrotropin in differentiated thyroid carcinoma: results of an international, randomized, controlled study. J Clin Endocrinol Metab **91:** 926–932.

5. Hänscheid H, Lassmann M, Luster M, Thomas SR, Pacini F, Ceccarelli C, Ladenson PW, Wahl RL, Schlumberger M, Ricard M, Driedger A, Kloos RT, Sherman SI, Haugen BR, Carriere V, Corone C, Reiners C 2006 Iodine biokinetics and dosimetry in radioiodine therapy of thyroid cancer: procedures and results of a prospective international controlled study of ablation after rhTSH or hormone withdrawal. J Nucl Med **47:**648–654.

6. Borget I, Remy H, Chevalier J, Ricard M, Allyn M, Schlumberger M, De Pouvourville G 2008 Length and cost of hospital stay of radioiodine ablation in thyroid cancer patients: comparison between preparation with thyroid hormone withdrawal and Thyrogen. Eur J Nucl Med Mol Imaging **35:**1457–1463.

7. Remy H, Borget I, Leboulleux S, Guilabert N, Lavielle F, Garsi J, Bournaud C, Gupta S, Schlumberger M, Ricard M 2008 ^{131}I effective half-life and dosimetry in thyroid cancer patients. J Nucl Med **49:**1445–1450.

8. Rosario PW, Borges MAR, Purisch S 2008 Preparation with recombinant human thyroid-stimulating hormone for thyroid remnant ablation with ^{131}I is associated with lowered radiotoxicity. J Nucl Med **49:**1776–1782.

9. Vallejo Casas JA, Mena Bares LM, Gálvez MA, Marlowe RJ, Latre Romero JM, Martinez-Paredes M 2011 Treatment room length-of-stay and patient throughput with radioiodine thyroid remnant ablation in differentiated thyroid cancer: comparison of thyroid-stimulating hormone stimulation methods. Nucl Med Commun **32:**840–846.

10. Tuttle RM, Brokhin M, Omry G, Martorella AJ, Larson SM, Grewal RK, Fleisher M, Robbins RJ 2008 Recombinant human TSH-assisted radioactive iodine remnant ablation achieves short-term clinical recurrence rates similar to those of traditional thyroid hormone withdrawal. J Nucl Med **49:**764–770.

11. Tuttle RM, Lopez N, Leboef R, Minkowitz SM, Grewal R, Brokhin M, Omry G, Larson S 2010 Radioactive iodine administered for thyroid remnant ablation following recombinant human thyroid stimulating hormone preparation also has an important adjuvant therapy function. Thyroid **20:**257–263.

12. Hugo J, Robenshtok E, Grewal R, Larson S, Tuttle RM 2012 Recombinant human thyroid stimulating hormone-assisted radioactive iodine remnant ablation in thyroid cancer patients at intermediate to high risk of recurrence. Thyroid **22:**1007–1015.

13. Schlumberger M, Catargi B, Borget I, Deandreis D, Zerdoud S, Bridji B, Bardet S, Leenhardt L, Bastie D, Schvartz C, Vera P, Morel O, Benisvy D, Bournaud C, Bonichon F, Dejax C, Toubert M-E, Leboulleux S, Ricard M, Benhamou E; Tumeurs de la Thyroide Refractaires Network for the Essai Stimulation Ablation Equivalence Trial

2012 Strategies of radioiodine ablation in patients with low-risk thyroid cancer. N Engl J Med **366:**1663–1673.

14. Mallick U, Harmer C, Yap B, Wadsley J, Clarke S, Moss L, Nicol A, Clark P, Path F, Farnell K, McCready R, Smellie J, Franklyn J, John R, Nutting C, Newbold K, Lemon C, Gerrard G, Abdel-Hamid A, Hardman J, Macias E, Roques T, Whitaker S, Vijayan R, Alvarez P, Beare S, Forsyth S, Kadalayil L, Hackshaw A 2012 Ablation with low-dose radioiodine and thyrotropin alfa in thyroid cancer. N Engl J Med **366:**1674–1685.

Address correspondence to:
James Magner, MD
Global Medical Affairs, Endocrinology
Genzyme Center, 7th Floor
500 Kendall Street
Cambridge, MA 02142

E-mail: james.magner@genzyme.com

J Clin Endocrin Metab. First published ahead of print October 22, 2009 as doi:10.1210/jc.2009-0869

ORIGINAL ARTICLE

Endocrine Care

Follow-Up of Low-Risk Differentiated Thyroid Cancer Patients Who Underwent Radioiodine Ablation of Postsurgical Thyroid Remnants after Either Recombinant Human Thyrotropin or Thyroid Hormone Withdrawal

R. Elisei, M. Schlumberger, A. Driedger, C. Reiners, R. T. Kloos, S. I. Sherman, B. Haugen, C. Corone, E. Molinaro, L. Grasso, S. Leboulleux, I. Rachinsky, M. Luster, M. Lassmann, N. L. Busaidy, R. L. Wahl, F. Pacini, S. Y. Cho, J. Magner, A. Pinchera, and P. W. Ladenson

Department of Endocrinology and Metabolism (R.E., E.M., L.G., A.P.), University of Pisa, 56124 Pisa, Italy; Institut Gustave Roussy and University of Paris-Sud XI (M.S., S.L.), 94805 Villejuif, France; Division of Nuclear Medicine (A.D., I.R.), University of Western Ontario, London, Ontario, Canada N6A 4G5; Department of Nuclear Medicine (C.R., M.Lu., M.La.), University of Wuerzburg, 97070 Wuerzburg, Germany; The Ohio State University (R.T.K.), Columbus, Ohio 43210; The University of Texas M. D. Anderson Cancer Center (S.I.S., N.L.B.), Houston, Texas 77030; University of Colorado Denver (B.H.), Aurora, Colorado 80045; Centre Rene Huguenin (C.C.), 92210 Saint Cloud, France; Division of Nuclear Medicine (R.L.W., S.Y.C.) and Division of Endocrinology and Metabolism (P.W.L.), Johns Hopkins University, Baltimore, Maryland 21287; Section of Endocrinology and Metabolism (F.P.), University of Siena, Siena 53100, Italy; and Genzyme Corp. (J.M.), Cambridge, Massachusetts 02142

Background: We previously demonstrated comparable thyroid remnant ablation rates in postoperative low-risk thyroid cancer patients prepared for administration of 3.7GBq ^{131}I (100 mCi) after recombinant human (rh) TSH during T_4 (L-T4) therapy *vs.* withholding L-T4 (euthyroid *vs.* hypothyroid groups). We now compared the outcomes of these patients 3.7 yr later.

Patients and Methods: Fifty-one of the 63 original patients (28 euthyroid, 23 hypothyroid) participated. Forty-eight received rhTSH and serum thyroglobulin (Tg) sampling. A ^{131}I whole-body scan was performed in 43 patients, and successful ablation was defined by criteria from the previous study. Based on the criterion of uptake less than 0.1% in thyroid bed, 100% (43 of 43) remained ablated. When no visible uptake instead was used, five patients (four euthyroid, one hypothyroid) had minimal visible activity. When the TSH-stimulated Tg criterion was used, only two of 45 (one euthyroid, one hypothyroid) had a stimulated Tg level greater than 2 ng/ml.

Results: No patient in either group died, and no patient declared disease free had sustained tumor recurrence. Nine (four euthyroid, five hypothyroid) had received additional ^{131}I between the original and current studies due to detectable Tg or imaging evidence of disease; with follow-up, all now had a negative rhTSH-stimulated whole-body scan and seven (three euthyroid, four hypothyroid) had a stimulated serum Tg less than 2 ng/ml.

Conclusions: In conclusion, after a median 3.7 yr, low-risk thyroid cancer patients prepared for postoperative remnant ablation either with rhTSH or after L-T4 withdrawal were confirmed to have had their thyroid remnants ablated and to have comparable rates of tumor recurrence and persistence. (*J Clin Endocrinol Metab* 94: 4171–4179, 2009)

ISSN Print 0021-972X   ISSN Online 1945-7197
Printed in U.S.A.
Copyright © 2009 by The Endocrine Society
doi: 10.1210/jc.2009-0869 Received April 28, 2009. Accepted August 21, 2009.

Abbreviations: CI, Confidence interval; DTC, differentiated epithelial thyroid cancer; rhTSH, recombinant human TSH; RxWBS, therapeutic WBS; Tg, thyroglobulin; Tg-Ab, Tg antibody; WBS, whole-body scanning.

4172 Elisei *et al.* rhTSH Follow-Up Ablation Study J Clin Endocrinol Metab, November 2009, 94(11):4171–4179

Postsurgical thyroid remnant ablation is a key element in treatment for selected differentiated epithelial thyroid cancer (DTC) patients (1, 2). In high-risk patients, nonrandomized trials have shown lower rates of tumor recurrence when adjunctive radioiodine is used (3–5). Ablation of remnant thyroid tissue also improves the accuracy of long-term patient monitoring with serum thyroglobulin (Tg) and radioiodine whole-body scanning (WBS) (6, 7). Because postoperative thyroid remnant ablation requires TSH activation of tissue, the traditional approach of preparation for radioiodine therapy has been to withhold thyroid hormone therapy to induce an endogenous TSH rise (1). Although this strategy is effective, it causes clinical hypothyroidism with unpleasant symptoms (8) and, in some settings, the need for longer hospitalization compared with patients prepared by recombinant human TSH (rhTSH) (9).

In a previous prospective randomized trial (10), we demonstrated comparable successful postsurgical ^{131}I thyroid remnant ablation rates in two groups of low-risk DTC patients who were prepared for administration of 3.7 GBq ^{131}I with either endogenous TSH stimulation induced by 4 or more weeks of thyroid hormone withdrawal or by rhTSH. Successful ablation was achieved in all patients in both groups, based on the primary prospectively defined criterion for thyroid remnant ablation: either no visible uptake or less than 0.1% thyroid bed uptake of the administered ^{131}I activity on imaging performed 8 months after therapy. Similarly, based on the secondary criteria of no visible uptake alone or a stimulated serum Tg level less than 2 ng/ml at 8 months, there were no significant differences between the hypothyroid and euthyroid patient groups. In the current study, we reexamined most patients from both of the original groups 3 or more years later to determine whether current TSH-stimulated testing confirmed that the comparability of thyroid remnant ablation success had persisted and whether there has been any difference in patients' clinical outcomes.

Subjects and Methods

Study objectives and design

This open-label study was designed to provide follow-up information about patients who had previously undergone postsurgical ^{131}I thyroid remnant ablation after preparation with either withdrawal of thyroid hormone therapy or rhTSH while euthyroid on thyroid hormone therapy, as has been previously described (10). Eight months later, all of these patients had undergone follow-up rhTSH-stimulated diagnostic WBS and serum Tg measurement. The current study involved patients from all nine sites that participated in the previous trial, including four centers in the United States, two in France, and one each in Italy, Germany, and Canada.

The primary objective of the study was to confirm, after a median follow up of 3.7 yr (range 3.4–4.4 yr), whether there was comparable persistence of thyroid remnant ablation in patients who had been prepared for 100 mCi (3.7 GBq) [131]I therapy by thyroid hormone withdrawal (hypothyroid group) *vs.* rhTSH administration while on L-T$_4$ therapy (euthyroid group). Secondary objectives of the study were: 1) to determine whether there were patients with clinically documented recurrences of thyroid cancer; 2) to assess the patients' current rhTSH-stimulated serum Tg concentrations, as an indicator of residual disease or normal thyroid tissue; and 3) to confirm the long-term safety of previous rhTSH exposures.

Study patients

In the original remnant ablation trial, 63 patients (61 with papillary thyroid cancer and two with follicular thyroid cancer) had been randomized to preparation for postthyroidectomy thyroid remnant ablation by one of the two methods. However, only 61 of these patients were eligible for recruitment to enroll in this follow-up study; one was ineligible due to the presence of lung metastases on a posttherapy scan in the earlier trial, and another had not received the full rhTSH dose in preparation for radioiodine therapy. For women of child-bearing potential, a negative serum human chorionic gonadotropin pregnancy test was required. Patients gave written informed consent for review of their medical records to capture medical information because the 8-month follow-up visit in the original study and to undergo additional diagnostic testing under this protocol.

Fifty-one of the 61 eligible patients (23 hypothyroid and 28 euthyroid) participated in the current follow-up study by providing their interim medical histories. The demographic, clinical, and histopathological features of these 51 patients are reported in Table 1. Features of the 10 patients (four euthyroid and six hypothyroid), who did not participate, principally due to the inconvenience of testing procedures or recent extensive routine diagnostic follow-up, did not differ from those of enrolled patients in the current study (Table 2). Thus, exclusion of these 10 patients did not result in any apparent bias. Because three of the 51 enrolled patients could not be given rhTSH for various reasons (*i.e.* breast-feeding in one case and rhTSH-stimulated testing having been recently performed for routine follow-up in two cases), 48 of the 51 enrolled patients (21 hypothyroid and 27 euthyroid) received rhTSH for diagnostic testing in this protocol. Among these 48 patients, 43 agreed to receive 4 mCi ^{131}I to perform the WBS. In 47 of the 48, serum Tg determinations were completed; in two of these 47 cases, they were uninterpretable because of the presence of serum Tg antibody (Tg-Abs) at a level interfering with Tg measurement (>30 U/ml). Thus, reliable rhTSH-stimulated Tg data were obtained in 45 patients (20 hypothyroid and 25 euthyroid).

Patients' median time of follow-up, which was defined as the period between earlier ^{131}I ablation and the date of signing the consent form for participating in the current follow-up study, was 3.7 yr (range 3.4–4.4 yr).

Assessments of outcome

To assess current status, patients underwent rhTSH-stimulated diagnostic WBS, static neck imaging, and serum Tg measurement. Recombinant TSH (rhTSH, TSH alfa, Thyrogen; Genzyme Corp., Cambridge, MA) was administered as 0.9 mg im per day for 2 consecutive days. The WBS and static neck imaging

J Clin Endocrinol Metab, November 2009, 94(11):4171–4179   jcem.endojournals.org   **4173**

TABLE 1. Demographic, clinical, and histopathological characteristics of study patients

Parameter	Hypothyroid group (n = 23)	Euthyroid group (n = 28)	Overall (n = 51)
Age at remnant ablation (yr)			
Mean (SD)	48 (13)	49 (12)	48 (12)
Median (range)	45 (24–67)	52 (24–71)	49 (24–71)
Gender, n (%)			
Female	18 (78)	23 (82)	41 (80)
Male	5 (22)	5 (18)	10 (20)
Race, (%)			
Caucasian	23 (100)	27 (96)	50 (98)
Black	0	1 (4)	1 (2)
Weight (kg)			
n	22	25	47
Mean (SD)	69.8 (14.0)	77.2 (18.3)	73.8 (16.7)
Median (range)	71.0 (46.0–95.0)	72.6 (50.2–121.0)	72.6 (46.0–121.0)
Height (cm)			
n	22	25	47
Mean (SD)	162 (9)	167 (9)	165 (10)
Median (range)	161 (145–182)	167 (149–186)	163 (145–186)
BMI (kg/m^2)			
n	22	25	47
Mean (SD)	26.7 (5.8)	27.4 (5.5)	27.1 (5.6)
Median (range)	26.8 (18.7–45.0)	25.9 (18.4–42.4)	26.2 (18.4–45.0)
Thyroid cancer type, n (%)			
Papillary	20 (87)	25 (89)	45 (88)
Follicular	0	0	0
Combined (considered papillary cancer patients)	3 (13%)	3 (11%)	6 (12%)
TNM			
T1	3 (13%)	7 (25%)	10 (20%)
T2	17 (74%)	19 (68%)	36 (71%)
T3	0	0	0
T4	3 (13%)	2 (7%)	5 (10%)
NX	1 (4%)	1 (4%)	2 (4%)
N0	12 (52%)	18 (64%)	30 (59%)
N1	6 (26%)	7 (25%)	13 (25%)
N1a	2 (9%)	1 (4%)	3 (6%)
N1b	2 (9%)	1 (4%)	3 (6%)
MX	3 (13%)	3 (11%)	6 (12%)
M0	20 (87%)	25 (89%)	45 (88%)
M1	0	0	0

BMI, Body mass index; TNM, tumor node metastasis.

were performed 48 ± 6 h after oral administration of 4 ± 0.4 mCi ^{131}I, which was given 24 ± 6 h after the second injection of rhTSH. All images were read by three independent nuclear medicine specialists, who were blinded to the original treatment. Static cervical images were assessed for uptake both visually and after quantification. If a majority of readers considered ^{131}I uptake to be visible in the thyroid bed, the percentage of administered ^{131}I activity then residing in the thyroid bed was calculated

TABLE 2. Characteristics of original study patients not enrolled in the current study

Patient	Age (yr)[a]	Sex	Thyroid cancer type	Original TNM
Former euthyroid group				
1	54	F	Follicular	T2NxMx
2	27	F	Papillary	T2N0M0
3	45	M	Papillary	T1N1M0
4	29	M	Papillary	T2N0M0
Former hypothyroid group				
5	37	F	Papillary/follicular	T1NxMx
6	32	F	Follicular	T2NxMx
7	52	F	Papillary	T2N0M0
8	47	F	Papillary	T2N0M0
9	33	F	Papillary	T2N0M0
10	62	M	Papillary	T2N0M0

TNM, Tumor node metastasis.

[a] Patient ages were defined at screening for the ablation study.

using the same standardized procedure applied in the 8-month follow-up assessments. The definition of successful ablation by scanning was no visible thyroid bed uptake or, if visible, less than 0.1% uptake in the thyroid bed (11).

Blood samples for Tg and TSH measurement were obtained on d 1 (before rhTSH administration) and d 5 (3 d after the second rhTSH injection). Circulating anti-Tg-Abs were also measured on d 1. Successful ablation was defined by the previously described criteria used in the original ablation study (10).

The general safety and tolerability of rhTSH were monitored through patient-reported adverse events and changes in laboratory assessments for routine chemical and hematological parameters. In addition, safety also was verified by changes in vital signs (including blood pressure, temperature, heart rate, and respiratory rate) and medical history or physical examination findings.

Laboratory measurements

Patients' blood was taken at the screening visit for measurement of TSH and free T_4 concentrations and independently measured at each respective study site using standard immunoassay procedures. Other blood samples were collected on d 1 and 5, immediately centrifuged, and stored at −20 C and then shipped to a central laboratory (Department of Endocrinology, University of Pisa, Pisa, Italy) for determinations of serum Tg and Tg-Ab levels.

Serum Tg determination was performed using the same immunometric assay (Diagnostic Products Corp., Los Angeles, CA) used in the previous ablation study. The functional sensitivity of this method was of 0.9 ng/ml, standardized against the certified reference material for human Tg (12). Tg assays were performed within 1 month from the receipt of samples. All of each patient's samples were analyzed in the same assay run.

Tg-Abs were measured with an immunoenzymometric assay (AIA PACK TgAb system; TOSOH Bioscence NV, Tessenderlo, Belgium). Samples with a potentially interfering level of Tg-Ab (*i.e.* >30 U/ml in the central laboratory) were excluded from final analyses of stimulated Tg values. To exclude further any possible interference of Tg-Ab, a second data analysis using a lower cutoff of interference (>5 U/ml) also was performed.

Although Tg released by cervical nodes with tumor or a distant metastasis could confound the Tg-based analysis of the elimination of normal thyroid remnant tissue, the data also were examined using a definition of successful ablation of a rhTSH-stimulated serum Tg level less than 2 ng/ml in the absence of interfering Tg-Abs. Yet another analysis of the rate of ablation using a stimulated serum Tg level less than 1 ng/ml was also performed.

Mean serum TSH and free T_4 concentrations were similar for both groups at screening. Although several TSH and free T_4 values were minimally out of range in patients in both groups, none of these abnormalities was considered clinically significant.

Biostatistical considerations

In this follow-up study, the study population was limited to the patients who completed the original remnant ablation study and consented to participate in the current follow-up study. The same noninferiority methodology used in the original study was again applied in the analysis of the ablation rates calculated using the criteria defined for the primary end point (10). In the present study, this statistical strategy was also applied for the interpre-

tation of the serum Tg values. Noninferiority was considered achieved if there was less than 20% difference between treatment groups (*i.e.* euthyroid group minus hypothyroid group), meaning that the lower bound of the 95% confidence interval (CI) was not more negative than −20%.

The standard $\alpha = 0.05$ was used to assess statistical significance. Missing or invalid data were not imputed. Patients were grouped according to their treatment assignments in the original study for comparison.

Results

Clinical outcomes

None of the 63 patients who participated in the original trial had died at the time of this follow-up study. Among the 51 patients enrolled in the current study, their interim medical histories revealed that nine patients (five hypothyroid and four euthyroid) had undergone additional ^{131}I treatments. Furthermore, two of them (one hypothyroid and one euthyroid) along with one additional patient who did not receive further ^{131}I treatments (former euthyroid) had been surgically treated for metastatic cervical lymph node disease identified by neck ultrasound and confirmed by fine-needle aspiration cytology; none of these patients' lesions were iodine avid (Table 3). In the previous study, these nine patients who required further treatment with additional ^{131}I had been considered ablated based on the criterion of absent neck radioiodine uptake, but none of the nine had definitive serum Tg evidence of absent thyroid tissue, due to either persistently detectable TSH-stimulated serum Tg (n = 5) or uninterpretable serum Tg due to the presence of potentially interfering Tg-Ab levels (n = 4). In one of these nine patients, there had been possible evidence of a small thyroid remnant by ultrasound, whereas in four patients there had been evidence of persistent thyroid bed or regional cervical lymph node metastases that had been shown at the posttherapeutic WBS (RxWBS). Similarly, the three patients who underwent surgery all had negative WBS but had detectable levels of serum Tg or interfering Tg-Ab and evidence of suspicious cervical adenopathy at neck ultrasound. In the current follow-up study, seven of the nine ^{131}I retreated patients underwent rhTSH stimulation, and all seven had a negative rhTSH-stimulated WBS, whereas two of these seven (one hypothyroid and one euthyroid) still had a rhTSH-stimulated serum Tg greater than 2 ng/ml, likely reflecting persistent tumor in cervical nodes. The other two of the nine ^{131}I retreated patients did not agree to undergo repeat rhTSH stimulation. None of the 51 patients in this follow-up study had been declared free of disease but then had suffered a tumor recurrence.

J Clin Endocrinol Metab, November 2009, 94(11):4171–4179   jcem.endojournals.org   **4175**

TABLE 3. Patients who received subsequent ^{131}I therapy following 8-month postablation testing

Treatment group	Sex/age	Original TNM	Total additional ^{131}I (mCi)	Comment	Stimulated Tg at 8 months control in the first study (ng/mL)	Neck uptake at 8 months control in the first study (%)
Euthyroid	F/47	T2N0M0	150	Tg-Ab positive; thyroid bed uptake (RxWBS)[a]	0.99	0.07
Euthyroid	M/37	T2N0M0	260	Physical exams, stimulated Tg and neck ultrasound suggestive of residual tumor; node biopsy: tumor; uptake in thyroid bed (two RxWBS)[a]	1.60	<0.004
Euthyroid	F/68	T2N1Mx	193	Bed uptake (RxWBS)[a]	0.99	0.015
Euthyroid	F/31	T1N0M0	150	Serum hypo-Tg: 7.4 ng/ml, and possible remnant (neck ultrasound)	3.70	0.005
Hypothyroid	F/65	T2N1M0	260	Serum hypo-Tg: 5.6 ng/ml	3.10	<0.013
Hypothyroid	F/75	T2NxM0	100	Serum hypo-Tg: 12.4 ng/ml	44.0	<0.009
Hypothyroid	F/40	T2N0M0	280	Serum hypo-Tg: 10 ng/ml	4.30	<0.006
Hypothyroid	F/43	T1N1M0	260	Tumor in neck (CT scan)	2.50	0.011
Hypothyroid	M/40	T4N0M0	251	Tg-Ab positive; tumor in neck (neck ultrasound); lymph node aspirations: tumor; pathological uptake in neck (RxWBS); PET scan positive for tumor[a]	32.0	<0.01

In addition to the radioiodine therapies given after the end of the initial ablation study, two of these nine patients (one hypothyroid and one euthyroid) had residual noniodine-avid metastatic lymph nodes identified by neck ultrasound and fine-needle aspiration cytology and excised by surgery. A third patient with neck node metastases not able to take up iodine (belonging to the euthyroid group) directly underwent surgery with no other ^{131}I treatments. TNM, Tumor node metastasis; CT, computed tomography.

[a] All of these RxWBS comments are referring to interval studies obtained outside the first study and this second follow-up study.

Persisting efficacies of thyroid remnant ablation after hypothyroidism and rhTSH

The long-term outcome of the original ablation procedure was analyzed in the 43 patients who completed both rhTSH-stimulated WBS and rhTSH-stimulated Tg testing in the current protocol. They included the above described nine patients who had received further treatments after the first study, which, of course, confounds the assessment of efficacy of the original ablation procedure. Considering all 43 patients who consented to scanning, based on the criterion of no visible uptake, or uptake less than 0.1% in the thyroid bed, (the predefined primary end point of the study), 100% of patients in both the hypothyroid and euthyroid groups remained ablated. It is worth noting that formal confidence intervals could not be calculated for these results because 100% of patients were ablated in the two groups. When the more strict but subjective criterion of no visible uptake was used, faint residual visible thyroid bed uptake was identified in five subjects (one hypothyroid and four euthyroid). Consequently, 94% of the hypothyroid and 84% of euthyroid patients were considered to have been persistently ablated by using that criterion, with no clinically significant difference between the two

groups (95% CI −23.2, 7.4) (Table 4). This indicates that this study was unable to prove noninferiority with regard to the no visible uptake end point, perhaps due to the small sample size, although the finding of trace thyroid bed uptake (which was quantitated to be very low in this study) is generally believed in most low-risk patients to be a finding of little or no clinical significance.

When the secondary end point of rhTSH-stimulated serum Tg was used as the criterion for successful ablation, 45 patients could be considered and all but two (one hypothyroid and one euthyroid) had rhTSH-stimulated Tg less than 2 ng/ml, corresponding to comparable ablation rates of 95 and 96%, respectively (95% CI −11.3, 13.3). When a more stringent rhTSH-stimulated serum Tg criterion, less than 1 ng/ml, was applied, all but four patients (two hypothyroid and two euthyroid) were considered to have been successfully ablated, corresponding to comparable ablation rates of 90 and 92%, respectively (95% CI −14.9, 18.9) (Table 4). Two patients (one hypothyroid and one euthyroid) had serum Tg-Ab levels greater than 30 U/ml that excluded them from the main Tg analyses. When the more stringent criterion of greater than 5 U/ml was used, nine patients (four hypothyroid and five euthyroid)

4176   Elisei *et al.*   rhTSH Follow-Up Ablation Study   J Clin Endocrinol Metab, November 2009, 94(11):4171–4179

TABLE 4. Comparison of 8-month and current study result for evaluable patients

	8-month postablation testing in original study		3- to 4-yr postablation testing in current study	
	Hypothyroid group (n = 30)	Euthyroid group (n = 33)	Former hypothyroid group (n = 21)	Former euthyroid group (n = 27)
Patients included in scan analysis/all original patients	28/30	32/33	18/21	25/27
Patients with no visible uptake or less than 0.1%/patients in scan analysis	28/28 (100%)	32/32 (100%)	18/18 (100%)	25/25 (100%)
Patients included in scan analysis/all original patients	28/30	32/33	18/21	25/27
Patients with no visible uptake/patients in scan analysis	24/28 (86%)	24/32 (75%)	17/18 (94%)	21/25 (84%)
Patients with serum Tg measured and no interfering TgAb/all original patients	21/30	24/33	20/21	25/27
Patients with serum Tg less than 2 ng/ml/all patients with Tg analyzed	18/21 (86%)	23/24 (96%)	19/20 (95%)	24/25 (96%)
Patients with serum Tg measured and no interfering TgAb/all original patients	21/30	24/33	20/21	25/27
Patients with serum Tg less than 1 ng/ml/all patients with Tg analyzed	18/21 (86%)	20/24 (83%)	18/20 (90%)	23/25 (92%)

were excluded. The findings and conclusions regarding comparable serum Tg evidence of ablation were not different when either cutoff was used (data not shown).

Comparison of the rhTSH-stimulated serum Tg in the present study with rhTSH-stimulated serum Tg values 8 months after radioiodine ablation in our original study showed that all patients with levels less than 1 ng/ml in the earlier study were confirmed to remain less than 1 ng/ml in the present. Only eight cases (four hypothyroid and four euthyroid) had a rhTSH-stimulated serum Tg above cutoff levels in the first study (five cases >2 ng/ml and three cases >1 ng/ml but <2 ng/ml). Three of these patients, although serum Tg positive, also had potentially interfering titers of Tg-Ab. Unfortunately, comparison of the two rhTSH-stimulated serum Tg values in these patients cannot be accurately performed because six of these patients were retreated. Consequently, both these retreatments and the reduction in level of interfering Tg-Ab antibodies alter the results of serum Tg measurement. In the sole patient from this cohort who had not been treated with radioiodine during the interim and who initially had no interfering

anti-Tg-Abs, the rhTSH-stimulated serum Tg decreased from 1.8 to less than 1 ng/ml.

Safety and tolerability of rhTSH

Retreatment with rhTSH for diagnostic testing during this follow-up study was well tolerated. One or more treatment emergent adverse events were reported by two patients (9%) in the former hypothyroid group and six patients (21%) in the former euthyroid group. Because all patients were euthyroid on T_4 when receiving rhTSH in this follow-up study, it was not clear how original treatment assignment more than 3 yr previously would have been relevant to the incidences of minor adverse events reported in this study. For all eight of these patients, no action or medications were prescribed for any of these adverse events and all patients recovered promptly and spontaneously.

Discussion

We previously demonstrated that the rates of successful postsurgical remnant ablation (determined 8 months after

J Clin Endocrinol Metab, November 2009, 94(11):4171–4179

[131]I treatment) in patients with low-risk DTC were similar whether patients were prepared for radioiodine therapy after rhTSH administration or thyroid hormone withdrawal (10). Besides a similar rate of ablation, a significantly better quality of life and lesser time lost from work has been documented in euthyroid patients prepared with rhTSH administration (13–15). In addition, the mean absorbed radiation dose to the blood, which can be considered as an indicator for bone marrow exposure, was lower than with comparable therapy in hypothyroid patients (11, 16). In the current study, we demonstrate that patients prepared with rhTSH and thyroid hormone withdrawal still have comparable rates of successful remnant ablation and have manifested similar clinical outcomes after approximately 4 yr of follow-up, which is the period with the highest risk of recurrent disease (3). Although the number of enrolled patients in this follow-up study was, of necessity, relatively small, statistical analysis of our results showed no difference in the rates of successful ablation between the two groups.

In the present study, all patients who were considered ablated at 8 months after radioiodine therapy according to the criterion of neck uptake being invisible or less than 0.1% of the administered activity were confirmed to have negative rhTSH-stimulated radioiodine scanning a median 3.7 yr later based on the same criterion. These results suggest that there is no need to repeat radioiodine scanning in these patients during their subsequent follow-up. When the criterion of TSH-stimulated serum Tg detectability was applied, the majority of patients similarly had no biochemical evidence of persisting thyroid tissue: 40 of 45 patients based on a stimulated Tg less than 1 ng/ml and 43 of 45 based on a stimulated Tg less than 2 ng/ml. Although there is an apparent increase in the successful ablation rate based on Tg criteria in this report *vs.* our original study, this difference is attributable to disappearance of Tg-Abs in several patients and to a modest decrease overall size of the study population. In fact, TSH-stimulated serum Tg testing performed several years after the remnant ablation revealed similar rates of cure, regardless of the preceding mode of TSH stimulation used to facilitate ablation.

Recently Tg assays with higher sensitivity than that used in the present work have been developed, and the question of whether a more sensitive Tg assay provides more clinically useful information than the Tg assay used after recombinant TSH stimulation is under investigation (17, 18). However, because consistency dictated our use of the same Tg assay as in the first study and its functional sensitivity was 0.9 ng/ml, we cannot comment on lower values with confidence.

Differentiated thyroid cancer recurrence is defined as the reappearance of tumor (either locally in thyroid bed, in neck nodes, or as distant metastatic disease) after a well-documented disease-free period. Such recurrences are becoming less common because of earlier primary treatment of thyroid cancer patients and more stringent criteria for definitive cure, *i.e.* undetectable TSH-stimulated serum Tg in the absence of interfering serum Tg-Abs, and negative cervical ultrasound in addition to negative radioiodine WBS (6, 7). In this study, we have shown that no patient had a definite recurrence of tumor in the sense that they had been declared disease free but then suffered tumor recurrence during the follow-up period. All patients with rhTSH-stimulated serum Tg less than 1 ng/ml at the 8-month evaluation in the original study again demonstrated a rhTSH-stimulated serum Tg less than 1 ng/ml in the present study. Although there are emerging data showing that patients with low detectable levels of rhTSH-stimulated serum Tg may avoid further treatment because the serum Tg may spontaneously decline over the time (19–21), we observed only one patient demonstrating this phenomenon, so we cannot draw any conclusion regarding this issue.

It is important to keep in mind that low stage of disease presentation was a criterion for inclusion in the original remnant ablation trial (10). All patients had been stage T2 or T4 with minor invasion of the thyroid capsule, N0-N1, and M0 or T0-T1, N1, and M0 (22). Furthermore, T_4 tumors were later considered ineligible because some participating centers routinely treated such patients with ^{131}I activities larger than 100 mCi or external radiotherapy. Consequently, the findings of this study, like its predecessor, may or may not apply to patients presenting with higher stages of disease.

In recent years, as serum Tg assay sensitivity has been progressively increased, it has become clear that when serum Tg remains undetectable after TSH stimulation in the absence of interfering serum Tg-Ab, its negative predictive value for subsequent disease recurrence is very high (20, 23), whereas persistently detectable serum Tg indicates persistence of functioning thyroid cells (24, 25). In contrast, the predefined criterion of no visible uptake or, if visible, less than 0.1% uptake is relevant for initial assessment in studies of the ablation of the normal thyroid remnant tissue because serum Tg could arise from tumor in cervical nodes. In our original study, 100% of the patients were considered successfully ablated based on this scan criterion, whereas a lower ablation rate (85–95%) was reported based on TSH-stimulated serum Tg testing. The ^{131}I treatments and/or surgery subsequently required for some patients in this study during follow-up prove that small amounts of residual either normal or malignant thyroid tissue may not be detected routinely using a 4 mCi ^{131}I diagnostic WBS as has been noted in other series (24, 25).

4178 Elisei *et al.* rhTSH Follow-Up Ablation Study

J Clin Endocrinol Metab, November 2009, 94(11):4171–4179

With the more stringent criterion of no visible uptake, ablation rates were found in the original study to be 86 and 75% in the hypothyroid and euthyroid groups, respectively, although the clinical meaning of trace thyroid bed uptake remains uncertain. Recall that for the original ablation study, radioiodine scanning had to be the primary end point because the goal of the study treatment was the elimination of the normal thyroid remnant tissue rather than the sterilization of all residual tumor in neck nodes. In other words, rhTSH plus ^{131}I was intended to eliminate the thyroid remnant, but this one-time use was not thought likely to eliminate all tumor cells, especially if there was no detectable uptake in tumor tissue or if located in nodes. As a matter of fact, most patients recognized as requiring subsequent treatment had a neck uptake less than 0.1% on WBS but had detectable serum Tg levels. This confirms the observation that serum Tg is a more sensitive test than a radioiodine scan to detect residual functioning thyroid cells, benign or malignant (26–28). However, the need for further treatments was unrelated to the mode of TSH stimulation for earlier remnant ablation because among the nine patients requiring ^{131}I retreatment, five originated from the hypothyroid group and four from the euthyroid group. These findings are similar to those of Tuttle *et al.* (29), who recently reported comparable clinical recurrence rates in 320 patients who earlier underwent radioiodine remnant ablation after rhTSH stimulation *vs.* 74 patients who were ablated after thyroid hormone withdrawal. Although the study by Tuttle *et al.* was retrospective and nonrandomized, the substantial number of thyroid cancer patients analyzed makes it valuable in supporting the comparability of the two methods.

In the present follow-up study, we showed that rhTSH can be safely administered to enhance ^{131}I uptake for remnant ablation in patients with low-risk DTC, with no long-term adverse effects observed over several years of follow-up. Although a number of the study patients received one or more cycles of rhTSH administration during the interim period to monitor their statuses, none developed apparent rhTSH-related adverse events of importance. This confirms the much larger clinical experience with repeated rhTSH use for diagnostic testing.

In conclusion, the current study performed a median 3.7 yr after postsurgical ^{131}I thyroid remnant ablation found no differences in the success of thyroid remnant ablative radioiodine therapy or clinical outcomes between patients prepared by endogenous TSH stimulation by withholding thyroid hormone therapy *vs.* exogenous rhTSH in the euthyroid state. There were no differences between the two approaches in eliminating thyroid remnants or in instances of residual disease detected. These findings confirm that rhTSH is an effective and safe alternative to thyroid hormone withdrawal in preparing low-risk DTC patients for the postsurgical thyroid remnant ablation. This study also confirms that rhTSH-stimulated serum Tg measurement is a highly sensitive indicator of residual disease or normal tissue and one that is superior to radioiodine scanning. Finally, we confirmed the long-term safety of repeated rhTSH exposures.

Acknowledgments

We thank all of our colleagues who contributed to this study, in particular C. Ceccarelli, D. Taddei, and F. Fragomeni (Department of Endocrinology and Metabolism, University of Pisa, Pisa, Italy); K. Evans (University of Colorado Denver, Aurora, Colorado); V. Carriere (Centre Rene Huguenin, Saint Cloud, France); M. Ricard (Institut Gustave Roussy and University of Paris-Sud XI, Villejuif, France); and M. Ewertz and W. Kasecamp (Johns Hopkins University School of Medicine, Baltimore, Maryland).

Address all correspondence and requests for reprints to: Rossella Elisei, Department of Endocrinology, University of Pisa, 56124 Pisa, Italy. E-mail: relisei@endoc.med.unipi.it.

This work was supported by Genzyme Corp.; it is registered with the number NCT00295763 on a public accessible database (www.clinicaltrials.gov).

Disclosure Summary: M.S., M. Lu, F.P., and P.W.L. are consultants for Genzyme Corp.; A.D. has received honoraria from Genzyme Corp. for consulting and teaching activities; J.M. is an employee of Genzyme Corp. The rest of the authors have nothing to disclose.

References

1. **Mazzaferri EL, Robyn J** 1996 Postsurgical management of differentiated thyroid carcinoma. Otolaryngol Clin North Am 29:637–662
2. **Schlumberger MJ** 1998 Papillary and follicular thyroid carcinoma. N Engl J Med 338:297–306
3. **Mazzaferri EL, Jhiang SM** 1994 Long-term impact of initial surgical and medical therapy on papillary and follicular thyroid cancer. Am J Med 97:418–428
4. **Mazzaferri EL** 1997 Thyroid remnant 131I ablation for papillary and follicular thyroid carcinoma. Thyroid 7:265–271
5. **Sawka AM, Thephamongkhol K, Brouwers M, Thabane L, Browman G, Gerstein HC** 2004 Clinical review 170: a systematic review and metaanalysis of the effectiveness of radioactive iodine remnant ablation for well-differentiated thyroid cancer. J Clin Endocrinol Metab 89: 3668–3676
6. **Cooper DS, Doherty GM, Haugen BR, Kloos RT, Lee SL, Mandel SJ, Mazzaferri EL, McIver B, Sherman SI, Tuttle RM** 2006 Management guidelines for patients with thyroid nodules and differentiated thyroid cancer. Thyroid 16:109–142
7. **Pacini F, Schlumberger M, Dralle H, Elisei R, Smit JW, Wiersinga W** 2006 European consensus for the management of patients with differentiated thyroid carcinoma of the follicular epithelium. Eur J Endocrinol 154:787–803
8. **Dow KH, Ferrell BR, Anello C** 1997 Quality-of-life changes in patients with thyroid cancer after withdrawal of thyroid hormone therapy. Thyroid 7:613–619
9. **Borget I, Remy H, Chevalier J, Ricard M, Allyn M, Schlumberger M, De Pouvourville G** 2008 Length and cost of hospital stay of radio-

J Clin Endocrinol Metab, November 2009, 94(11):4171–4179   jcem.endojournals.org   **4179**

iodine ablation in thyroid cancer patients: comparison between preparation with thyroid hormone withdrawal and thyrogen. Eur J Nucl Med Mol Imaging 35:1457–1463

10. Pacini F, Ladenson PW, Schlumberger M, Driedger A, Luster M, Kloos RT, Sherman S, Haugen B, Corone C, Molinaro E, Elisei R, Ceccarelli C, Pinchera A, Wahl RL, Lebouilleux S, Ricard M, Yoo J, Busaidy NL, Delpassand E, Hanscheid H, Felbinger R, Lassmann M, Reiners C 2006 Radioiodine ablation of thyroid remnants after preparation with recombinant human thyrotropin in differentiated thyroid carcinoma: results of an international, randomized, controlled study. J Clin Endocrinol Metab 91:926–932

11. Hänscheid H, Lassmann M, Luster M, Thomas SR, Pacini F, Ceccarelli C, Ladenson PW, Wahl RL, Schlumberger M, Ricard M, Driedger A, Kloos RT, Sherman SI, Haugen BR, Carriere V, Corone C, Reiners C 2006 Iodine biokinetics and dosimetry in radioiodine therapy of thyroid cancer: procedures and results of a prospective international controlled study of ablation after rhTSH or hormone withdrawal. J Nucl Med 47:648–654

12. Feldt-Rasmussen U, Profilis C, Colinet E, Black E, Bornet H, Bourdoux P, Carayon P, Ericsson UB, Koutras DA, Lamas de Leon L, DeNayer P, Pacini F, Palumbo G, Santos A, Schlumberger M, Seidel C, Van Herle AJ, De Vijlder JJ 1996 Human thyroglobulin reference material (CRM 457). 1st part: assessment of homogeneity, stability and immunoreactivity. Ann Biol Clin (Paris) 54:337–342

13. Mernagh P, Campbell S, Dietlein M, Luster M, Mazzaferri E, Weston AR 2006 Cost-effectiveness of using recombinant human TSH prior to radioiodine ablation for thyroid cancer, compared with treating patients in a hypothyroid state: the German perspective. Eur J Endocrinol 155:405–414

14. Schroeder PR, Haugen BR, Pacini F, Reiners C, Schlumberger M, Sherman SI, Cooper DS, Schuff KG, Braverman LE, Skarulis MC, Davies TF, Mazzaferri EL, Daniels GH, Ross DS, Luster M, Samuels MH, Weintraub BD, Ridgway EC, Ladenson PW 2006 A comparison of short-term changes in health-related quality of life in thyroid carcinoma patients undergoing diagnostic evaluation with recombinant human thyrotropin compared with thyroid hormone withdrawal. J Clin Endocrinol Metab 91:878–884

15. Borget I, Corone C, Nocaudie M, Allyn M, Iacobelli S, Schlumberger M, De Pouvourville G 2007 Sick leave for follow-up control in thyroid cancer patients: comparison between stimulation with thyrogen and thyroid hormone withdrawal. Eur J Endocrinol 156:531–538

16. Luster M, Sherman SI, Skarulis MC, Reynolds JR, Lassmann M, Hänscheid H, Reiners C 2003 Comparison of radioiodine biokinetics following the administration of recombinant human thyroid stimulating hormone and after thyroid hormone withdrawal in thyroid carcinoma. Eur J Nucl Med Mol Imaging 30:1371–1377

17. Iervasi A, Iervasi G, Ferdeghini M, Solimeo C, Bottoni A, Rossi L, Colato C, Zucchelli GC 2007 Clinical relevance of highly sensitive Tg assay in monitoring patients treated for differentiated thyroid cancer. Clin Endocrinol (Oxf) 67:434–441

18. Rosario PW, Purisch S 2008 Does a highly sensitive thyroglobulin (Tg) assay change the clinical management of low-risk patients with thyroid cancer with Tg on T_4 <1 ng/ml determined by traditional assays? Clin Endocrinol (Oxf) 68:338–342

19. Kloos RT, Mazzaferri EL 2005 A single recombinant human thyrotropin-stimulated serum thyroglobulin measurement predicts differentiated thyroid carcinoma metastases three to five years later. J Clin Endocrinol Metab 90:5047–5057

20. Castagna MG, Brilli L, Pilli T, Montanaro A, Cipri C, Fioravanti C, Sestini F, Capezzone M, Pacini F 2008 Limited value of repeat recombinant human thyrotropin (rhTSH)-stimulated thyroglobulin testing in differentiated thyroid carcinoma patients with previous negative rhTSH-stimulated thyroglobulin and undetectable basal serum thyroglobulin levels. J Clin Endocrinol Metab 93:76–81

21. Baudin E, Do Cao C, Cailleux AF, Leboulleux S, Travagli JP, Schlumberger M 2003 Positive predictive value of serum thyroglobulin levels, measured during the first year of follow-up after thyroid hormone withdrawal, in thyroid cancer patients. J Clin Endocrinol Metab 88:1107–1111

22. Sobin LH, Fleming ID 1997 TNM classification of malignant tumors, fifth edition (1997). Union Internationale Contre le Cancer and the American Joint Committee on Cancer. Cancer 80:1803–1804

23. Mazzaferri EL, Robbins RJ, Spencer CA, Braverman LE, Pacini F, Wartofsky L, Haugen BR, Sherman SI, Cooper DS, Braunstein GD, Lee S, Davies TF, Arafah BM, Ladenson PW, Pinchera A 2003 A consensus report of the role of serum thyroglobulin as a monitoring method for low-risk patients with papillary thyroid carcinoma. J Clin Endocrinol Metab 88:1433–1441

24. Pacini F, Lippi F, Formica N, Elisei R, Anelli S, Ceccarelli C, Pinchera A 1987 Therapeutic doses of iodine-131 reveal undiagnosed metastases in thyroid cancer patients with detectable serum thyroglobulin levels. J Nucl Med 28:1888–1891

25. Pineda JD, Lee T, Ain K, Reynolds JC, Robbins J 1995 Iodine-131 therapy for thyroid cancer patients with elevated thyroglobulin and negative diagnostic scan. J Clin Endocrinol Metab 80:1488–1492

26. Cailleux AF, Baudin E, Travagli JP, Ricard M, Schlumberger M 2000 Is diagnostic iodine-131 scanning useful after total thyroid ablation for differentiated thyroid cancer? J Clin Endocrinol Metab 85:175–178

27. Mazzaferri EL, Kloos RT 2002 Is diagnostic iodine-131 scanning with recombinant human TSH useful in the follow-up of differentiated thyroid cancer after thyroid ablation? J Clin Endocrinol Metab 87:1490–1498

28. Pacini F, Capezzone M, Elisei R, Ceccarelli C, Taddei D, Pinchera A 2002 Diagnostic 131-iodine whole-body scan may be avoided in thyroid cancer patients who have undetectable stimulated serum Tg levels after initial treatment. J Clin Endocrinol Metab 87:1499–1501

29. Tuttle RM, Brokhin M, Omry G, Martorella AJ, Larson SM, Grewal RK, Fleisher M, Robbins RJ 2008 Recombinant human TSH-assisted radioactive iodine remnant ablation achieves short-term clinical recurrence rates similar to those of traditional thyroid hormone withdrawal. J Nucl Med 49:764–770